UTERINE CONTRACTILITY

SERONO SYMPOSIA, USA

FERTILIZATION IN MAMMALS
Edited by Barry D. Bavister, Jim Cummins, and Eduardo R. S. Roldan

GAMETE PHYSIOLOGY
Edited by Ricardo H. Asch, Jose P. Balmaceda, and Ian Johnston

GLYCOPROTEIN HORMONES: Structure, Synthesis, and Biologic Function
Edited by William W. Chin and Irving Boime

THE MENOPAUSE: Biological and Clinical Consequences of Ovarian Failure: Evaluation and Management
Edited by Stanley G. Korenman

NEUROENDOCRINE REGULATION OF REPRODUCTION
Edited by Samuel S. C. Yen and Wylie W. Vale

UTERINE CONTRACTILITY: Mechanisms of Control
Edited by Robert E. Garfield

UTERINE CONTRACTILITY

Mechanisms of Control

Edited by

ROBERT E. GARFIELD

McMaster University Health Sciences Center
Hamilton, Ontario, Canada

Serono Symposia, USA
Norwell, Massachusetts

Proceedings of the Symposium on Uterine Contractility: Mechanisms of Control, sponsored by Serono Symposia, USA, held March 17–20, 1990, in St. Louis, Missouri

© 1990 Serono Symposia, USA
100 Longwater Circle
Norwell, Massachusetts 02061

ISBN: 1-878601-05-9

Printed in the United States of America

SYMPOSIUM ON UTERINE CONTRACTILITY

Scientific Committee

Robert E. Garfield, Ph.D., *Chairman*
Hamilton, Ontario, Canada

Robert H. Hayashi, M.D.
Ann Arbor, Michigan

James M. Roberts, M.D.
San Francisco, California

Melvyn S. Soloff, Ph.D.
Toledo, Ohio

Organizing Secretary

L. Lisa Kern, Ph.D.
Serono Symposia, USA
100 Longwater Circle
Norwell, Massachusetts

Preface

The Serono conference and this subsequent volume represent the efforts of many to understand the mechanisms that control the cellular events of the uterus and how to manipulate them in the laboratory and clinic. It is appropriate that we focus on uterine contractility as it is the essential feature of labor and delivery, a process termed *parturition*. Normal labor is characterized by the forceful myometrial contractions that are required to expel the contents of the pregnant uterus. Clearly, uterine contractility is a major medical issue as either the absence of labor or preterm labor can lead to significant problems.

The idea for a meeting on uterine contractility was born on the streets of Brussels several years ago as Jim Roberts, Mel Soloff, and I strolled along enjoying the beautiful sites. We were taking a break from a similar conference, and we contemplated a future meeting with a slightly different emphasis. Since that time, much has happened, and we were very pleased when Serono agreed to sponsor this meeting. Bob Hayashi was added to the organizing committee sometime later to assist in the clinical aspects of the meeting.

The site and date of the meeting were chosen to correspond with the Annual Meeting of the Society of Gynecologic Investigation in which many speakers and guests also participate. Perhaps the location was also significant for it was in St. Louis that Arpad Csapo lived and worked. Certainly, no conference on uterine contractility can ever be conducted without some inclusion of Csapo's ideas. Considering that Csapo worked with some very crude tools by today's standards, his conclusions were remarkable. Above all, Csapo taught us that labor is more than simply an increase in contractile stimulants at term, a view that some have still failed to grasp. He recognized that some events eventually convert the uterus into an active and reactive organ at the end of pregnancy. This concept continues to dominate the theories of the control of uterine contractility, and it was supported by many of the papers at the Serono symposium.

In the meeting we attempted to explore the underlying basis for uterine contractions, the electrical activity. We were very fortunate to have Dr. Jean Marshall and Dr. Jean Mironneau. Both have contributed much to our understanding of the electrophysiology of the myometrium.

We were all sad that Sir Alexander Turnbull could not join us, but we were delighted that he prepared a manuscript for this volume. We know we would have benefited tremendously by his presence.

It was a privilege for me to be chairman and coordinator of the Serono conference on uterine contractility. The organizing committee was a great help, and I appreciate the support they gave me. I also want to thank Dr. Lisa Kern and other members of the Serono Symposia, USA organization. They did an outstanding job with everything. Finally, many thanks to the speakers—those who presented posters and all those who attended the conference. The meeting was a huge success with participants and guests from many countries around the world. I am confident that our gathering and this book will contribute much to our continued search for the factors involved in the control of uterine contractility.

R. E. Garfield

Contents

ELECTRICAL SIGNALS AND UTERINE CONTRACTILITY

1

Relation Between Membrane Potential and Spontaneous Contraction of the Uterus

Jean M. Marshall

Department of Medicine, Rhode Island Hospital/Brown University School of Medicine, Providence

I n the myometrium, as in other smooth muscles, contraction is initiated when the concentration of free, ionized calcium increases inside the cell. This free so-called activator calcium may come from intracellular storage sites, principally the sarcoplasmic reticulum, or from the extracellular space. Calcium influx occurs via receptor-operated channels, activated by hormones, neurotransmitters, drugs, and other agents and via potential-operated channels, activated by changes in membrane potential.

The most important source of activator calcium for the spontaneous, myogenic contractions of the uterus is extracellular calcium. This calcium enters through the potential-operated channels. Calcium entry is minimal at the resting membrane potential but increases when the membrane is depolarized, culminating in the production of the action potential. Thus membrane electrical events play an important role in the regulation of calcium influx and thereby contraction. Within this framework, the changes in membrane potentials and their relation to spontaneous contractions during pregnancy will be considered first, and then the changes in membrane potentials and spontaneous contractions in the different muscle layers during pregnancy will be compared. Most of the examples are taken from experiments on myometrial segments isolated from the rat, with a few examples from the human. More extensive accounts of this material appear in two excellent recent reviews (1, 2).

MEMBRANE POTENTIAL AND CONTRACTION DURING PREGNANCY

During the course of pregnancy the resting membrane potential declines as a consequence of the changing hormonal environment and the stretch imposed on the myometrium by the developing fetus. The resting potential is defined as the maximal level of membrane polarization reached during the quiescence between periods of spontaneous activity. In the longitudinal myometrium of the rat, for example, the resting potential falls from a level of around –60mV at midterm (as measured with an intracellular electrode relative to the extracellular fluid) to near –45mV at term.

These changes in resting potential are accompanied by alterations in the pattern of action-potential discharge. At midpregnancy, when the resting potential is relatively high, the electrical activity is very irregular, consisting of small, local depolarizations that frequently fail to reach threshold for generation of an action potential; when they do reach threshold, they produce action potentials of varying heights and frequencies. Propagation of the action potential from one cell to the other over the muscle is poor, as a result of the high level of the resting membrane potential and the paucity of cell-to-cell junctions, the so-called gap junctions believed to be the site of current spread within the muscle (see Chapter 3). As a result of this erratic pattern and restricted propagation of the action potentials, the contractions are small and infrequent.

As pregnancy progresses and the resting potential declines, generation of action potential becomes more regular and cell-to-cell propagation improves, culminating in the regular, rhythmic, spontaneous activity that appears just before and during delivery. At this time several types of electrical activity underlie the contractile patterns. One of these is the *slow wave*, characterized by slow depolarizations of the membrane followed by repolarization back to the resting level. When the depolarization phase of the slow wave reaches a critical threshold, a second, much faster depolarization occurs, the *pacemaker* or *generator potential*. The pacemaker potential generates the action potential. The rate of depolarization of the pacemaker potential determines the frequency of discharge of the action potentials.

The frequency of action potential discharge within the individual cells and the number of cells activated determine the *force of contraction;* the higher the frequency, the greater the force. The number of cells activated is determined by the propagation of the action potential from cell to cell. At term propagation is rapid and uniform throughout the muscle primarily due to an increase in the number of gap junctions and also as a result of the decrease in the level of the resting potential. Consequently, large numbers of cells are activated and this enhanced recruitment augments the force of contraction. The *duration of contraction* is determined by the duration of the train of action potentials, which, in turn, is related to the duration of the depolarization phase of the slow wave—that is, the period of time that the membrane potential remains in the critical threshold range. The *rate of contraction* is determined by the rate of the slow wave.

The mechanism underlying the slow wave is not clear. One suggestion is that it is related to the oscillatory activity of an electrogenic sodium pump analogous to that observed in the circular muscle of the gut. The pacemaker potential and the depolarization phase of the action potential are believed to be related to an inward calcium current flowing through the potential-operated channels. The pacemaker potential and the action potentials are abolished in calcium-free solutions and in the presence of calcium channel blockers. Is the calcium carried inward during the action potential sufficient to initiate a contraction? Although the kinetics of the calcium currents during the action potential have never been measured in the myometrium, measurements in isolated smooth muscle cells from the urinary bladder and arterioles indicate that calcium entry during a single action potential transiently (about 1 sec) increases intracellular calcium to about 1 μM. Since much of the calcium entering the cell is buffered by uptake into intracellular storage sites, a sustained increase of calcium to at least 2–3 μM inside the cell would probably be needed for the strong, rhythmic contractions of the uterus at term. An increase of this magnitude might be accomplished by the repetitive trains of action potentials that are synchronous with each contraction and determine its magnitude and duration.

Membrane Potential and Contraction in Different Muscle Layers

The features described thus far concern the behavior of the longitudinal myometrial layer. Some years ago Osa and Katase (3) noted that there were qualitative differences in the behavior of the longitudinal and circular layers of the myometrium. One of the most prominent of these differences was the contour of the action potential in the circular muscle and the changes it undergoes during pregnancy. These characteristic differences are most easily demonstrated in the uterus of rodents, where the two muscle layers are morphologically distinct and can be surgically separated reasonably well.

In contrast to longitudinal muscle, whose electrical activity consists of bursts of spike-type action potentials of varying frequencies, the electrical activity of circular muscle consists of single, plateau-type action potentials during most of gestation. Contractions accompanying the plateau-type action potentials are small, and many action potentials are not associated with contractions. Synchronization between electrical activity and contraction begins early on the day of expected delivery at a time when several single spikes appear on the plateau. Later on this day all electrical activity abruptly ceases, coincident with a sudden increase in level of the resting membrane potential that transiently interrupts the gradual decline that occurs during the previous days. Shortly thereafter the membrane potential again decreases and trains of repetitive spike-type action potentials appear. During delivery the electrical activity consists of repetitive spike bursts synchronous with large, regular contractions; a pattern almost identical to that of the longitudinal muscle. Both the plateau-type action potentials and the repetitive spike trains in circular muscle are abolished when extracellular calcium ions are absent or in the presence of a calcium channel blocker.

The asynchrony between the plateau-type action potentials and contractions in the circular muscle that occurs during most of gestation results principally from the limited propagation of the action potentials within the muscle. Just before and during delivery, when repetitive spike trains appear along with synchronization between electrical activity and contraction, the contractile force also increases in circular muscle. The latter results from improved propagation of the action potentials, thereby recruiting more cells into activity and from an increase in spike frequency within each individual muscle cell.

The electrophysiological and contractile differences between the circular and longitudinal muscle layers suggest that there is little interaction between the two layers during most of gestation. At term, however, when the behavior of the two layers is similar, an interaction might occur. This possibility has been tested by arranging a muscle strip containing both muscle layers so that the electrical activity of one layer is recorded simultaneously with the contractions of the other layer (4). Under these circumstances there is a 1:1 coordination of the electrical activity of the circular layer with the contractions of the longitudinal and vice versa in a muscle strip isolated from a rat just before or during delivery. At earlier times in gestation no such coordination is present. The morphological pathways for the conduction of the action potential between the two muscle layers may reside in the regions of the myometrial wall where light micrographs have shown strands of circular muscle invading the longitudinal (R. E. Garfield, personal communication). If the number of gap junctions within these connecting strands increases dramatically at the end of gestation, as noted in the two muscle layers, this would enhance the electrical coupling between the two layers and promote the coordination of the activity between them.

The functional significance of the coordination of activity between the two muscle layers remains to be established, but one can speculate as follows. The weak, irregular contractions of the circular muscle that is located primarily in the interplacental regions might cause a tonic constriction of this muscle and prevent the movement of the fetuses toward the cervix. The longitudinal muscle, although uniformly distributed over both placental and nonplacental regions, is relatively inactive and has extensive areas of conduction block during early and midpregnancy. As the activity of the circular muscle becomes more organized and the fetuses grow, the constrictions between the fetuses become less obvious and disappear during the quiescent period of the circular muscle on the day of expected delivery. When labor begins, the coordinated activity of both muscle layers might function to move the fetuses toward the cervix, the contractions of the longitudinal muscle shortening the entire uterine horn and the contractions of the circular muscle pushing along the individual fetuses.

Differences in the patterns of discharge of action potential and contraction have also been noted in strips of human myometrium taken from the isthmic portion of the uterus in the final trimester of pregnancy at the time of cesarean section (5). One type of action potential has prominent plateau and is synchronous with a large contraction whose duration is determined by the duration of the plateau. Another type of electrical activity consists of single spikelike potentials that initiate contractions of much smaller amplitude and duration than those initiated by the plateau-type potentials. These differences are not apparent in isthmic myometrial segments taken from uteri at term. At this time the electrical activity consists of slow waves and bursts of spikes that initiate large regular contractions reminiscent of the activity of the rat myometrium during delivery. The electrical activity at all times during gestation is abolished in calcium deficient solutions and in the presence of calcium channel blockers (5).

REFERENCES

1. Parkington HC, Coleman HA. The role of membrane potential in the control of uterine motility. In: Carsten ME, ed. The cellular basis of uterine function. New York: Plenum Press, 1990:194-248.
2. Kao CY. Electrophysiological properties of uterine muscle. In: Wynn RM, Jollie WP, eds. The biology of the uterus. New York: Plenum Press, 1989:403-53.
3. Osa T, Katase T. Physiological comparison of the longitudinal and circular muscles of the pregnant rat uterus. Jpn J Physiol 1975;25:153-64
4. Tomiyasu BA, Chen CJ, Marshall JM. Comparison of the activity of circular and longitudinal myometrium from pregnant rats. Clin Exp Pharmacol Physiol 1988;15:647-56.
5. Kawarabayashi T, Ikeda M, Sugimori H, Nakano H. Spontaneous electrical activity and effects of noradrenaline on pregnant human myometrium recorded by the single sucrose-gap method. Acta Physiol Hung 1986;67:71-82.

2

Ion Channels and Excitation-Contraction Coupling in Myometrium

Jean Mironneau

Laboratoire de Physiologie Cellulaire et Pharmacologie Moléculaire,
INSERM JF 88-13, Bordeaux, France

T he ion channels involved in the generation of electrical signals can be separated in two different groups. Ligand-gated ion channels are opened in response to activation of an associated receptor. Typical channels of this type include the nonspecific ion channel associated with the nicotonic acetylcholine receptor (1), and, in smooth muscle, the nonspecific channels that are opened by activation of muscarinic receptors (2) or ATP receptors (3–5). Activation of ligand-gated ion channels mediate local increases in ion conductance, producing depolarization or hyperpolarization of the membrane. In contrast, voltage-sensitive ion channels mediate rapid, voltage-gated changes in ion conductance during action potentials in excitable cells. In smooth-muscle cells, the action potential is largely dependent on an increase in calcium conductance. The calcium entering cells during action potential serves as the primary intracellular second messenger for the electrical signal generated in the plasma membrane, and initiates excitation-contraction coupling and multiple calcium-activated biochemical processes. In addition, voltage-gated ion channels can be regulated by receptor-dependent processes, including protein phosphorylation and interaction with GTP-binding proteins.

This chapter focuses on the different ion channels that have recently been described in myometrial cells: (*a*) voltage-gated sodium channels, (*b*) voltage-gated calcium channels and modulation by oxytocin, and (*c*) ATP-activated cation channels.

Acknowledgments: This work was supported by grants from Etablissement Public Régional d'Aquitaine, Ministère de la Recherche et de la Technologie, Fondation pour la Recherche Médicale, and Association Française contre les Myopathies, France. We thank Nathalie Biendon for her excellent secretarial assistance.

VOLTAGE-GATED SODIUM CHANNELS

Characterization of sodium channels has been advanced through the use of the selective sodium channel blockers, saxitoxin (STX) and tetrodotoxin (TTX). It is now clear that mammalian sodium channels are encoded by a multigene family (6) and show different functional properties in different tissues. The most widely known difference is that TTX-sensitive sodium channels in nerve and skeletal muscle are blocked by nanomolar concentrations of the neurotoxins (7, 8), whereas TTX-resistant sodium channels in cardiac muscle and noninnervated skeletal muscle can be blocked only by micromolar concentrations of the neurotoxins (9, 10).

In myometrial smooth muscle cells, sodium-dependent action potentials (TTX-resistant) were first reported using the microelectrode technique (11). More recently, TTX-sensitive sodium currents have been described in freshly dissociated cells from pulmonary artery (12) and myometrium of pregnant rats (13). However, no complete biochemical analysis has been made for the presence of sodium channels in myometrial smooth muscle using radioligand experiments.

Equilibrium Binding of [^{3}H]STX to Myometrial Membranes.   The specific binding of [^{3}H]STX to its receptor was proportional to the concentration of myometrial membranes from 0.05 mg of protein/ml to 0.40 mg of protein/ml. A Scatchard plot of the specific binding component indicates the existence of both high- and low-affinity binding sites. The dissociation constants (K_D) and maximal binding capacities (B_{max}) were $K_D = 0.53 \pm 0.11$ nM and $B_{max} = 39 \pm 5$ fmol/mg of protein for the high-affinity site, and $K_D = 27 \pm 6$ nM and $B_{max} = 350 \pm 45$ fmol/mg of protein for the low-affinity binding site (n = 6).

Properties of the High-Affinity Binding Site for [^{3}H]STX.   The properties of the high-affinity [^{3}H]STX site were examined using 0.4 nM [^{3}H]STX. Under these conditions, about 80% of the signal originated from binding to the high-affinity binding sites and 20% from binding to the low-affinity binding sites. Increasing concentrations of unlabeled STX or TTX gradually inhibited the [^{3}H]STX binding. The inhibition constant values (K_i) for STX and TTX were 0.18 ± 0.02 and 0.94 ± 0.04 nM, respectively (n = 4). The Hill coefficients were close to 1, indicating that the drugs bound to a single binding site.

Properties of the Low-Affinity Binding Site for [^{3}H]STX.   The properties of the low-affinity [^{3}H]STX site were examined using 15 nM [^{3}H]STX. Under these conditions, about 80% of the total bound ligand was associated with the low-affinity binding site. Increasing concentrations of unlabeled neurotoxins gradually inhibited [^{3}H]STX binding to the low-affinity binding sites. The inhibition constant values (K_i) for STX and TTX were 55 ± 9 nM (n = 3) and 1.2 ± 0.4 µM (n = 3), respectively. The Hill coefficients were close to 1, suggesting that the neurotoxins bound to a single binding site.

Patch-Clamp Identification of Veratridine-Activated Current.   In short-term primary cultures, it has been shown that voltage-gated sodium channels can be revealed by external applications of neurotoxins such as veratridine and sea anemone toxins (11). When 100 µM veratridine was applied in the bath solution to a voltage-clamped myometrial cell, the inward calcium channel current elicited by a positive voltage pulse was progressively inhibited within 2 to 3 min. After the pulse, there was a standing inward tail current representing a population of veratridine-modified channels that did not close at −80 mV. The tail current decayed to zero within several seconds. In the continuous presence of external veratridine, the tail current was recorded without a noticeable variation in amplitude for 5 to 10 min.

Ion Selectivity of the Veratridine-Activated Current. Plotting the maximal tail current (measured 5 ms after returning to the holding potential) against the test potentials showed that the current-voltage relationship was linear. Reversal potentials were determined when the sodium electrochemical gradient was altered by replacing external or internal sodium. The experimental points were closely distributed along a straight line with a slope of 1, as expected for a pure sodium conductance. The amplitude of the current appeared to be related only to the extracellular sodium concentration as it was recorded in the absence of external calcium.

Inhibition of Veratridine-Activated Sodium Current. Both STX and TTX applied for 5 min reduced the amplitude of the sodium current in a concentration-dependent manner. The concentrations of STX and TTX inhibiting 50% of the maximal current (IC_{50}) were estimated to be 1.4 ± 0.3 and 8.8 ± 0.2 nM, respectively (n = 5). The slope factor of the concentration-response curves was about 0.6, suggesting that the neurotoxins have multiple sites of interaction in myometrial membrane.

Conclusion. The apparent dissociation constant of STX measured by electrophysiology does not correspond to the K_D of [^{3}H]STX for both high- and low-affinity membrane receptors. These observations suggest that the high- and low-affinity receptors for STX identified by binding experiments could reflect the existence of two different subtypes of STX-sensitive sodium channels, which could correspond to slightly different membrane proteins. Recently, Pidoplichko (14) reported that two types of sodium currents recorded from ventricular cells can be distinguished by their sensitivity to TTX (K_D = 80 nM and 7 µM). Unequivocal answers to these molecular questions will require more detailed electrophysiological and biochemical experiments in smooth muscle. However, it is now clear that mammalian sodium channels are encoded by a multigene family and that separate genes encode for high- and low-affinity STX receptors (6).

VOLTAGE-GATED CALCIUM CHANNELS

A number of calcium entry blockers, including nifedipine, nicardipine, diltiazem, verapamil, and gallopamil have been shown to inhibit uterine contractions after intravenous and/or per os administration. The species have included the rat, rabbit, sheep, monkey, and human (15). The dihydropyridines are the most potent and selective inhibitors of uterine tension development among the calcium entry blockers and therefore are of considerable interest for both therapeutic and experimental purposes. In cardiac cells the concentrations of dihydropyridines, which give rise to half-maximal electrophysiological responses, are several orders of magnitude greater than the dissociation constant values determined from radioligand binding (16–18). Recent electrophysiological experiments in vascular and visceral smooth muscle cells have demonstrated a voltage dependence of dihydropyridine antagonist action, and this has been postulated to account for the differences between the binding affinities and the dissociation constants determined from the pharmacological effects of these drugs (19, 20).

Number of Inward Calcium Channel Currents in Single Myometrial Cells

Recent studies (21–24) have indicated that vascular and visceral smooth-muscle cells contain two distinct kinds of calcium channels. In a given cell type, the two types of calcium channels (T and L channels) have different selectivity, single-channel conductance, and pharmacology. Furthermore, T-type channels are inactivated by steady-state holding potentials to about −40 mV, while L-type channels need much more positive holding potentials for steady-state inactivation.

We examined whether the inward current in single rat myometrial cells might be composed of two components by applying depolarizing test pulses to various test potentials from two different holding potentials. In 85% of cells used, neither change in kinetics of inactivation nor shift in the peak current was observed between the two families of currents (n = 125). Thus, in our experimental conditions much evidence suggests that the calcium channel current appears to be mainly a L-type inward current: (*a*) Equimolar replacement of barium for calcium induces an increase in the peak current and a decrease in the inactivation rate. (*b*) Residual inward currents were recorded at the end of the pulses. (*c*) Membrane potential for midinactivation was about −40 mV. However, in 15% of cells tested, two components of calcium channel currents could be separated by variations in holding potential (25).

Effects of (+)Isradipine on the Calcium Channel Current

As in various structures, it was found that T-type channel currents were insensitive to (+)isradipine (a dihydropyridine derivative) blockade while L-type channel currents were fully inhibited with low concentrations of (+)isradipine. To study the mechanism of blockade of the calcium channel current with (+)isradipine in more detail we used different protocols to assess the relative contribution of initial, conditioned, and tonic blockade of calcium channels. First, when voltage clamp depolarization was applied at a frequency of 0.05 Hz, the inhibition induced by 20 nM (+)isradipine reached $50 \pm 5\%$ (n = 7) within 5 min. Second, isradipine (20 nM) was applied during a rest period of 5 min and blockade was assessed as the difference between peak current in the control and the first pulse after drug exposure. The calcium channel current was inhibited by $48 \pm 6\%$ (n = 4), indicating that the blockade was not dependent on the number of voltage depolarizations applied at 0.05 Hz. Because hyperpolarizing the membrane to −90 mV for 1 min restored the inward current, we can assume that the blockade was largely initial.

Third, in order to investigate whether (+)isradipine bound with a higher affinity to the inactivated state of the calcium channel, we studied the effect of (+)isradipine blockade on the steady-state inactivation curve of the calcium channel current. From the shift in the inactivation curve, it is possible to estimate the dissociation constant for (+)isradipine binding in the resting and inactivated state by using the approach described by Bean (16), assuming one-to-one binding of drug to the resting and inactivated states. The dissociation constant for binding to the inactivated state (K_i) can be calculated using the equation $\Delta Vh = k \, Ln(1 + [Isr]/K_i)/(1 + [Isr]/K_r)$, where ΔVh is the shift of the midpoint of the steady-state availability curve, k is the slope factor of the inactivation curve, [Isr] is the (+)isradipine concentration used, and K_r is determined as the potency of (+)isradipine for the resting calcium channel. With $\Delta Vh = 24$ mV, k = 5.7 mV, $K_r = 23$ nM and [Isr] = 20 nM, we found $K_i = 130$ pM.

Determination of the Dissociation Constant for (+)[^{3}H]Isradipine on Myometrial Membranes

As the potency of (+)isradipine blockade changed with the holding potential in a manner consistent with a very high binding to the inactivated state of the calcium channel and a much weaker binding to the resting state, it was of interest to verify whether the K_i we determined quantitatively was similar to the dissociation constant of the high-affinity binding site for (+)isradipine determined with radioligand binding studies. Scatchard analysis of the specific binding of (+)[^{3}H]isradipine resulted in a linear plot, thereby indicating specific binding to a single class of sites. The dissociation constant, K_D, was 100 ± 10 pM, and the maximal binding capacity, B_{max}, was 95 ± 5 fmol/mg of protein (n = 8). The Hill plot was linear with a slope of 0.93.

Modulation of Calcium Channels by Oxytocin

It is well known that oxytocin increases the frequency and the force of spontaneous contractions of the uterus. This effect has been correlated with an increase in calcium current (26) and a release of calcium from intracellular stores. The concentration of oxytocin receptors in myometrium depends on the steroid concentration, because estrogens are capable of causing an increase in oxytocin receptor concentration and progesterone antagonizes the estrogen effect (27).

In the absence of estrogens in the culture medium, oxytocin (0.2 nM) produced a small increase of the maximal calcium current elicited from a holding potential of –40 mV. The current stimulation was estimated to be 10–15% (n = 10). In contrast, when isolated cells from pregnant rats at 18 days' gestation were cultured with 1 μM diethylstilbestrol (DES) for 12 h, the increase in calcium current induced by 0.2 nM oxytocin reached $55 \pm 8\%$ (n = 5) as shown in Figure 1. Oxytocin markedly increased the amplitude of the calcium current at all potentials, but did not influence the reversal potential—the potential at which the current was maximal—and the threshold potential. Thus, the analysis may be confined to possible changes in calcium conductance or inactivation parameters. Since the

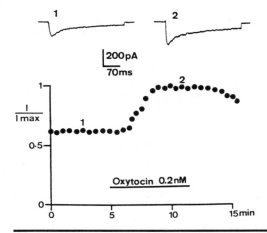

Fig. 1.   Effects of oxytocin on calcium channel current evoked by depolarizations to 0 mV from a holding potential of −40 mV in isolated myometrial cells, and time-course of the peak inward current during application of 0.2 nM oxytocin in a cell cultured with 1 µM diethylstilbestrol for 15 h. Currents are expressed as a fraction of their maximal values. *Inset:* Current traces correspond to number on the curves; external solution contained 10 nM barium.

steady-state inactivation curve of the calcium current was similar in control and in the presence of 0.2 nM oxytocin, it is assumed that oxytocin acts by increasing the maximal calcium conductance of myometrial cells.

Conclusion

The dihydropyridine blockade of calcium channel current in vascular and visceral cells is enhanced by depolarizing the holding potential. We found in myometrial cells not only that (+)isradipine bound to the closed, available state of calcium channels, but also that it had a high affinity for the inactivated state. At the resting state, where most calcium channels were thought to be in the closed, available state, we found an IC_{50} of about 20 nM, which was fairly low compared to the IC_{50} found in cardiac cells (IC_{50} = 400 nM[18]) Assuming one-to-one binding of (+)isradipine to the resting and inactivated state, we calculated a dissociation constant for binding to the inactivated state (K_i) of about 100 pM. This value is similar to the dissociation constant obtained from both equilibrium binding and kinetic experiments in isolated membranes.

These results indicate that low concentrations of dihydropyridine can affect the contractility of the uterus. Although the resting membrane potentials in intact tissues of rat myometrium and portal vein were similar (about −45 mV), the potency of isradipine blockade for the resting state of the L-type calcium channel was much greater in vein. A K_r value of 0.15 nM with (+)isradipine was reported for the resting calcium channel in rat portal vein cells (19), which is about 3–5 times lower than the value reported in myometrium. This observation suggests that the membrane potential is not the sole determinant of dihydropyridine binding affinities in smooth muscles.

Oxytocin increases the L-type calcium current of myometrial cells, an effect that was more pronounced in DES-treated cells. However, the transduction mechanisms for agonist-induced increase in calcium current remain to be studied.

LIGAND-GATED NONSPECIFIC CHANNELS

ATP has received increasing attention, because it has effects similar to activation of nonadrenergic, noncholinergic nerves in various smooth muscles, including uterus (28). Evidence has accumulated indicating that ATP is involved in the physiological regulation of nonvascular smooth muscle tone through liberation from "purinergic" nerve endings. In uterine smooth muscles, ATP shows different actions depending on the hormonal condition. In pregnant rat myometrium, applications of ATP in the range of 10 µM to 1 mM caused phasic and tonic contractions (29). In the estrogen-treated rat myometrium, the generation of phasic contraction was less frequent and the amplitude of tonic contractions was much smaller than in the pregnant one.

The ability of ATP to release internal Ca has been demonstrated for a variety of smooth muscle cells (30, 31). The Ca release has been related to the production of inositol triphosphate through activation of P_2 receptors by ATP.

Ionic mechanisms underlying electrical responses of pregnant rat myometrial smooth muscle cells to ATP have not been thoroughly investigated. We focused on the ATP-activated Ca-independent conductance in single myometrial cells maintained in short-term primary culture (4).

Electrophysiological Effects of ATP

Bath application of 1 mM ATP in a single cell maintained at a holding potential of −70 mV, produced a sustained inward current. Responses to ATP of about 200 pA in amplitude were recorded in 96% of the cells obtained from pregnant rats at 19 days' gestation. As previously reported (29), the response of myometrial cells to ATP is modified during gestation. In order to determine whether the decrease in ATP response is due to the increase in estrogenic impregnation during pregnancy, we studied the effect of estrogen pretreatment of isolated cells in primary culture. Isolated cells from pregnant rats at 19 days' gestation were cultured with 10 µM diethylstilbestrol (DES) for 15 h. The mean peak amplitude of the ATP-induced inward current recorded at −70 mV was strongly reduced to about 20% of control.

A pressure ejection pulse of 1 mM ATP (for 2 s) produced a response that was fast in onset and had a short time to peak. The latency (interval between start of pressure ejection and onset of inward current) was less than 100 ms in all cells tested. Furthermore, it was possible to obtain several similar responses to ATP in a cell without any decline in the amplitude of the response.

The concentration-response relationship can be fitted well by assuming that a receptor needs to bind one ATP molecule at a single site to activate current. From the fitted curve, the interpolated concentration for half-activation of the conductance is about 0.6 mM. If the free-acid form of ATP was the only effective form of ATP, the recorded concentration for half-activation of the conductance would correspond to a value of 0.09 mM ATP^{4-}.

Ionic Selectivity of I_{ATP}

With a reversal potential close to 0 mV, it is to be expected that ATP activates either a chloride or a nonspecific cationic conductance. We tried to determine which ions carry I_{ATP} by changing the ionic composition of the internal and external solutions. In order to test whether chloride ions were involved in I_{ATP}, we substituted most of the extracellular chloride with aspartate. With this low external chloride concentration (49 mM), the chloride equilibrium potential was calculated to be about +30 mV. However, in these experimental conditions, the apparent reversal potential of I_{ATP} remained close to 0 mV; indicating that it was very unlikely that chloride was involved in I_{ATP}. Investigating quantitatively the role of sodium entry in I_{ATP}, we found that the relationship between the reversal potential of I_{ATP} and the sodium equilibrium potential was linear, but it differed from the predicted curve for a purely sodium conductance. It is interesting that there was a measurable, although very small, inward current remaining with an extracellular solution containing only 2 mM Na$^+$ representing 3%–5% of the inward current recorded in the presence of 137 mM Na$^+$. This little inward current could still be recorded when sodium ions were substituted with choline (in the presence of 0.1 mM atropine), suggesting that it could be carried by divalent cations.

We also studied the effect of extracellular sodium substitutions with cesium and potassium. The ability of cesium, potassium, and sodium to carry large currents with identical reversal potential through the ATP-activated conductance pathway demonstrates that this conductance is cation selective but with little discrimination between at least sodium, potassium, and cesium ions.

Effects of Divalent Cations on I_{ATP}

In order to determine whether divalent cations were permeable through the conductance activated by 1 mM ATP, we investigated the effects of increasing concentrations of barium on I_{ATP}. The amplitude of the ATP response was gradually decreased when the barium concentration was raised from 2.5 mM to 10 mM. It may be possible that in the presence of increasing concentrations of divalent cations, the concentration of ATP in the free-acid form would be reduced to subthreshold levels owing to barium chelation. In order to verify whether ATP in the free-acid form was the effective ligand, we investigated the effects of divalent cation substitution (at the concentration of 2.5 mM) on the amplitude and the reversal potential of I_{ATP}. Substitution of barium ions with calcium, magnesium, and cobalt ions gradually depressed the amplitude of I_{ATP}. As the theoretical order for ATP chelation is Co > Mg > Ca > Ba, we tend to believe that ATP in the free-acid form may be the effective ligand for activation of purinoceptors in rat myometrial cells. This characteristic does not seem to be a general feature of purinergic receptors in smooth-muscle cells since in an isotonic calcium solution (110 mM) a large inward current through the ATP-activated conductance is recorded in single ear artery smooth-muscle cells with micromolar concentrations of ATP (3).

Pharmacology of the Response to ATP

The ability of other phosphorylated derivatives of adenosine to activate the ATP conductance was tested. Adenosine, AMP, and ADP failed to elicit any measurable current, suggesting that the receptors were of P_2 type.

Conclusion

In myometrium, ATP binds to P_2-receptors and activates a nondesensitizing conductance that is cation selective and estrogen sensitive but that does not appear to discriminate strongly between at least sodium, potassium, and cesium ions. The cellular mechanism underlying the ATP-elicited conductance is calcium independent. The other possibilities would be either a direct control of a channel closely linked to a ligand receptor or the generation of a chemical second messenger. It is quite possible that the ATP-activated conductance involves a chemical second messenger, since onset kinetics of I_{ATP} were relatively fast (< 100 ms) and, furthermore, I_{ATP} did not undergo any desensitization. However, we found that oxytocin, acetylcholine, isoproterenol, prostaglandin E_2, phorbol esters, and caffeine were ineffective in eliciting a comparable increase in membrane conductance. These possibilities remained to be explored in more detail.

EXCITATION-CONTRACTION COUPLING IN MYOMETRIUM

In myometrium, it has been shown that contraction is dependent on both calcium influx through voltage-dependent calcium channels and calcium release from intracellular stores (32, 33). Furthermore, activation of voltage-gated sodium channels by neurotransmitters and hormones as well as ATP-activated nonspecific cation channels may produce membrane depolarizations. These depolarizations may, in turn, activate the calcium channels and initiate the contractile response.

Important questions remain to be answered about the functional roles of the different types of ion channels in myometrium. Because of the importance of electrical signaling in information transmission in smooth muscle cells, in the action of many classes of pharmacological agents, and in regulation of ion channels by neurotransmitters and hormones, development of a detailed understanding of the mechanisms of electrical excitability will continue to be a major goal in cellular and molecular physiology.

REFERENCES

1. Sobel A, Hofler J, Heidman T, Changeux JP. Structural and functional properties of the acetylcholine regulator. In: Ceccarelli B, Clementi F, eds. Advances in cytopharmacology, vol 3. New York: Raven Press, 1979:191-6.
2. Benham CD, Bolton TB, Lang RJ. Acetylcholine activates an inward current in single mammalian smooth muscle cells. Nature 1985;316:345-7.

3. Benham CD, Tsien RW. A novel receptor-operated Ca^{2+}-permeable channel activated by ATP in smooth muscle. Nature 1987;328:473-88.

4. Honoré E, Martin C, Mironneau C, Mironneau J. An ATP-sensitive conductance in cultured smooth muscle cells from pregnant rat myometrium. Am J Physiol 1989;257:C297-305.

5. Friel D. An ATP-sensitive conductance in single smooth muscle cells from the rat vas deferens. J Physiol (Lond) 1988;401:361-80.

6. Rogart RB, Cribbs LL, Muglia LK, Kephart DD, Kaiser MW. Molecular cloning of a putative tetrodotoxin-resistant rat heart Na^+ channel isoform. Proc Natl Acad Sci USA 1989;86:8170-4.

7. Paponne P. Voltage-clamp experiments in normal and denervated mammalian skeletal muscle fibres. J Physiol (Lond) 1980;306:377-410.

8. Benoit E, Corbier A, Dubois JM. Evidence for two transient sodium currents in the frog mode of Ranvier. J Physiol (Lond) 1985;361:339-60.

9. Renaud JF, Kazazoglou T, Lombet A, Chicheportiche R, Jaimovich E, Romey G, Lazdunski M. The Na^+ channel in mammalian cardiac cells. J Biol Chem 1983;258:8799-805.

10. Guo X, Uehara A, Ravindran A, Bryan SH, Hall S, Moczydloski E. Kinetic basis for insensitivity to tetrodotoxin and saxitoxin in sodium channels of canine heart and denervated rat skeletal muscle. Biochem 1987;26:7546-56.

11. Amédée T, Renaud JF, Jmari K, Lombet A, Mironneau J, Lazdunski M. The presence of Na^+ channels in myometrial smooth muscle cells is revealed by specific neurotoxins. Biochem Biophys Res Comm 1986;137:675-81.

12. Okabe K, Kitamura K, Kuriyama H. The existence of a highly tetrodotoxin sensitive Na channel in freshly dispersed smooth muscle cells of the rabbit main pulmonary artery. Pflügers Arch 1988;411:423-8.

13. Ohya Y, Sperelakis N. Fast Na^+ and slow Ca^{2+} channels in single uterine muscle cells from pregnant rats. Am J Physiol 1989;257:C408-12.

14. Pidoplichko VI. Two different tetrodotoxin-separable inward sodium currents in the membrane of isolated cardiomyocytes. Gen Physiol Biophys 1986;6:593-604.

15. Hollingsworth M, Downing S. Calcium entry blockers and the uterus. Med Sci Res 1988;16:1-16.

16. Bean B. Nitrendipine block of cardiac calcium channels: high-affinity binding to the inactivated state. Proc Natl Acad Sci USA 1984;81:6388-92.

17. Kokubun S, Prod' Hom B, Becker C, Porzig H, Reuter H. Studies on Ca channels in intact cardiac cells: voltage-dependent effects and cooperative interactions of dihydropyridine enantiomers. Mol Pharmacol 1987;30:571-84.

18. Hamilton S, Yatani A, Brush K, Schwartz A, Brown A. A comparison between the binding and electrophysiological effects of dihydropyridines on cardiac membranes. Mol Pharmacol 1987;31:221-31.

19. Dacquet C, Pacaud P, Loirand G, Mironneau C, Mironneau J. Comparison of binding affinities and calcium current inhibitory effects of a 1, 4-dihydropyridine derivative (PN 200-110) in vascular smooth muscle. Biochem Biophys Res Comm 1988;152:1165-72.

20. Loirand G, Mironneau C, Mironneau J, Pacaud P. Two types of calcium currents in single smooth muscle cells from rat portal vein. J Physiol (Lond) 1989;412:333-49.

21. Loirand G, Pacaud P, Mironneau C, Mironneau J. Evidence for two distinct calcium

channels in rat vascular smooth muscle cells in short-term primary culture. Pflügers Arch 1986;407:566-8.

22. Sturek M, Hermsmeyer K. Calcium and sodium channels in spontaneously contracting vascular muscle cells. Science 1986;233:475-8.

23. Benham C, Hess T, Tsien R. Two types of calcium channels in single smooth muscle cells from rabbit ear artery studied with whole-cell and single-channel recordings. Circ Res 1987;61:I10-6.

24. Yoshino M, Someya T, Nishio A, Yabu H. Whole-cell and unitary Ca channel currents in mammalian intestinal smooth muscle cells: evidence for the existence of two types of Ca channels. Pflügers Arch 1988;411:229-31.

25. Honoré E, Amédée T, Martin C, Dacquet C, Mironneau C, Mironneau J. Calcium channel current and its sensitivity to (+)isradipine in cultured pregnant rat myometrial cells. Pflügers Arch 1989;414:477-83.

26. Mironneau J. Effects of oxytocin on ionic currents underlying rhythmic activity and contraction in uterine smooth muscle. Pflügers Arch 1976;363:113-8.

27. Soloff MS. Regulation of oxytocin action at the receptor level. In: Bottari S, Thomas JP, Vokaer A, Vokaer R, eds. Uterine contractility. Paris: Masson, 1984:261-4.

28. Burnstock G. Purinergic nerves. Pharmacol Rev 1972;24:509-81.

29. Osa T, Maruta K. The mechanical response of rat myometrium to adenosine triphosphate in Ca-free solution. Jpn J Physiol 1987;37:515-31.

30. Phaneuf S, Berta P, Casanova J, Cavadore JC. ATP stimulates inositol phosphate accumulation and calcium mobilization in primary culture of rat aortic myocytes. Biochem Biophys Res Comm 1987;143:454-60.

31. Tawada Y, Furukawa KI, Shigekawa M. ATP-induced calcium transient in cultured rat aortic smooth muscle cells. J Biochem 1987;102:1499-509.

32. Mironneau J. Excitation-contraction coupling in voltage-clamped uterine smooth muscle. J Physiol (Lond) 1973;233:127-41.

33. Lalanne C, Mironneau C, Mironneau J, Savineau JP. Contractions of rat uterine smooth muscle induced by acetylcholine and angiotensin II in Ca^{2+}-free medium. Br J Pharmacol 1984;81:317-26.

3

Intercellular Coupling and Modulation of Uterine Contractility

R. E. Garfield, T. Tabb, and G. Thilander

Departments of Biomedical Sciences and Obstetrics/Gynecology,
McMaster University, Hamilton, Ontario, Canada

T he myometrium is extremely active mechanically during labor at the end of gestation. The onset and progression of frequent and synchronous activity are required to forcefully expel the fetus. Conversely, the absence of these vigorous contractions and the prevailing state of relative quiescence and asynchrony are believed to be indispensable for implantation of the fertilized ovum and nourishment of the developing fetus during pregnancy. The observation that gap junctions are present in large numbers between myometrial cells during parturition is thought to be significant with regard to the control and coordination of uterine contractility. In this brief review, we outline some of the salient features of the ways gap junctions are involved in the modulation of myometrial contractility.

IMPORTANCE OF COUPLING

Uterine muscle, the myometrium, is composed of a multitude of small smooth-muscle cells usually aligned in two muscle layers (1). The number of myometrial cells in the human uterus at term is estimated at 200 billion cells, with the size of each fusiform cell about 5–10 μm in diameter and about 200 μm long (2). Considering the structure of the uterus and the number of cells, it follows that some mechanism must exist for the tissue to contract rhythmically and forcefully. Also evident is that phasic or cyclical patterns of contractile activity of the uterus cannot be accounted for by the stimulation or inhibition from the nervous or endocrine systems.

Potential force generation in any muscle tissue is a function of the cross-sectional area and the number of contractile units. Changes therefore, in either muscle mass or alterations in the mechanism of excitation to recruit more muscle cells contribute greatly to the generation of forceful contractions. Total uterine mass increases approximately 20-fold during gestation mainly due to hypertrophy and hyperplasia of the muscle cells. Similarly, in nonpregnant animals, the myometrium enlarges after estrogen treatment, though not to the same extent as during pregnancy. These increases in mass cannot account for the phasic and intense contractions of the uterus, however.

When the force of spontaneous uterine contractions, as recorded in vitro, is normalized to a cross-sectional area of the tissue, the magnitude of the uterine contractions is greater near term than in early pregnancy. However, when the same comparisons are made after treatment with some contractile agonists (i.e., KCl or carbachol), maximal stimulation generally produces the same force per cross-sectional area at any time of pregnancy (3). The latter observations suggest that the force-generating potential of the muscle cells does not change at different times during pregnancy (see also reference 2). Thus, the contractile units do not vary their inherent properties markedly during pregnancy, but according to Laplace's theorem, the force developed by the entire uterus has the ability to significantly increase, because of the enlargement of the muscle. In other words, the capacity for a contraction is great at term but we cannot explain the forces of labor by the changes in individual muscle cells.

While the concept of mass versus force is useful in understanding contractions of striated muscle, it is not normally applicable to contractions of the uterus. It would be unusual for all the muscle cells of the uterus to contract simultaneously. Normally contractions of the preterm uterus are local, asynchronous, and fail to generate effective force. At term, for the successful expulsion of the fetus, the contractions become increasingly more frequent, synchronous, and intense to produce powerful propulsive contractions similar to the peristaltic movement of the intestine. The mechanisms that control the inactivity of the myometrium during early pregnancy and the conversion to the active state of labor are fundamental to our understanding of uterine contractility. Especially important is the mechanism by which the myometrium recruits contractile units to produce a forceful contraction.

The basis for a uterine contraction lies in the electrical and chemical changes that occur within the muscle cells (see Chapters 1 and 2). Phasic contractile activity is a direct consequence of the underlying electrical activity of the muscle cells (4, 5). The sequence of contraction and relaxation of the myometrium results from the cyclic depolarization and repolarization of the muscle cell membranes known as spikes or action potentials (4-6). The driving force for myometrial contractility is thought to be provided by propagated action potentials (Fig. 1) that arise from pacemaker regions (4-6). As in other excitable tissues, the action potential in uterine smooth muscle results from voltage- and time-dependent changes in membrane ionic permeabilities (the ionic theory of excitation). The depolarizing phase of the spike is due to an inward current carried mainly by Ca^{++} ions but also by Na^+ ions. The outward current, causing repolarization, is carried by K^+ ions and consists of a fast (voltage-dependent) and a slow (Ca^{++} activated) component (6). The frequency and intensity of contractions are directly proportional to the regularity and duration of action potentials in each muscle cell and the total

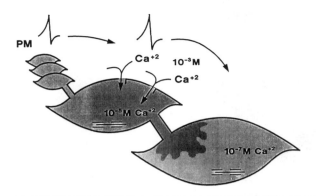

Fig. 1. A group of myometrial cells interconnected by low-resistance pathways. Action potentials, as recorded with microelectrodes, are initiated in pacemaker cells (PM) and propagate to coupled cells. As the action potential passes, it increases Ca^{++} ions intracellularly from $10^{-7}M$ to $10^{-5}M$ to produce a contraction.

number of cells that are active (4, 5). The contractile event of uterine smooth muscle is initiated by a rise in the intracellular free ionized Ca^{++} to approximately $10^{-5}M$ from a resting level of about $10^{-7}M$ (Figs. 1 and 2) (6). The source of this activator Ca^{++} is extracellular (Ca^{++} ions that flow into the cell down their electrochemical gradient in response to a change in membrane permeability) or intracellular (Ca^{++} ions released from intracellular storage sites) or a combination of both (6). Conversely, a reduction of intracellular free Ca^{++} (either as a result of efflux into the extracellular space or re-uptake into intracellular storage sites) terminates contraction (4–8). Therefore, the mechanism that controls the propagation of action potentials between muscle cells from pacemaker regions indirectly regulates the availability of intracellular Ca^{++} ions.

In the myometrium, an action potential depolarization opens voltage-dependent Ca^{++} channels allowing Ca^{++} ions to enter the muscle cell and interact with the myofilaments (Fig. 1). The Ca^{++} ions from a single action potential can initiate a twitch contraction (Fig. 2) (4–6). However, when action potentials are repetitively discharged (for example, in spike bursts) the contraction amplitude is increased because the intracellular level of free Ca^{++} is increased and because the increments in tensions triggered by individual spikes can summate. When action potentials are discharged at a rate higher than about 1 cycle per second, a fused tetanic type contraction is generated (4). Thus, the frequency and duration of spike discharge can control the contraction height and duration, respectively (4, 5). In this way, the frequency of pacemaker discharge determines the rate and intensity of uterine contractions. However, increases in contractile force in the muscle may be achieved by a more or less synchronous stimulation of large areas of the myometrium by increases in conduction of action potentials, as opposed to a faster

Pacemaker   Electrical Activity   Mechanical
                                              Event

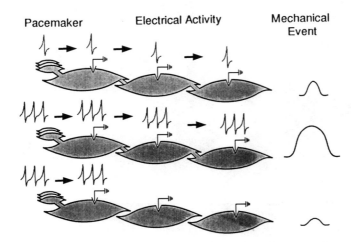

Fig. 2. Electrical and mechanical activity in three groups of cells. The frequency, duration, and magnitude of the contractions are proportional to the frequency of action potentials generated by pacemakers, the number of action potentials produced in each cell, and the number of cells involved in the contractile event. A single propagated action potential produces a weak contraction *(top group)*. Bursts of conducted action potentials result in a much greater contraction *(middle group)*. The consequence of conduction block or failure to propagate is also a reduction in contraction *(bottom group)*.

rate of stimulation of individual cells (see Fig. 2) (4–6). The ability of muscle cells to propagate action potentials is related to the resting membrane potential (about −45 mV), the ability of ions to pass through the membranes, as well as the extent of intercellular coupling. Cells more easily elicit action potentials when they are more positive and nearer their threshold. Conversely, action potentials develop more difficultly when cells are more negative (hyperpolarized) (4, 5). Therefore, the level of excitability of the muscle cells as well as the extent of electrical coupling between the cells significantly influence the ability of the muscle to contract. Intrinsic substances from either the endocrine, nervous, and immune systems or from the application of pharmacological agents which either change the membrane potential, initiate pacemaker activity, influence ionic exchange, or modulate electrical propagation, can have important consequences.

Despite a variety of experimental approaches, most investigators of myometrial contractility have ultimately concluded that propagation of electrical signals between muscle cells plays a major role in the excitation-contraction process (1–20). Most also have found that electrical coupling is greatest during parturition and is either higher or lower, respectively, after estrogen or progesterone treatment of nonpregnant animals (2, 4, 13, 20). However, it has only been recently that the essentials of cell-to-cell conduction have been realized.

BASIS OF PROPAGATION

Electrical interaction between myometrial cells implies the existence of intercellular low-resistance pathways for current spread. Initial observations of the crayfish giant motor synapse started research into intercellular coupling when it was noted that electrical current injected into one cell could alter the electrical potential of an adjacent cell without delay (21). These studies were followed by structural investigations that showed certain membrane specializations in the intercellular region, now termed gap junctions, could be responsible for electrical interaction (22). Gap junctions are now acknowledged as the sites of electrical and metabolic coupling in all types of cells (23–29).

Gap junctions (Figs. 3 and 4) are intercellular channels that link cells to their neighbors by allowing the passage of inorganic ions and small molecules. They have been found between cells in every tissue and organ examined and are ubiquitous in the animal kingdom. In the electron microscope they appear in regions of close apposition between cells as zones of paired, parallel membranes, of unusually smooth outline, separated by a narrow space of constant width about 2 nM—the "gap" (23–29). Both negative staining and freeze-fracture show that these regions

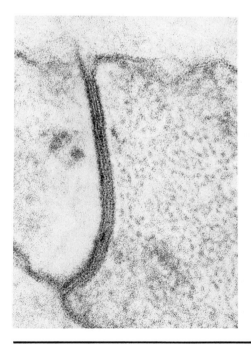

Fig. 3. High magnitude electron micrograph (246,000×) of a gap junction between two myometrial cells. Note lined appearance and central "gap" between the membranes. (From Garfield RE, Blennerhassett MG, Miller SM, Control of myometrial contractility: role and regulation of gap junctions, Oxford Rev 1988;10:436–90.)

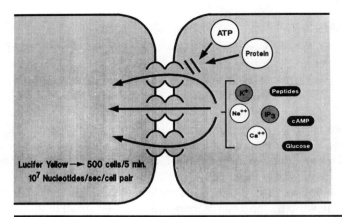

Fig. 4. Model of two cells coupled together by gap-junction channels. Shown are small current-carrying ions (CA^{++}, NA^{++}, K^+, and also Cl—not indicated), metabolites, and second messengers (glucose, peptides, cAMP, and IP_3) that are capable of passing between cells via the 2 nM diameter channels. The movement of larger molecules (proteins, ATP, etc.) is restricted. Two examples of rapid diffusion of substances are displayed in the left cell (see text for details).

have characteristic membrane particles present in each contributing membrane, that meet in register at regularly spaced intervals along the gap (22). Each cell of the pair contributes a set of particles, with one particle termed a hemichannel or connexon,* and two together forming one intercellular channel. While connexons, like other membrane proteins, can move laterally in the fluid membrane, unpaired connexons are not functional, and gap junctions seem to be formed only when these particles aggregate into characteristic, roughly circular plaques. The mechanism for this is not known, nor whether functional channels can occur between single pairs of connexons.

In excitable cells, electrical coupling via the gap junctions allows transmission of action potentials by local circuit current flow. The net junctional resistance is determined by the number of channels, the mean open time of each channel, and perhaps the predominant conductance state. Regulation of cell coupling in any of these ways will determine the rate of electrical propagation and the extent of electrical coordination. In excitable and nonexcitable cells, gap junctions appear to be composed of ionic channels, with large unitary conductance of 120–165 pS, that undergo spontaneous openings and closings and discriminate poorly between cations and anions (23–29). The rate of transition between states is rapid, and it is suggested to be due to conformational change in the channel macromolecule. In tissues where the number of gap junctions is modulated in response to extracellular stimuli, for example, steroid hormones and the uterus (see below) or glucose

---

*Note that *connexon* refers to the hemichannel, while the term *connexin* (discussed later in this chapter) indicates one of six proteins of the connexon.

stimulation of pancreatic β-cells (30), the increase probably occurs by insertion of single particles, which then aggregate. When the gap-junction number decreases, either particles disperse into the surrounding membrane or the intact junctional membrane is taken into the cytoplasm by one cell, as an annular gap junction (24). In general, modulation of gap junction area occurs over a time measurable in hours, which corresponds with the approximately 5-h half-life of the liver gap-junction protein (31).

The rapid closure of gap junctions is necessary to isolate healthy cells from damaged neighbors, to prevent the loss of small cytoplasmic components, and also apparently to allow rapid adjustment of coupling levels to changing circumstances. Experimentally, cell coupling can be rapidly and reversibly blocked or enhanced with modulation of permeability occurring within seconds to minutes, according to the following, apparently independent mechanisms: (a) intracellular Ca^{++} and intracellular pH, (b) intracellular cAMP and phosphorylation, and (c) transjunctional voltage. In addition, there are a number of pharmacological agents that act either through modulation of gap junction number or permeability (29).

In all tissues, a second consequence of gap junctions is the variation in metabolic coupling—that is, the number and size of metabolites and second messengers to pass between cells (Fig. 4). Gap junctions act as molecular filters, allowing not only current-carrying ions, but also hydrophilic molecules that are smaller than the channel diameter to pass from cell to cell (23–32). As judged by passage or obstruction of fluorescently labeled molecules, the upper limit is between 1.6 nm and 2.0 nm in mammalian cells, which would permit spherical molecules of roughly 1000 MW to pass. Thus, monovalent and divalent ions, small peptides, IP_3 and cyclic nucleotides may pass, but not larger molecules such as proteins and ATP (Fig. 4). This exchange of small substances could serve in homeostasis and, interestingly, to convey signals intercellularly.

Analysis of the rates of intercellular transfer of small molecules via gap junctions clearly indicates a functionally important level of communication can occur. The fluorescent probe Lucifer Yellow (MW 440), when injected into one cell of the mouse dermis, passes into more than 500 surrounding cells in less than 5 min (33). In a cell culture system combining two mutant fibroblast strains, one incapable of synthesizing purine nucleotides and the other incapable of synthesizing thymidine nucleotides, growth occurs at the normal rate of the wild-type strain as a result of nucleotide exchange occurring at a rate greater than 10^7 nucleotides per second per cell pair (27). The consequences of increased gap junctional area in smooth muscle of the uterus at parturition are therefore immense (see below), allowing coordination of metabolism and facilitation of homeostasis as well as mechanical coordination via increased electrical coupling.

Myometrial gap junctions have been well characterized both by structural and functional studies (34–46). These studies show that when gap junctions and contractility are increased or decreased, there are concommitent changes in accompanying electrical and metabolic coupling as evidenced by alterations in (a) space constant, (b) tissue impedance, (c) velocity of action potential conduction, (d) distance of action potential propagation, (e) metabolic cooperation, (f) input resistance, (*g*) dye transfer, and (*h*) glucose diffusion (40, 41, 43, 45, 46). Similarly, opening and closing of the gap junction channels by changing their permeability results in conditions either favorable or unfavorable, respectively, for coupling. These studies indicate that gap junctions are the structural correlate of the site coupling in the myometrium. However, there are difficulties with all the above studies because they were performed in vitro. Gap junctions form spontaneously in vitro in preterm tissues and the tissues may lack substances that keep the few junctions closed (see below; also 36, 40, 46). Therefore, all of the above measurements on preterm tissues are probably overestimated and the differences between preterm versus parturient tissues are greater than noted. The increase in the junctions may also account for the fact that myometrial tissues from preterm animals conduct action potentials and contract vigorously in vitro but not in vivo (46).

CHANGES IN COUPLING DURING PREGNANCY

Myometrial gap junctions increase between myometrial cells immediately prior to the onset of labor and provide the intercellular pathways that permit the synchronization of ionic and molecular activities during parturition (see reference 43). The increase in the junctions has been found consistently whether labor occurs at term or preterm and in all species that we and others have studied. Figure 5 shows the

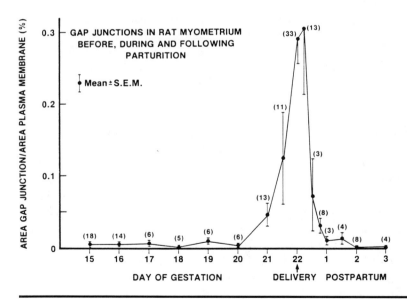

Fig. 5. Area of gap junction in the rat myometrium from day 15 of gestation to 3 days postpartum. Note that the area begins to rise on day 21, is at its highest level during delivery, and then declines sharply following delivery. (From Garfield RE, Blennerhassett MG, Miller SM, Control of myometrial contractility: role and regulation of gap junctions, Oxford Rev 1988;10:436–90.)

area of gap junctions in the rat myometrium during late pregnancy, delivery at term, and postpartum. The increase in gap-junction area begins about 24 h prior to delivery, reaches maximal values during delivery when the muscle activity is greatest, and then declines rapidly to preterm levels in the immediate postpartum period. The increase in gap junction area (from less than 0.01% of plasma membrane surface area preterm to 0.3% during labor) represents increases in both the number (from about 10/cell to 1000/cell) and sizes (from 80 nM to 250 nM) of the junctions. The increase in the junctional area is particularly apparent in rats (34, 35, 38, 44) and rabbits (42), whereas guinea pigs, sheep, and perhaps humans (see reference 43) differ slightly in that higher numbers of gap junctions have been demonstrated earlier in gestation.

The development of the junctions and preterm delivery has been investigated following ovariectomy, after estrogen, prostaglandin, antiprogesterone treatments (35, 39, 43, 47), and intrauterine infection with *Eschericia coli* (unpublished data). Furthermore, these studies also show that if the junctions are prevented from forming under the same circumstances, by manipulating the hormones, then labor and delivery are either delayed or prevented. These multiple correlation studies demonstrate that the junctions are dynamic and transitory structures whose presence is obligatory for the events of term or preterm labor. No known exception to this phenomenon has been recognized, and for this reason gap junctions appear to be necessary for labor. However, the fact that their increase does not always lead to labor indicates that their presence alone is not sufficient for labor. The latter has been shown following antiprogesterone treatments (47).

Recently, clones for the cDNA encoding the gap-junction proteins (connexins) from several tissues have been made. The cDNAs for the liver connexin (connexins 32 and 26), heart and myometrium (connexin 43), and endometrium (connexins 26 and 21) have been prepared (48–51). The cDNA's to connexin 43 have been used to study the expression of the gap-junction mRNA in heart and myometrium during pregnancy and after estrogen treatment of nonpregnant rats (50, 51). In addition, antibodies to the connexin 43 protein (predicted to have a sequence of 382 amino acids) have been raised to portions of the protein (50, 51). Immunocytochemical studies with the antibodies confirm that the gap junctions increase dramatically in the rat uterus during labor (Fig. 6) and are low during earlier stages of pregnancy (50, 51) (Fig. 7). Furthermore, immunoblots using the cDNA's show that the connexin 43 mRNA rises in the myometrium immediately prior to delivery in the myometrium, but not in the heart (51). These studies add valuable information to our knowledge of myometrial gap junctions and the control of contractility and labor. They also show that the same gap-junction protein may be modulated differently in tissues that are responsive and nonresponsive to hormone.

MECHANISMS THAT CONTROL MYOMETRIAL GAP JUNCTIONS

Labor in most species is preceded and accompanied by changes in steroid hormones, prostaglandins, and other substances (2, 52–54). Many studies suggest that

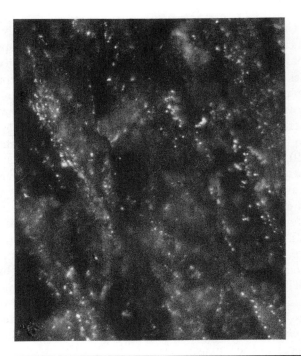

Fig. 6. Light micrograph (1000×) of myometrial tissue from delivering rat uterus after staining with antibodies to connexin 43. Note the abundance of bright fluorescent spots which represent gap junctions. (From Garfield RE, Hertzberg EL, Cell-to-cell coupling in the myometrium: Emil Bozler's prediction, in: Sperelakis N, Wood JD, eds, Frontiers in smooth muscle research, New York: Wiley-Liss, 1990:673–81.)

the changes in the levels of uterine hormones and prostaglandins that occur with labor regulate the myometrial gap junctions (43). Thus, these studies show how alterations in hormones can be translated to a structural change in the muscle cells favoring conditions for improved propagation and contraction. We have proposed three sites for the regulation of myometrial gap junctions: two relatively slow processes requiring hours that control the presence of the junctions, through their synthesis and degradation, and a rapid system (seconds or minutes) that controls the gating of gap-junction channels (Fig. 8). These processes will be considered below.

Control of the Synthesis and Degradation

The changes in the steroid hormones that occur before labor (an increase in estrogen and a fall in progesterone) are thought to be responsible for activating the synthesis of the myometrial gap junctions through a genomic mechanism, at least in rodents (34–47). Evidence that progesterone suppresses the junctions is sug-

Fig. 7. Light micrograph (1000×) of myometrial tissue from rat uterus at day 18 of gestation after staining with connexin 43 antibodies. Note the lack of staining as compared to Figure 6. (From Garfield RE, Hertzberg EL, Cell-to-cell coupling in the myometrium: Emil Bozler's prediction, in: Sperelakis N, Wood JD, eds, Frontiers in smooth muscle research, New York: Wiley-Liss, 1990:673–81.)

gested from the following observations: (*a*) Progesterone normally declines in rats and rabbits at term prior to the development of gap junctions and labor. If progesterone levels are maintained by injections of the hormone, animals do not develop junctions and they do not go into labor. (*b*) Ovariectomy leads to premature progesterone withdrawal, appearance of junctions and labor. Progesterone treatment after ovariectomy prevents all three effects. (*c*) Progesterone will inhibit the estrogen induced development of the junctions in nonpregnant animals. (*d*) Antiprogesterone compounds induce preterm delivery and development of the junctions, and progesterone receptor agonists with high affinity will prevent these effects. (*e*) Progesterone will suppress gap-junction development in vitro providing estrogen is present.

Because steroid hormones are known to react mainly, if not exclusively, through binding to cytoplasmic and nuclear receptors to control protein synthesis (55), we have proposed that progesterone suppresses the presence of the junctions by regulating the gene that codes for the gap-junction protein. Inhibitors of protein synthesis effectively block the synthesis of the junctions in vitro and in

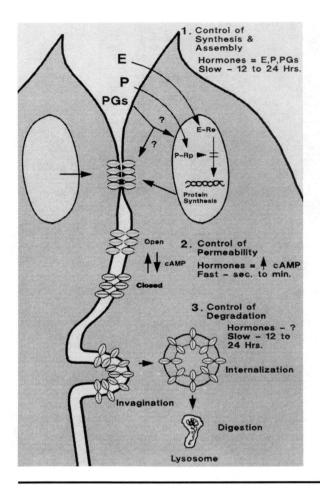

Fig. 8. Schematic illustration of two myometrial cells showing sites for the control of the synthesis, permeability, and degradation of the junctions. Estrogen (E), progesterone (P), and the prostaglandins (PGs) regulate site 1. An increase in cAMP closes the junctions (site 2). Degradation of the junctions involves invagination, internalization, and digestion (site 3).

vivo, supporting the view that this step is involved in the formation of large numbers of the junctions (56).

Estrogens promote the synthesis of gap junctions in the myometrium and in other target tissues that possess steroid receptors (see reference 43). That estrogens stimulate the formation of gap junctions is provided by the following observations: (a) Estrogens rise prior to labor, and injections of estrogens into pregnant animals stimulate the premature appearance of gap junctions and labor. (b) Injections of estrogens into immature and mature ovariectomized rats induces gap junctions. (c) Estrogens promote gap junctions in tissues incubated in vitro.

(*d*) Antiestrogen compounds such as tamoxifen prevent the estrogens from stimulating the increase in gap junctions (57). (*e*) mRNA extracted from estrogen-treated rats induces the formation of gap junctions in cells that normally lack gap junctions (56). We contend that estrogen may stimulate the synthesis of gap junctions by interacting with its receptor and stimulating the specific genome responsible for coding for the gap-junction protein. The ability of estrogen to control the synthesis of other proteins in this fashion has been proposed (55).

The ability of inhibitors of prostaglandin synthesis, such as indomethacin and meclofenamate, to alter the area of gap junctions in the myometrium indicates that the prostaglandins and/or leukotrienes are also in some way involved in the control of the junctions. The manner in which the metabolites of arachidonic acid influence the junctions must be complex, because in some conditions prostaglandin inhibition reduces gap junctions (36) and in other conditions it stimulates their presence (57). We have suggested that (*a*) there may be a prostaglandin that normally suppresses the junctions until term; (*b*) lipoxygenase products may stimulate junctions; and/or (*c*) prostaglandins may regulate levels of the steroid receptors. Further study is required to identify the metabolite(s) and their mode of action on gap junctions.

The disappearance of gap junctions following delivery is accompanied by a profound inability of the muscle to contract spontaneously and a decrease in the capacity of the uterus to respond to stimulation. These result from the lack of action potentials to propagate, a decrease in the excitability of the muscle, a change in the number of excitatory receptors, an involution of the muscle cells and connective tissues, and a general remodeling of the entire uterus. The receding numbers of gap junctions is the effect of the destruction of the junctions by an internalization process involving endocytosis and digestion (36), such as occurs in other tissues (24), and of the reduction in the synthetic processes that regulate the synthesis of the junctions (see Fig. 8). It remains to be resolved what mechanisms and hormones might control the degradation process. Clearly, this is an important system, because an inhibition of breakdown of the junctions would be expected to prolong their presence and function, whereas stimulation of their destruction should have the opposite effects.

Control of Permeability of the Junctions

The extent of functional coupling occurs independently of changes in structural coupling in a wide variety of cell types (26, 29). These observations suggest that changes in junctional permeability may result from alterations in the gap-junction connexons, such as an all-or-none closure or dilation of the cell-to-cell channel, leading to a state of either decreased or enhanced coupling, respectively. Examples of modulation of junctional permeability by hormones, neurotransmitters, and many different agents have been described in practically all types of cells. That the permeability of the junctions and, therefore, the extent of functional coupling in the myometrium may be regulated by endogenous mechanisms is an exciting possibility. Improved functional coupling would be expected to promote greater electrical and contractile synchrony in the myometrium and lead to an enhanced rate of intrauterine pressure development and more effective labor. Alternatively, contractility when gap junctions are closed would be the same as in the absence of the junctions and lead to reduced synchrony, ineffective labor, and a prolongation of pregnancy. It is likely that substances which control permeability are different from those that regulate the presence of the junctions. Regulation of openness of the gap junction channels is intriguing because this method of uncoupling is rapid (seconds, see above), while regulation of the presence of the junctions is slow (hours). Thus, treatments to alter the junctions might be targeted at either an immediate (i.e., control of junctional conductance) or delayed effect (i.e., control of the number of junctions) to alter labor (Fig. 8).

We have used the diffusion of deoxyglucose between cells to study the influence of several agents on coupling in the myometrium of parturient rats (40). Similar studies have been completed measuring input resistance in myometrial cells (3, 43). Our studies suggest that the permeability of the junctions in the parturient myometrium is influenced by intracellular Ca^{++}, pH, and cAMP (40–42). Both elevated intracellular Ca^{++} produced by the calcium ionophore A23187 and lowered pH from treatment with the substituted benzyl ester, σ-nitrobenzyl acetate, reduced the longitudinal distribution and apparent diffusion coefficient of deoxyglucose in the parturient myometrium (41).

Elevated cAMP as a consequence of treatment with dibutyryl- or 8-bromo-cAMP significantly reduces cell-to-cell diffusion of deoxyglucose in the myometrium, and this can be mimicked by inhibiting phosphodiesterase activity with theophylline or by stimulating adenylate cyclase with forskolin (41). That cAMP may play a role in regulating functional coupling in the myometrium is significant in that relaxin, prostacyclin (PI_2), and β_2-adrenoceptor agonists appear to influence labor and parturition through inhibitory effects on the myometrium by elevating intracellular cAMP. Moreover, porcine relaxin, carbacyclin (a stable PGI_2 analog), and isoproterenol (a nonspecific β-adrenoceptor agonist) decreased deoxyglucose diffusion (41). These data suggest that there are specific receptor and secondary messenger-mediated physiological mechanisms for controlling gating of the gap-junction channels in the myometrium. The cAMP-mediated uncoupling mechanism may be involved in maintaining pregnancy in instances of premature junction formation and/or in species such as the guinea pig, sheep, and possibly human, in which low, but significant numbers of gap junctions are present throughout pregnancy. Perhaps the high levels of relaxin and prostacyclin observed in preterm pregnant animals act to elevate intracellular cAMP and close the junctions to prevent synchronous and forceful activity in the myometrium.

Whether junctional permeability in the myometrium can be enhanced by circulating hormones is unresolved at this time. Perhaps oxytocin or stimulatory prostaglandin increases cell-to-cell communication between uterine smooth muscle cells either through a direct interaction with the gap junctions or, as noted above, by reversing the inhibition of coupling produced by relaxin and/or prostacyclin. Below, we consider how other agonists and antagonists (in addition to those noted above) interact with myometrial cells to influence their contractile function.

RELATIONSHIP TO OTHER CONTROL SYSTEMS

Agents that stimulate or inhibit the myometrium to contract or relax, respectively, can influence the muscle cells in a number of different ways that may or may not directly affect the gap junctions. However, these agents do not work independently of the gap junctions and the propagation of action potentials. As noted above, the influx and efflux of Ca^{++} ions in the muscle cells during the passage of the action potentials, and the opening of voltage-dependent Ca^{++} channels, are responsible for the cyclical increases and decreases in tension. This mechanism can be modified by endogenous or exogenous hormones, neurotransmitters, and other agonists and antagonists to either increase of decrease the excitability of the muscle and thereby raise or lower the ability of action potentials to propagate. Thus, the effects of excitatory and inhibitory agents are only superimposed upon the driving force that is supplied by the propagation of action potentials (Fig. 9).

Each myometrial cell is thought to contain many systems that regulate the influx of Ca^{++} and other ions (6). The systems involved in the control of raising

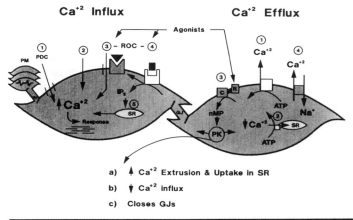

Fig. 9. The influx and efflux pathways for Ca^{++} ions shown in two separate cells coupled together via gap junctions and to a pacemaker (PM). Although both pathways exist within every myometrial cell, they are illustrated separately to emphasize the importance of the junctions. Shown are many different mechanisms for influencing the levels of internal Ca^{++} ions to contract (i.e., potential-dependent channels [PDC]; receptor-operated channels [ROC]; IP_3 generation; release from sarcoplasmic reticulum [SR], or inhibit (i.e., receptor–R=C-mediated nucleotide–nMP and protein kinase interaction, uptake into sarcoplasmic reticulum, extrusion from the cell by active and passive mechanisms, and closure of gap junctions). The most important mechanism involved in phasic contractions is the opening of PDC during passage of the action potential. Gap junctions are involved in regulating both contraction and inhibition. The effects of agonists that effect contractility are only superimposed upon the ability of action potentials to propagate between cells.

intracellular Ca^{++} levels include (a) voltage- or potential-dependent channels (see above); (b) passive influx; (c) receptor-operated channels, which may or may not be coupled to the generation of IP_3; and (d) release from sarcoplasmic reticulum (Fig. 9). The voltage-dependent channels are the primary source of activator Ca^{++} ions. The propagation of action potentials from pacemaker regions are essential for activating these channels. Without intercellular coupling, either from the absence of gap junctions or their closure, action potentials would not propagate and the myometrium would not contract phasically.

Contractile agonists can interact with the above systems and others in an almost unlimited number of ways to increase Ca^{++} inside the muscle cells and effect contraction. The most common action might be through effects on receptor-operated channels. However, in general, the effects of these agents are to increase the membrane potential or the ability of action potentials to propagate and thereby increase the excitability of the muscle cells. In this fashion, action potentials propagate more easily between cells because the membrane potential is closer to its threshold. Contractile agonists do not, by themselves, drive the myometrium to contract, but in higher concentrations some may produce sustained contractions with or without action potentials.

An example of the effects of a contractile agonist is demonstrated in the action of oxytocin. Oxytocin binds to specific receptors to increase Ca^{++} influx by (a) inhibiting Ca^{++} extrusion by the suppression of Ca^{++}-ATPase (the Ca^{++} pump), (b) opening Ca^{++} channels, and (c) stimulating IP_3, which releases internally stored Ca^{++} ions (6, 58). Kao (6) has described a 4-fold action of oxytocin on the myometrium: (a) initiation of spike discharge in quiescent preparations, (b) increase in frequency of burst discharge, (c) increase of spikes in any burst, and (d) increase in amplitude of action potential. However, oxytocin's net action is to raise intracellular levels of CA^{++} and thereby depolarize the cells (4, 5) or it may act to facilitate opening of voltage-dependent ion channels during the process of excitation by action potentials (6, 58). Increased action-potential propagation resulting from depolarization and its other effects is the basis by which oxytocin acts to increase contractility. It does not by itself produce contractions independent of the underlying electrical activity. Nor does oxytocin initiate labor separate from that of propagated action potentials.

The actions of other stimulants are probably similar to oxytocin. Marshall (5) has proposed that carbachol depolarizes myometrial cells like oxytocin. The effects of the prostaglandins are not well known, but they also may operate through the same mechanisms. However, prostaglandins have varied effects, some producing relaxation and others contractions in the myometrium. In addition, prostaglandins have immediate and delayed effects. As noted above, prostaglandins seem to be involved in the formation of gap junctions. Therefore, the delayed contractile effects of prostaglandins could be mediated through the stimulation of gap-junction synthesis (57), and their immediate action may be similar to that of oxytocin.

The efflux, or lowering, or intracellular Ca^{++} ions is regulated by mechanisms that extrude Ca^{++} (Ca^{++} pump and Na^+-Ca^{++} exchange system) and those that promote its uptake into the sarcoplasmic reticulum (Fig. 9). These systems can be affected indirectly by extrinsic substances through actions on receptors to stimulate the formation of secondary messengers to influence the mechanical event (59). However, when considering these mechanisms and the effects of various agents, a distinction should be made between inactivity of the muscle and relaxation. Inactivity of the myometrium occurs during periods of the absence of action potentials, whereas relaxation follows and is dependent upon a contraction. Agents that contribute to inactivity will encourage further quiescence in an inactive tissue and relax a contracted tissue, but agents that only "relax" a tissue may not inhibit contractions. Similarly, substances that increase Ca^{++} efflux during a contraction will induce relaxation, but substances that increase inactivity need not influence Ca^{++} efflux.

Studies of isolated tissues show that in the complete absence of nerves and contractile agents, the myometrium periodically contracts and relaxes (4, 5). Therefore, neither contraction nor relaxation are dependent on external stimuli. Contraction or relaxation can each be prompted by various agents, but these mechanisms are not obligatory for these processes.

Inactivity results from the lack of conducted action potentials and it is promoted by decreases in coupling among cells, pacemaker activity, and excitability of the muscle cells. Substances that close gap junctions, decrease their number, and suppress the generation of the action potential inhibit the active events and thereby affect contractility. Most agents that promote quiescence probably do so by preventing activity of the myometrium, not by acting to "relax" the muscle cells. Thus, these agents act as contractile antagonists, but their action is not mediated in the classical sense through a blockage of receptors.

Most studies have shown that the most responsive element of these contractile antagonists is the modulation of spike activity (4, 6). Generally, β-noradrenergic agents act to hyperpolarize the myometrial tissues by increasing K^+ conductance and Ca^{++} efflux or sequestration. Their net action then, is opposite to that of contractile agonists in that they inhibit the ability of action potentials to spread through the tissue.

However, probably the most important action of the β-agonists, and other substances that raise cAMP, is not the change in the membrane potential or effects on the efflux of Ca^{++} but on the closure of the gap junctions between the myometrial cells (see above, Fig. 9). That the effects of the β-agonists are to shut the junctions and thereby decrease the ability of action potentials to propagate between cells is disclosed in the diffusion studies discussed above. These agents therefore promote the inactivity of the myometrium rather than relaxation. These conclusions are also based on the observations that β-agonists, at lower concentrations, cause a cessation of spiking activity without an appreciable hyperpolarization (6). Furthermore, the claim that β-agonists increase K^+ conductance has not been detected by Kao (6). This evidence supports the hypothesis that the main action of the β-agonists may be to decrease the permeability of the junctions.

REFERENCES

1. Garfield RE. Myometrial ultrastructure and uterine contractility. In: Bottari S, Thomas JP, Vokaer A, Vokaer R, eds. Uterine contractility. New York: Masson, 1984:81-109.
2. Csapo AI. Force of labor. In: Iffy L, Kamientzky HA, eds. Principles and practice of obstetrics and perinatology. New York: John Wiley and Sons, 1981:761-99.
3. Garfield RE, Beier S. Increased myometrial responsiveness to oxytocin during term and preterm labor. Am J Obstet Gynecol 1989;161:454-61.
4. Marshall JM. Regulation of activity in uterine smooth muscle. Physiol Rev 1962;42:213-27.
5. Marshall JM. The physiology of the uterus. In: Norris HJ, Hertig AT, Abell MR, eds. The uterus. Baltimore: Williams and Wilkins, 1973:89-109.
6. Kao CY. Electrophysiological properties of uterine smooth muscle. In: Wynn RM, Jollie WP, eds. Biology of the uterus. 2d ed. New York: Plenum Press, 1989:403-54.
7. Kuriyama H. Recent studies on the electrophysiology of the uterus. In: Progesterone and the defence mechanism of pregnancy. Ciba Foundation Study Group, vol. 9. Boston: Little, Brown, 1961:51-70.
8. Kuriyama H. Excitation-contraction coupling in various visceral smooth muscles. In: Bulbring E, Brading AF, Jones AW, Tomita T, eds. Smooth muscle: an assessment of current knowledge. London: Edward Arnold, 1981:171-97.
9. Abe Y. The hormonal control and the effects of drugs and ions on the electrical and mechanical activity of the uterus. In: Bulbring E, Brading AF, Jones AW, Tomita T, eds. Smooth muscle: an assessment of current knowledge. London: Edward Arnold, 1970:396-417.
10. Bozler E. Electrical stimulation and conduction of excitation in smooth muscle. Am J Physiol 1938;122:616-23.
11. Bozler E. Influence of estrone on the electric characteristics and motility of uterine muscle. Endocrinology 1941;29:225-7.
13. Csapo AI. Defence mechanism of pregnancy. In: Progesterone and the defence mechanism of pregnancy. Ciba Foundation Study Group, vol. 9. Boston: Little, Brown, 1961:1-27.
14. Carsten ME. Regulation of myometrial composition, growth and activity. In: Assali NS, ed. Biology of the uterus, vol 1. New York: Academic Press, 1968:355-423.
15. Csapo AI, Kuriyama H. Effects of ions and drugs on cell membrane activity and tension in the postpartum rat myometrium. J Physiol (Lond) 1963;165:575-92.
16. Mironneau J. Relationship between contraction and transmembrane ionic current in voltage-clamped uterine smooth muscle. In: Bulbring E, Shuba MF, eds. Physiology of smooth muscle. New York: Raven Press, 1976a:175-83.
17. Mironneau J, Savineau J-P. Effects of calcium ions on outward membrane currents in rat uterine smooth muscle. J Physiol (Lond) 1980;302:411-25.
18. Osa T. An interaction between the electrical activities of longitudinal and circular smooth muscles of pregnant mouse uterus. Jpn J Physiol 1974;24:189-203.
19. Osa T, Ogasawara T, Kato S. Effects of magnesium, oxytocin and prostaglandin $F_{2\alpha}$ on the generation and propagation of excitation in the longitudinal muscle of rat myometrium during late pregnancy. Jpn J Physiol 1983;33:51-67.
20. Saldivar JT, Melton CE. Effect in vivo and in vitro of sex steroids on rat myometrium. Am J Physiol 1966;211:835-43.

21. Furshpan EJ, Potter DD. Transmission at the giant motor synapses of the crayfish. J Physiol 1959;145:289-325.

22. Revel J-P, Karnovsky M. Hexagonal array of subunits in intercellular junctions of the mouse heart and liver. J Cell Biol 1967;33:C7-C12.

23. Hooper ML, Subak-Sharpe JH. Metabolic cooperation between cells. Int Rev Cytol 1981;69:45-104.

24. Larsen WJ. Biological implications of gap junction structure, distribution and composition: a review. Tissue Cell 1983;15:645-71.

25. McNutt NS, Weinstein RS. The ultrastructure of the nexus. A correlated thin section and freeze-cleave study. J Cell Biol 1970;47:666-88.

26. Peracchia C. Structural correlates of gap junction permeation. Int Rev Cytol 1980;66:81-146.

27. Pitts JD, Finbow ME. The gap junction. J Cell Sci Suppl 1986;4:239-66.

28. Revel J-P, Nicholson BJ, Yancey SB. Chemistry of gap junctions. Annu Rev Physiol 1985;47:263-79.

29. Spray DC, Bennett MVL. Physiology and pharmacology of gap junctions. Am J Physiol 1985;47:281-303.

30. Meda P. Merrelet A, Orci L. Increase of gap junctions between pancreatic B-cells during stimulation of insulin secretion. J Cell Biol 1979;82:441-8.

31. Fallon RF, Goodenough DA. Five hour half-life of mouse liver gap junction protein. J Cell Biol 1981;90:521-6.

32. Saez JC, Connor JA, Spray DC, Bennett MVL. Hepatocyte gap junctions are permeable to the second messenger, inositol 1,4,5-trisphosphate, and to calcium ions. Proc Natl Acad Sci USA 1988;86:2708-12.

33. Kam E, Melville L, Pitts JD. Patterns of junctional communication in skin. J Invest Derm 1986;87:748-763.

34. Garfield RE, Sims S, Daniel EE. Gap junctions: their presence and necessity in myometrium during gestation. Science 1977;198:958-60.

35. Garfield RE, Sims SM, Kannan MS, Daniel EE. Possible role of gap junctions in activation of myometrium during parturition. Am J Physiol 1978;235:C168-79.

36. Garfield RE, Merrett D, Grover AK. Gap junction formation and regulation in myometrium. Am J Physiol 1980b;239:C217-28.

37. Garfield RE, Hayashi RH. Appearance of gap junctions in the myometrium of women during labor. Am J Obstet Gynecol 1981;140:254-60.

38. Garfield RE, Puri CP, Csapo AI. Endocrine, structural and functional changes in the uterus during premature labor. Am J Obstet Gynecol 1982;142:21-7.

39. Garfield RE, Baulieu EE. The antiprogesterone steroid RU486: a short pharmacological and clinical review with emphasis on the interruption of pregnancy. Baillierer Clin Endocrinol Metabolism 1987;1:207-21.

40. Cole WC, Garfield RE, Kirkaldy JS. Gap junctions and direct intercellular communication between rat uterine smooth muscle cells. Am J Physiol 1985;249:C20-31.

41. Cole WC, Garfield RE. Evidence for physiological regulation of gap junction permeability. Am J Physiol 1986; 251:C411-20.

42. Demianczuk N, Towell M, Garfield RE. Myometrial electrophysiologic activity and gap junctions in the pregnant rabbit. Am J Obstet Gynecol 1984;149:485-91.

43. Garfield RE, Blennerhassett MG, Miller SM. Control of myometrial contractility: role and regulation of gap junctions. Oxford Rev 1988;10:436-90.

44. Puri CP, Garfield RE. Changes in hormone levels and gap junctions in the rat uterus during pregnancy and parturition. Biol Reprod 1982;27:967-75.
45. Sims SM, Daniel EE, Garfield RG. Improved electrical coupling in uterine smooth muscle is associated with increased gap junctions at parturition. J Gen Physiol 1982;80:353-75.
46. Miller SM, Garfield RE, Daniel EE. Improved propagation in myometrium associated with gap junctions during parturition. Am J Physiol 1989;256:C130-41.
47. Garfield RE. Effects of antiprogesterone compounds on uterine contractility. In: Proceedings of the symposium on hormone antagonists for fertility regulation. Bombay: Indian Society for the Study of Reproduction and Fertility and the World Health Organization's Special Programme of Research, Development and Research Training in Human Reproduction, 1988:63-85.
48. Paul DL. Molecular cloning of cDNA for rat liver gap junction protein. J Cell Biol 1986;103:123-34.
49. Beyer EC, Paul DL, Goodenough DA. Connexin43: a protein from rat heart homologous to a gap junction protein from liver. J Cell Biol 1987;105:2621-9.
50. Beyer EC, Kistler J, Paul DL, Goodenough DA. Antisera directed against connexin43 peptides react with a 43-dK protein localized to gap junctions in myocardium and other tissues. J Cell Biol 1989;108:595-605.
51. Risek B, Guthrie S, Kumar N, Gilula NB. Modulation of gap junction transcript and protein expression during pregnancy in the rat. J Cell Biol 1990;110:269-82.
52. Fuchs A-R. Hormonal control of myometrial function during pregnancy and parturition. Acta Endocrinol Suppl 1978;221:1-70.
53. Challis JRG, Lye SJ. Parturition. In: Clarke JR, ed. Oxford Rev 1986;8:61-129.
54. Casey ML, MacDonald PC. Initiation of labor in women. In: Huszar G, ed. The physiology and biochemistry of the uterus in pregnancy and labor. Boca Raton, FL: CRC Press, 1986:155-61.
55. Gorski J, Gannon F. Current models of steroid hormone action: a critique. Annu Rev Physiol 1976;38:425-50.
56. Dahl G, Azarina R, Werner R. De novo construction of cell-to-cell channels. In Vitro 1980;16:1068-75.
57. MacKenzie LW, Garfield RE. Hormonal control of gap junctions in the myometrium. Am J Physiol 1985;248:C296-308.
58. Edwards E, Good DM, Granger SE, et al. The spasmogenic action of oxytocin in the rat uterus—comparison with other agonists. Br J Pharmacol 1986;88:899-908.
59. Riemer RK, Roberts JM. Endocrine modulation of myometrial response. In: Huszar G, ed. The physiology and biochemistry of the uterus in pregnancy and labor. Boca Raton, FL: CRC Press, 1986:53-71.
60. Garfield RE, Hertzberg EL. Cell-to-cell coupling in the myometrium: Emil Bozler's prediction. In: Sperelakis N, Wood JD, eds. Frontiers in smooth muscle research. New York: Wiley-Liss, 1990:673-81.

CONTRACTILITY AND CALCIUM

4

Regulation of Smooth-Muscle Contractility: Ca++ and Myosin Phosphorylation

R. Ann Word,[1] James T. Stull,[2] Kristine E. Kamm,[2] and M. Linette Casey[1,3]

Departments of Obstetrics-Gynecology,[1] Physiology,[2] Biochemistry,[3] and The Cecil H. & Ida Green Center for Reproductive Biology Sciences, The University of Texas Southwestern Medical Center, Dallas

U terine smooth muscle belongs to a broad class of smooth muscles termed *phasic smooth muscle*. Phasic smooth muscle is characterized by generation of action potentials, spontaneous contractile activity that is independent of extrinsic innervation, and the presence of gap junctions that serve to electrically couple adjoining myocytes. In contrast, tonic smooth muscle is dependent on extrinsic innervation and is characterized by a maintained contractile response during depolarization. Whereas there are intrinsic differences in the contractile responsiveness among various smooth muscles, the regulation of contraction by myosin light-chain phosphorylation is applicable to all smooth-muscle types and of central importance in the biochemical regulation of relaxation and contraction.

It is well established that a number of hormones and neurotransmitters affect cellular functions by regulating cytoplasmic Ca^{++} concentration. An increase in the concentration of cytoplasmic Ca^{++}, as a primary second messenger, and binding of Ca^{++} to calmodulin, results in activation of a number of Ca^{++}-dependent cellular processes, including smooth-muscle contraction. The regulation of actin-myosin interactions in smooth muscle by Ca^{++} is more complex than that in skeletal or cardiac muscle, where contraction is effected by Ca^{++} binding to troponin on thin filaments. The preponderance of biochemical evidence indicates that Ca^{++}-dependent myosin phosphorylation serves an obligatory role in regulation of smooth muscle contraction, although additional mechanisms for Ca^{++} regulation are not entirely excluded (1).

Muscle contraction occurs as a result of the cyclic interaction of myosin with actin filaments. Myosin, composed of two heavy-chain subunits (200 kD) and two pairs of light-chain subunits (20 and 17 kD), is arranged in its hexameric form into thick filaments. Each heavy chain consists of an α-helical carboxy-terminal region

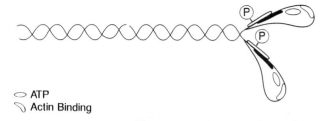

○ ATP
↘ Actin Binding

Fig. 1. Schematic drawing of the myosin phosphorylation system. Myosin is composed of two heavy-chain subunits arranged in rod-shaped, α-helical coils that end in globular head projections. Two types of light-chain subunits are bound to the neck region of each myosin head. Phosphorylation of one type of light-chain subunit (the regulatory light chain) is indicated by the circled P. Myosin phosphorylation is catalyzed by Ca++/calmodulin-dependent myosin light-chain kinase and dephosphorylation by myosin light-chain phosphatase.

and an amino-terminal globular head region that contains an actin-binding site, an ATP hydrolysis site, and one each of the two types of light chain (Fig. 1). The tail regions of the heavy chains intertwine to form the backbone of the bipolar thick filaments from which the two head regions protrude and interact with filamentous actin to form a cross-bridge. Muscle myosin is an actin-activated MgATPase (2). Whereas phosphorylation of the regulatory light chain in skeletal muscle is manifested as a potentiation of isometric twitch tension (3), myosin light-chain phosphorylation in smooth muscle is obligatory for actin-activated MgATPase activity and thereby initiation of contraction (4).

We will discuss the role of the specific phosphorylation of myosin by the Ca++/calmodulin-dependent enzyme myosin light-chain kinase in regulation of smooth-muscle contraction. Other chapters in this book focus on specific aspects of signal-transduction mechanisms and hormonal regulation of uterine smooth-muscle contractility.

BIOCHEMICAL PROPERTIES OF CONTRACTION

The scheme generally accepted to be necessary and sufficient for the biochemical activation of smooth-muscle contraction is phosphorylation of the 20 kD regulatory light chain of myosin (Fig. 2). Cytoplasmic Ca++ is believed to be the primary determinant for regulation of myosin light-chain phosphorylation. The increase in cytoplasmic free Ca++ via influx of extracellular Ca++ or through mobilization of intracellular Ca++ stores can be induced by two distinct mechanisms of excitation-contraction coupling: (*a*) electromechanical coupling, mediated through depolarization of the surface membrane by action potentials or high K+ solutions; and (*b*) pharmacomechanical coupling, a mechanism by which agents mediate an increase in the intracellular Ca++ concentration independent of cell surface membrane potentials. Pharmacomechanical coupling may involve Ca++ influx via receptor-

BIOCHEMICAL CASCADE FOR RECEPTOR STIMULATED MYOSIN PHOSPHORYLATION

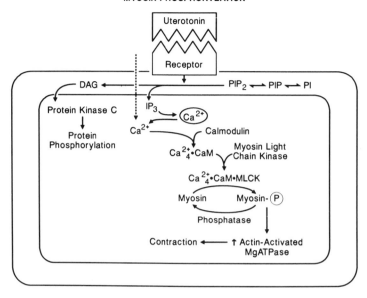

Fig. 2. A general scheme for regulation of uterine smooth-muscle contraction. Uterotonin binding to its receptor leads to (*a*) the hydrolysis of phosphoinositides and formation of the second messengers diacylglycerol (DAG) and inositol 1,4,5-trisphosphate (IP$_3$) or (*b*) influx of extracellular CA++ via receptor-operated Ca++ channels. These events result in an increase in cytoplasmic Ca++ concentrations, activation of the calmodulin-dependent myosin light-chain kinase, and phosphorylation of myosin light chain.

operated Ca++ channels or by receptor-mediated inositol trisphosphate formation and release of Ca++ from intracellular stores in the sarcoplasmic reticulum.

In relaxed conditions, the free cytoplasmic Ca++ concentration is low (110–150 nM). Thus, very little Ca++ is bound to calmodulin, and myosin light-chain kinase is minimally activated, resulting in low amounts of phosphorylated myosin light chain. Initially, smooth-muscle cells are stimulated to contract by an agonist binding to its receptor or by electrical depolarization, both of which result in an increase in the cytoplasmic Ca++ concentration. Ca++ binds to calmodulin, forming a Ca++/calmodulin complex (5). The second step of the Ca++-dependent activation involves Ca++/calmodulin binding to myosin light-chain kinase, thus activating the enzyme through conformational change. Myosin light-chain kinase catalyzes the phosphorylation of the 20 kD light-chain subunit of myosin. Myosin light-chain phosphorylation results in activation of actomyosin MgATPase, initiating cross-bridge cycling and mechanical output (i.e., force generation and muscle shortening) (6–8). Sequestration or extrusion of Ca++ from the cell results in inactivation of myosin light-chain kinase followed by dephosphorylation of myosin light chain by myosin light-chain phosphatase, inactivation of myosin MgATPase, and relaxation of smooth muscle.

Dephosphorylation of myosin light chain by myosin light-chain phosphatase is also important in the regulation of smooth-muscle contractility. The structure, function, and mechanism of regulation of myosin light-chain kinase is well defined (9). In contrast, the structure, function, and regulation of myosin light-chain phosphatase is uncertain (10). Smooth muscle, like many tissues, contains a number of protein phosphatases, most of which have broad and overlapping substrate specificities. At present, it is not clear whether a specific phosphatase is responsible for the dephosphorylation of myosin light chain in intact tissue. The extent of myosin light-chain phosphorylation correlates with force generation and reflects the respective activities of myosin light-chain kinase and myosin light-chain phosphatase in a given muscle.

PHYSIOLOGIC STATES OF CONTRACTION

Many investigators have demonstrated that force generation is dependent on myosin phosphorylation. Confirmatory evidence has accumulated from experiments with purified proteins, permeabilized muscle preparations, and intact tissue (11). The development of a physiologic preparation for the study of the rapid and synchronous activation of tracheal smooth-muscle cells via release of neurotransmitter was instrumental in establishing the kinetic properties of the force–myosin light-chain phosphorylation relationship (6). In this preparation, electrical stimulation of bovine trachealis muscle results in the release of acetylcholine from parasympathetic-cholinergic nerve fibers and activation of muscarinic receptors on smooth-muscle cells. At various times after stimulation, muscle strips were frozen with a rapid-release electronic freezing device and analyzed for myosin light-chain phosphorylation. After stimulation, there is a latency of 500 ms prior to the increases in force, stiffness, and myosin light-chain phosphorylation (7). Thereafter, myosin light chain is phosphorylated from levels of 0.04 to 0.80 mol phosphate per mol light chain by 3.5 sec. With continuous neural stimulation of tracheal smooth muscle for prolonged periods and after maximal responses are obtained, there is an apparent decrease in the cytoplasmic Ca^{++} concentration with a reduction in the extent of myosin light-chain phosphorylation and maximal shortening velocity (Fig. 3). Similarly, Ca^{++}-dependent phosphorylase a activation decreased with time in tracheal smooth muscle. This phase of contraction (force maintenance) is characterized by relatively low levels of myosin light-chain phosphorylation and maximal velocity of shortening (Fig. 3). A similar relationship between myosin light-chain phosphorylation and force development has been described in the estrogen-primed rat uterus (12). Stimulation with KCl in the presence of an elevated extracellular Ca^{++} concentration (10 mM) leads to rapid increases in myosin light-chain phosphorylation (to levels of 0.46 mol phosphate per mol light chain in <20 sec). By 2 min, myosin light-chain phosphorylation decreases to 0.28 mol phosphate per mol light chain.

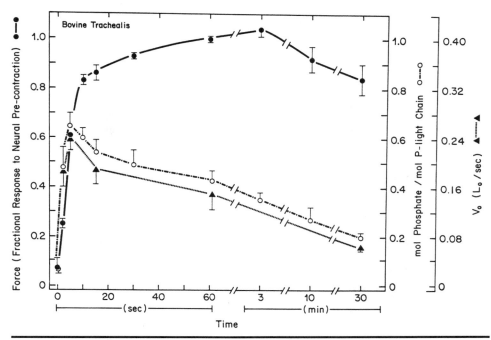

Fig. 3.   Time-course of force, myosin light-chain phosphorylation, and maximal shortening velocity (V_0) in neurally stimulated strips of tracheal muscle. For measurement of light-chain phosphorylation, strips were frozen during rest or at indicated times between 2 sec and 30 min of stimulation. Force at time of freezing is expressed as a fraction of force obtained with a maximal neural precontraction ($P < 0.01$). (From Kamm KE, Stull JT, Activation of smooth muscle contraction: relation between myosin phosphorylation and stiffness, Science 1986;232:280–2, with permission.)

In spontaneous phasic contractions of human uterine smooth muscle, we find that myosin light-chain phosphorylation increases from 0.10 to 0.49 mol phosphate per mol light chain within 10% of the time required to develop the maximal force of spontaneous contractions (Fig. 4). Increased levels of light-chain phosphorylation are maintained until peak contractile force is reached, at which time myosin light-chain phosphorylation decreases and the muscle relaxes.

As presented in Figure 3, force is maintained despite relatively low levels of myosin light-chain phosphorylation in tonic smooth muscle (for example, bovine trachealis). This maintenance of force has been attributed to myosin-actin cross-bridges ("latch bridges") that are composed of actin and attached, yet dephosphorylated, myosin. Latch bridges do not cycle, but are able to maintain force due to a slow rate of detachment from actin (8). It is likely that latch bridges do not accumulate during the phasic contractions of uterine smooth muscle. Thus, alter-

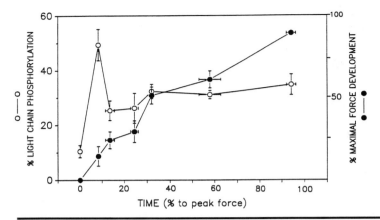

Fig. 4. Temporal relationship between myosin light-chain phosphorylation and force development in spontaneous contractions of human uterine smooth-muscle strips. For measurement of light-chain phosphorylation, strips were frozen during rest or at indicated times. Time is expressed as a fraction of time required for maximal force development. Force at time of freezing is expressed as a fraction of force obtained at maximal peak amplitude of contraction.

ations in contractile force generated during spontaneous contractions reflect alterations in the extent of myosin light-chain phosphorylation.

CELLULAR INDEXES OF CONTRACTION

Typical values for myosin light-chain phosphorylation in noncontracting smooth muscle are 0.1 mol phosphate per mol light chain. Stimulation with agonists or KCl results in an increase in myosin light-chain phosphorylation prior to development of maximal force. Addition of pharmacologic agents that interfere with the Ca^{++}-dependent activation of myosin light-chain kinase (i.e., calmodulin antagonists and Ca^{++} channel blockers) results in a decrease in the extent of phosphate incorporation into the light chain and proportionate decreases in isometric force (13).

It is important to understand the cellular processes involved in myosin light-chain kinase activation. Intracellular determinants dictate a positively cooperative activation of myosin light-chain kinase at Ca^{++} concentrations less than 1 µM. These determinants include (a) the requirement for Ca^{++} occupancy of three to four binding sites in calmodulin for activation, (b) a high molar ratio of calmodulin to kinase, (c) a high cellular content of calmodulin (10–40 µM) and kinase (1 µM) (the concentrations of calmodulin and kinase are 10,000- and 1,000-fold greater, respectively, than the dissociation constant of Ca^{++}/calmodulin for myosin light-chain kinase), and (d) an increase in the affinity for Ca^{++} when calmodulin binds to the kinase.

In resting myometrial smooth-muscle cells in culture, the cytoplasmic free

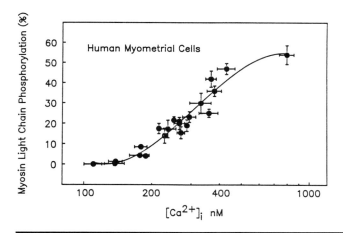

Fig. 5. Ca++ activation of myosin light-chain phosphorylation in human myometrial smooth-muscle cells. Each point represents the mean ± SEM of values obtained from 6 or more cell samples. (From MacKenzie LW, Word RA, Casey ML, Stull JT, Myosin phosphorylation in myometrial smooth muscle cells, Am J Physiol 1990;27:C92–8, and Word RA, Kamm KE, Stull JT, Casey ML, Endothelin increases cytoplasmic calcium and myosin phosphorylation in human myometrium, Am J Obstet Gynecol 1990 [in press], with permission.)

Ca++ concentration is 120–150 nM (Fig. 5). Stimulation by agonists (oxytocin, prostaglandins E_2 and $F_{2\alpha}$, angiotensin II, and endothelin) or by the Ca++ ionophore, ionomycin, results in an increase in the cytoplasmic free Ca++ concentration and extent of light-chain phosphorylation (Table 1 and Fig. 5) (14, 15). Maximal concentrations of free cytoplasmic Ca++ that are achieved in response to ionophore (1–3 µM) are much greater than those achieved in response to other agents (200–300 nM). The quantitative relationship between cytoplasmic Ca++ concentrations and myosin light-chain phosphorylation is similar, irrespective of the stimulating agent. In unstimulated human myometrial cells, the levels of light-chain phosphorylation are low (0.04 mol phosphate per mol light chain), as expected for a Ca++-dependent reaction. When cytoplasmic Ca++ concentrations increase above 150 nM, light-chain phosphorylation increases, with maximal phosphorylation of 0.54 mol phosphate per mol light chain (Fig. 5). Half-maximal activation of phosphorylation occurs at an intracellular Ca++ concentration of 300 nM. Based on the Hill coefficient of approximately 3 for the relationship between light-chain phosphorylation and cytoplasmic free Ca++ concentration, there is apparent positive cooperativity. Thus, small increases in cytoplasmic free Ca++ lead to increases in myosin light-chain phosphorylation.

As presented in Table 1, prostaglandins E_2 and $F_{2\alpha}$, oxytocin, and endothelin effect a significant increase in cytoplasmic free Ca++ and myosin light-chain phosphorylation in human myometrial cells. The increase in Ca++ and light-chain phosphorylation correlate with the effectiveness of these agents in stimulating contractile responses in human uterine smooth-muscle strips in vitro

Table 1. Effect of various physiologic agonists on [Ca^{++}]$_i$ and myosin light-chain phosphorylation in cultured human myometrial smooth-muscle cells.

Treatment	[Ca^{++}]$_i$ (nM)	Myosin Light-Chain Phosphorylation (%)
Control	121 ± 5	3.7 ± 2.5
PGF$_{2\alpha}$ (10^{-8}M)	$165 \pm 8^*$	$14.5 \pm 1.4^*$
PGE$_2$ (10^{-8}M)	$220 \pm 15^*$	$20.0 \pm 1.1^*$
Oxytocin (2×10^{-8}M)	$180 \pm 10^*$	$18.0 \pm 1.0^*$
Angiotensin II (10^{-7}M)	$199 \pm 12^*$	$22.8 \pm 4.0^*$
Endothelin (10^{-7}M)	$297 \pm 12^*$	$36.0 \pm 2.0^*$

Source: Data obtained from MacKenzie LW, Word RA, Casey ML, Stull JT, Myosin phosphorylation in myometrial smooth muscle cells, Am J Physiol 1990;27:C92–8, and Word RA, Kamm KE, Stull JT, Casey ML, Endothelin increases cytoplasmic calcium and myosin phosphorylation in human myometrium, Am J Obstet Gynecol 1990 (in press).

Human myometrial smooth-muscle cells were treated with test agents and [Ca^{++}]$_i$ was determined at 15 sec.

*P < 0.02 compared with control using two-tailed Student's t test.

(unpublished data). We find that human uterine smooth-muscle strips obtained from nonpregnant women at the time of hysterectomy contract rhythmically at a rate of 0.18 ± 0.02 per minute. Spontaneous activity is characterized by phasic increases in isometric force (peak amplitude, 266 ± 24.6 g/cm^2), whereas uterotonic agents act to increase contractile frequency, force amplitude, and duration of contraction. For example, in strips of longitudinal muscle treated with endothelin (10^{-8}M), contractile frequency increases from spontaneous activity of 0.24 to 1.0 contractions per minute (Fig. 6). Contractile force increases and duration of con-

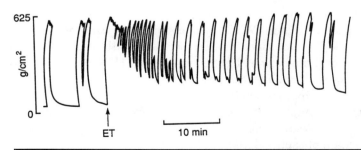

Fig. 6. Effect of endothelin (10^{-8}M) on contraction of human myometrial uterine smooth muscle. Uterine smooth-muscle strips from the longitudinal layer of uteri were obtained from premenopausal women at the time of hysterectomy for benign disease. The amplitude of contraction is correlated directly with force; a scale of force normalized to tissue cross-sectional area is provided.

traction is prolonged in response to endothelin (15). These contractile responses are presumably due to increases in cytoplasmic Ca^{++} concentrations and myosin light-chain phosphorylation. Alterations in the myometrium that accompany pregnancy result in an increased responsiveness to various uterotonins. For example, at term, increased myometrial responsiveness to oxytocin is effected by an increase in oxytocin receptors (16). Additional investigations with human myometrial smooth muscle are needed to establish cellular mechanisms associated with altered contractile states during parturition.

SUMMARY

In summary, the Ca^{++}-dependent phosphorylation of myosin light chain is an important regulatory step in the initiation of smooth-muscle contraction. The intracellular Ca^{++} concentration is a primary determinant for myosin light-chain phosphorylation; thus, cellular mechanisms by which intracellular Ca^{++} levels are regulated are important in smooth-muscle contractility.

REFERENCES

1. Kamm KE, Stull JT. Regulation of smooth muscle contractile elements by second messengers. Annu Rev Physiol 1989;51:299-313.
2. Hartshorne DJ, Gorecka A. Biochemistry of the contractile proteins of smooth muscle. In: Bohr DF, Somlyo AP, Sparks Jr. HV, eds. Handbook of physiology. The cardiovascular system, vol. 2. Vascular smooth muscle. Bethesda, MD: Am Physiol Soc, 1980:93-120.
3. Stull JT, Nunnally MH, Moore RL, Blumenthal DK. Myosin light chain kinase and myosin phosphorylation in skeletal muscle. In: Weber G, ed. Advances in enzyme regulation. 23rd ed. New York: Permagon Press, 1985:123-40.
4. Kamm KE, Stull JT. The function of myosin and myosin light chain kinase phosphorylation in smooth muscle. Annu Rev Pharmacol Toxicol 1985;25:593-620.
5. Cox JA. Interactive properties of calmodulin. Biochem J 1988;249:621-9.
6. Kamm KE, Stull JT. Myosin phosphorylation, force, and maximal shortening velocity in neurally stimulated tracheal smooth muscle. Am J Physiol 1984;249:C238-47.
7. Kamm KE, Stull JT. Activation of smooth muscle contraction: relation between myosin phosphorylation and stiffness. Science 1986;232:280-82.
8. Hai C-M, Murphy RA. Cross-bridge phosphorylation and regulation of latch state in smooth muscle. Am J Physiol 1988;254:C99-106.
9. Stull JT, Nunnally MH, Michnoff CH. Calmodulin-dependent protein kinases. In: The enzymes. New York: Academic Press, 1986:113-6.
10. Cohen P. The structure and regulation of protein phosphatases. Annu Rev Biochem 1989;58:463-508.
11. Kamm KE, Leachman SA, Michnoff CH, et al. Myosin light chain kinases and kinetics of myosin phosphorylation in smooth muscle cells. In: Siegman MJ, Somlyo AP Stephens NL, eds. Regulation and contraction of smooth muscle. New York: Liss, 1987;245:183-93.
12. Haeberle JR, Hott JW, Hathaway DR. Regulation of isometric force and isotonic shortening velocity by phosphorylation of the 20,000 dalton myosin light chain of rat uterine smooth muscle. Pflügers Arch 1985;403:215-99.

13. Asano M, Stull JT. Effects of calmodulin antagonists on smooth muscle contraction and myosin phosphorylation. In: Hidaka H, Hartshorne DJ, eds. Calmodulin antagonists and cellular physiology. Orlando, FL: Academic Press, 1985:225-60.

14. MacKenzie LW, Word RA, Casey ML, Stull JT. Myosin phosphorylation in myometrial smooth muscle cells. Am J Physiol 1990;27:C92-8.

15. Word RA, Kamm KE, Stull JT, Casey ML. Endothelin increases cytoplasmic calcium and myosin phosphorylation in human myometrium. Am J Obstet Gynecol 1990 (in press).

16. Soloff, MS. The role of oxytocin in the initiation of labor and oxytocin-prostaglandin interactions. In: McNellis D, Challis JRG, MacDonald PC, Nathaniels PW, Roberts JM, eds. The onset of labor: cellular and integrative mechanisms. Ithaca, NY: Perinatology Press:87-110.

5

Ca⁺⁺ Regulation in Smooth Muscle

Gary G. Spencer, Islam Khan, and Ashok K. Grover

Department of Biomedical Sciences, McMaster University,
Health Science Centre, Hamilton, Ontario, Canada

SMOOTH-MUSCLE CONTRACTILITY

S mooth muscle (SM) is the contractile apparatus present in the muscular walls of the uterus, blood vessels, airways, urogenital tract, and the gastrointestinal tract (1). The properties of SM vary depending on its location and function in the body. As a result, the mechanisms controlling SM contractility range from hormonal or neurogenic to myogenic, and the relative contribution of each also varies. In all these mechanisms, however, contractility is ultimately controlled by regulating the intracellular calcium ion level, $[Ca^{++}]_i$, which triggers a cascade of events leading to muscle contraction (1, 2).

Besides being the primary messenger for contraction activation, Ca^{++} plays other important physiological roles within the cell. Calcium sometimes acts as a second messenger by activating various proteins (i.e., Ca^{++} binding proteins) (3, 4) and ion channels, which in turn mediate various effects within the cell (3, 5). Calcium is also required for cell division and repair, enzyme activity, and immune function (6). Because of the importance of Ca^{++} in regulating cellular activity, the $[Ca^{++}]_i$ is maintained within a narrow range, and all the Ca^{++} movements are tightly regulated.

Ca⁺⁺ MOVEMENTS

Sources and Sinks

One major source of intracellular Ca^{++} is the extracellular fluid. The ratio of extracellular to intracellular Ca^{++} ion concentration is 10,000:1 (i.e., extracellular Ca^{++} is >1 mM; $[Ca^{++}]_i$ is 0.1:10µM) (7). Thus, minor changes in the permeability of the plasma membrane (PM) result in Ca^{++} entering the cell along its electrochemical gradient, causing significant fluctuations in $[Ca^{++}]_i$. Considerable amounts of Ca^{++} are also sequestered in intracellular stores, such as the endoplasmic reticulum (ER, alias sarcoplasmic reticulum [SR]). Other intracellular organelles such as the mitochondria, Golgi vesicles, and lysosomes appear to be less important in storing Ca^{++} and thus have not been widely studied (4).

Ca^{++} Movements During Contraction

For contraction to occur $[Ca^{++}]_i$ may be raised to greater than 1 μM (7). As mentioned above, one major reservoir of Ca^{++} is located extracellularly. Most of the Ca^{++} enters the cell by passive diffusion through voltage-operated Ca^{++} channels (VOC), receptor-operated Ca^{++} channels (ROC) or perhaps other mechanisms, such as stretch-activated Ca^{++}-permeable channels found in amphibian SM cells (8). Ca^{++} may also leak into the cell or be transported in via the Na^+–Ca^{++} exchanger (4).

VOC are present in both excitable and nonexcitable cells (3). Evidence for VOC stems from studies on Ca^{++} entry, contractility experiments, and studies on membrane currents including patch clamps. Three types of Ca^{++} channels have been identified: L, T, and N (4). They have different properties due to their different sensitivities to transmembrane potentials. These channels are blocked differentially by antagonists, which include tertiary amines such as verapamil, dihydropyridines, benzothiazepines, and other agents. Ion channels (e.g., K-channels), electrogenic ion pumps (e.g., the ouabain-sensitive Na^+ K-pump), and membrane exchangers (e.g., the Na^+–Ca^{++} exchanger) all contribute to the membrane potential and thus to the opening and closing of the various VOC (9). The entry of Ca^{++} through VOC or ROC may increase the $[Ca^{++}]_i$, which in turn opens Ca^{++}-activated K-channels resulting in hyperpolarization of the PM and the further opening of VOC (9). As well, it is proposed that intracellular Ca^{++} may itself stimulate the further entry of Ca^{++} into the cell (5, 10).

The presence of ROCs has remained controversial for some time (7). They were postulated to be present when agonists were observed to cause the entry of $[45]Ca^{++}$ into SM cells followed by contraction, without changing the membrane potential (9). Previously, however, other factors that might have contributed to Ca^{++} entry were not adequately controlled. This and the lack of suitable selective antagonists for ROC lead one to question their existence. Now evidence for ROCs is stronger since they are being verified using patch-clamp studies on cell-attached and membrane-excised patches (11).

Some workers have proposed that ROC are opened indirectly by agonists such as histamine, NE, vasopressin, angiotensin, thrombin, and bradykinin (9). These actions however, may be due to changes in membrane permeability resulting from receptor-induced changes in the inositol phosphate pathway or other metabolic processes.

Extracellular Ca^{++} is not the only Ca^{++} source available for contraction. Sufficient amounts of Ca^{++} are stored by and can be released from intracellular stores for this purpose (2, 4, 12, 13). IP_3 may play a key role in SM and nonmuscle cells in mobilizing Ca^{++} from intracellular stores by binding to a receptor coupled to a cation channel via a G-protein (9, 14). Experiments in Ca^{++}-free media have indicated that agonists such as vasopressin and α 1-adrenergic agonists can stimulate the production of the intracellular messenger inositol 1,4,5-triphosphate (IP_3), followed by the release of Ca^{++} from the ER (2). This intracellular nonmitochondrial store is also sensitive to ATP, Ca^{++}, caffeine, and ryanodine (12, 15, 16). Ca^{++} released from either intracellular or extracellular sources appears to potentiate the further release of Ca^{++} from the ER (i.e., Ca^{++}-induced Ca^{++} release) (9). Caffeine induces Ca^{++} release, but this process does not appear to involve a G-protein as with IP_3, and it is more readily blocked by procaine. Thus, two types of Ca^{++} release channels are postulated to exist in smooth-muscle ER: those sensitive to Ca^{++}, caffeine, and ATP, and those sensitive only to IP_3 (16, 17). For a review, see Fleischer and Inui (12).

It has been proposed that in nonmuscle cells the IP_3-sensitive Ca^{++} store may be a new organelle termed the *calciosome*, and not the ER. The reason is that the distribution of the ER markers (i.e., cytochrome P-450, sulfatase C, and glucose-6-phosphatase) did not correspond to the distribution of this IP_3-sensitive organelle (19, 20). One may question, however, if we have yet found a highly reliable marker for the ER. Thus, the calciosome proposal requires further confirmation.

Ca⁺⁺ Movements During Relaxation

$[Ca^{++}]_i$ must be reduced to less than 0.1 μM in order for SM to relax. Reducing $[Ca^{++}]_i$ is a more complex process than increasing it. Major mechanisms for reduction of $[Ca^{++}]_i$ involve transport of Ca^{++} against its own electrochemical gradient and are discussed in the next section. Calcium binding to proteins or to the inner surface of the PM and other intracellular membranes may also play some role (4). Though Ca^{++} binding proteins mostly function in signal processing, proteins such as calsequestrin aid in sequestering Ca^{++} once it is inside intracellular organelles, thus allowing for the further uptake of Ca^{++} (21). In the cytoplasm, however, Ca^{++} binding proteins lead to only small overall reductions in $[Ca^{++}]_i$, since this process is limited by the total amount of protein present and their affinity for Ca^{++} (3). A more efficient way of reducing the Ca^{++} concentration is either by moving it across the PM and out of the cell or by sequestering it into intracellular organelles like the ER or SR.

An electrogenic Na^+–Ca^{++} exchanger present in the PM may also contribute to reduction of $[Ca^{++}]_i$ (4, 22). Its contribution to Ca^{++} movement varies from tissue to tissue, being most active in heart, brain, and nervous tissue (4). The exchanger is nonvectorial and electrogenic, at least in cardiac muscle, with a stochiometry of >3 Na^+/Ca^{++}. In SM, this exchange process has also been reported in myometrium, mesenteric artery, aorta, and gastrointestinal tract (7). The activity of the Na^+–Ca^{++} exchanger in SM is much lower than in the heart. As with the mitochondrial system, however, the Ca^{++} affinity of the exchanger is too low to account for the submicromolar levels of Ca^{++} (i.e., 0.1–1 μM) observed in SM cells under normal conditions (4). Even in the presence of ATP, acidic phospholipids, and controlled proteolysis, the apparent K_m is never reduced to a low enough level. Thus, even though the extrusion of Ca^{++} through PM may be thermodynamically favorable, its kinetic properties do not favor it as a major Ca^{++} extrusion mechanism. Therefore, the reduction and fine tuning of $[Ca^{++}]_i$ appear to be through Ca^{++}-pumps localized in the membranes of the ER and PM.

Ca++-PUMPS

One observation confirming the presence of Ca++-pumps was that isolated membrane vesicles could sequester Ca++ from media containing submicromolar [Ca++] in the presence of ATP (7). Also, sufficient Ca++ could be sequestered to account for the observed transmembrane Ca++ concentration gradient, which was abolished on addition of the Ca++-ionophores A23817, X537A, and ionomycin. This uphill Ca++ transport was insensitive to azide and was not dependent on the presence of Na+, thus ruling out mitochondrial uptake and the Na+–Ca++ exchanger, respectively. All of this evidence has implicated the Ca++-pump, which has now been identified in skeletal, cardiac, smooth, and nonmuscle tissue as an enzyme that requires Ca++ and Mg++ for using the chemical energy of ATP hydrolysis to transport Ca++.

Skeletal Muscle Sarcoplasmic Reticulum

Reaction Cycle. In the process of coupling ATP hydrolysis to the transport of Ca++ into the SR, the internal membrane Ca++-pump protein alternates between two conformational states designated E_1 and E_2 (23, 24). These forms have different affinities for Ca++, Mg++, and ATP, which are required for pump activity. The first step in the E_1-E_2 pumping cycle involves the cooperative binding of two Ca++ ions to high-affinity sites (K_m 0.1–1 μM) on the E_1 form of the enzyme (25, 26). One or possibly both of these high-affinity sites are composed of the carboxylate or carboxamide side chains of 6 amino acid residues—Glu309, Glu771, Asn796, Thr799, Asp800, and Glu908—located near the center of the transmembrane domain of the Ca++-pump (27, 28). Pro308 and Pro803 may also be involved in the structure of the high-affinity Ca++ binding sites (29). Ca++ binding converts the enzyme into a form that is rapidly phosphorylated by ATP (26). Phosphorylation results in an acylphosphoprotein intermediate as the γ-phosphate of ATP is transferred to an aspartyl residue (Asp351) in the catalytic site of the enzyme (30). This occurs in the presence of Mg++, resulting in the formation of an Ca++-enzyme-Mg++ ATP complex (31).

Mg++ also promotes the next step, in which the enzyme undergoes a conformational change in translocating Ca++ across the membrane. This transition involves the movement of peptide segments between hydrophobic and hydrophilic environments as indicated by time-resolved X-ray diffraction, fluorescence, and photolabeling (26). This altered form of the enzyme, now called E_2, has a lower affinity for Ca++ (K_m = 2 mM). Thus Ca++ is released, further altering the protein conformation (25). This form can now interact with water, causing the hydrolysis and liberation of both Mg++ and P_i, and the interconversion of the enzyme back to the E_1 form (31, 32). For every ATP hydrolyzed, the skeletal muscle SR Ca++-pump transports 2 Ca++ ions and has a turnover of 10^3 min^{-1}, which is accelerated by the binding of ATP at the low-affinity regulatory ATP binding site (23).

The ATP binding site was originally located as lysine 515 by examining the binding of fluorescein isothiocyanate (FITC), which blocks the binding of ATP (33). When lysine was altered by site-directed mutagenesis and the protein expressed in

Cos-1 cells, however, there was a reduction in Ca^{++} transport, but this effect was not as dramatic as was expected. Instead Asp351 and Lys352 appear to be critical for Ca^{++} transport and Ca^{++}-dependent phosphorylation by ATP (31). Thus ATP binding may require a tertiary structure in which three residues are in close proximity (35).

Examining the conservation of amino acids between different cation-transporting ATPases, and testing their importance using site-directed mutagenesis, shows GLY233 and Pro312 to be important for E_1 to E_2 conformational changes (29, 36). Thus, a conformational change occurs at every step in the reaction cycle, thus leading to vectorial and chemical specificity of the coupled reactions (25, 37). Interactions between the Ca^{++}-pump, its lipid environment, Ca^{++}, ATP, Mg^{++}, and other ions are currently under investigation. Thus, the scheme outlined in Figure 1 is our simplified interpretation of a very complex scheme.

Structure, Localization, and Function.   The cDNA and the gene for rabbit skeletal muscle SR Ca^{++}-Mg^{++}-ATPase have been cloned, and the structure of the Ca^{++}-pump is known in some detail at the molecular level (38). The structure of the Ca^{++}-pump has been predicted from electron micrographs, X-ray diffraction, and hydropathy analysis of the pump's primary structure. Confirmation of these predictions has been obtained from studies of protease digestion and site-directed mutagenesis (29, 36, 39).

The Ca^{++}-pump contains 10 transmembrane stretches with 40%–50% of the Ca^{++}-pump peptide mass located inside the hydrophobic core of the membrane (26). A large portion of the enzyme protrudes from the cytoplasmic side and is responsible for binding to Ca^{++} and ATP. The pump has a stalk region composed of

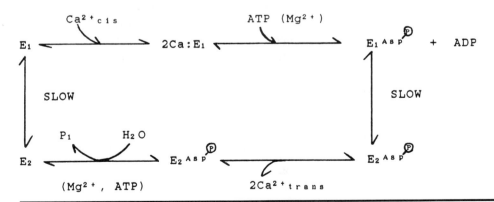

Fig. 1.   Proposal for reaction cycle of the internal membrane and plasma membrane calcium-pump protein. The subscript "cis" denotes the membrane side from which Ca^{++} is transported, and the subscript "trans" denotes the membrane side to which Ca^{++} is pumped. Compounds written in brackets may or may not be present when the reaction occurs.

amphipatic helixes, which are involved in the handling of bound Ca^{++} following ATP utilization (28). The stalk region connects 3 cytoplasmic globular domains to the transmembrane sequences. These globular regions include the nucleotide, transduction, and phosphorylation domains, which are highly interactive (38).

The skeletal muscle Ca^{++}-pump has been identified in fast-twitch and slow-twitch skeletal muscle, localized predominantly in the membrane of the SR. Initial studies indicated that these two pumps might be similar. Antibody cross-reactivity studies revealed that although some epitopes of the fast-twitch skeletal muscle Ca^{++}-pump are similar to epitopes on the slow-twitch/cardiac Ca^{++}-ATPase, others are quite different (40–42). Proteolytic digestion studies and various molecular cloning techniques have also confirmed these differences (43). Examination of rabbit cDNA and genomic DNA confirmed that the fast-twitch and slow-twitch/cardiac SR Ca^{++}-ATPases are encoded by two different genes (43, 44). Identity between the fast-twitch and slow-twitch Ca^{++}-pump protein sequences was 84%.

The Ca^{++}-pump from adult and neonate fast-twitch muscles differ in their C-terminal sequence as well (45). The difference arises from a developmentally regulated alternate splicing event in which a penultimate 42-bp exon is spliced out of the neonatal form but retained in the adult form (45). As a result of this, the C-terminus glycine of the adult form is replaced by 8 highly charged amino acid residues, thus forming the neonatal isoform (46). Both isoforms have since been expressed in Cos-1 cells, but their Ca^{++} affinities and Ca^{++} transport activities are similar (34). Thus, the functional significance of their different carboxyl-terminal sequences is not known.

Regulation. In slow-twitch skeletal muscle the internal Ca^{++}-pump is regulated by phospholamban, which inhibits the pump when bound but is released when phosphorylated (12, 40, 47, 48, 49). Phospholamban phosphorylation may occur via a cAMP-dependent, Ca^{++}-calmodulin-dependent, cGMP-dependent or a Ca^{++}-phospholipid-dependent protein kinase. Release of phospholamban increases the affinity for Ca^{++}, thus stimulating the pump. Phospholamban has been purified, cloned, and sequenced (12). Surprisingly, phospholamban is not present in fast-twitch skeletal muscle, although the fast-twitch SR Ca^{++}-pump does contain the phospholamban binding domain (45, 48). Possibly a phospholamban-like protein may yet be identified.

The skeletal muscle SR Ca^{++}-pump is also modulated by the phospholipid environment that is needed for pump activity (50). Because of the length of the chain and the degree of unsaturation of phosphatidylcholine, phosphatidic acid, and lysophosphatidylcholine, these phospholipids result in maximal pump activity. Hydrophobic compounds, such as triphenylphosphine and diphenylamine, inhibit the Ca^{++}-pump in the forward and reverse reactions by interacting with hydrophobic domains of the Ca^{++}-pump protein (51). Their hydrophobicity determines their access and resulting effectiveness in interacting with the pump.

The pump is also inhibited by cyclopiazonic acid (52, 53). AlF_4- is a universal inhibitor of SR, ER, and PM transport ATPases because it interacts with their phosphate-binding site in a manner similar to that of vanadate (52).

Cardiac Tissue

Structure, Localization, Regulation.   The structure of the Ca^{++}-pump located in cardiac tissue (i.e., I_c) is identical to that in slow-twitch skeletal muscle (38). The heart may also contain an alternately spliced isoform, I_s (see below). As yet, the location of these isoforms within cardiac tissue has not been determined. It is possible that their different carboxyl-terminal sequences function in targeting these isoforms within the cell since I_s contains a potential glycosylation site not contained in I_c (54).

Both of these Ca^{++}-pump isoforms are regulated by phospholamban. Pump stimulation has been demonstrated using monoclonal antibodies against phospholamban and by limited proteolytic treatment (12). It is also assumed but not established that the same factors modulating the activity of I_c modulate the activity of I_s. The different carboxyl-terminal sequences may, however, result in differential regulation.

Erythrocytes

Structure and Localization.   Erythrocytes contain Ca^{++}-pumps in their PM constituting less than 0.05% of the total PM protein (4). Though the erythrocyte Ca^{++}-pump has only been partially sequenced, amino acid similarity and hydropathy profile comparison suggest that the transmembrane organization of the PM Ca^{++}-pump is similar to that described previously for the SR Ca^{++}-pump (55). This is also true for the other surface membrane Ca^{++}-ATPases.

The PM Ca^{++}-pump is approximately 30 kD larger than the SR Ca^{++}-pump, with the homology between the two being no closer than that between other membrane transport ATPases (i.e., Na^+, K-pump, H-pump, etc.) (56). The PM Ca^{++}-pump has a 90-kD domain that appears to be the central part required for hydrolyzing ATP, forming phosphorylated intermediates, transporting Ca^{++}, remaining associated with the membrane, and mediating Ca^{++}-dependent regulation (57). The remaining 50-kD peptide fragment can be trimmed from the amino end without noticeably affecting the enzyme function. This 50-kD fragment is not present in the SR Ca^{++}-pump, and its role is not yet known. Some isoforms of the PM Ca^{++}-pump also have a potential phosphorylation site for the cAMP-dependent protein kinase (Ser-1178) situated downstream (C-terminal) from the calmodulin binding site (55). Both of these sites are in the 9-kD carboxy-terminal fragment identified in proteolytic digestion studies (57). Thus the carboxy terminus region in the PM pump is known as the *regulatory region*. The PM Ca^{++}-pump from kidney and brain has been cloned, but it is not known how similar it is to the erythrocyte Ca^{++}-pump except in the highly conserved calmodulin binding domain.

A region that is conserved in both the PM and internal membrane Ca^{++}-pump is a hydrophobic region containing the FITC binding site and the region where the acylphosphate intermediate is formed (23, 55). Other highly conserved regions include those important for ion specificity and the binding and transport of Ca^{++} ions across the membrane.

Reaction Cycle.   The reaction cycle for the PM Ca^{++}-pump is similar to the reaction cycle for the SR Ca^{++}-pump in skeletal muscle except only 1 Ca^{++} ion may be transported per ATP hydrolyzed instead of 2 as reported for the SR Ca^{++}-pump (23, 24). In terms of substrate specificity, though both enzymes have higher affinity for ATP than for any other nucleotides, the PM Ca^{++}-pump appears to be more selective (23). The SR and the PM Ca^{++}-pump also differ in their ability to catalyze the reverse reaction (23). Reversal of the pump uses the energy of the $[Ca^{++}]$ gradient to form ATP from ADP and P_i. For the SR pump, the Ca^{++}, ADP, and P_i concentration can be altered such that the rate of ATP synthesis approaches the rate of the forward reaction (23). The backward reaction of the PM Ca^{++}-pump, however, can only be increased to a rate that is 0.05%–1% of the forward reaction (23).

Regulation.   As stated above, the PM Ca^{++}-pump contains a regulatory domain that mediates the effects of Ca^{++}-calmodulin binding and phosphorylation by the cAMP-dependent protein kinase. The Kd for calmodulin binding to the pump is in the nanomolar range only when at least three of its four Ca^{++} binding sites are occupied (23). Ca^{++}-calmodulin binding increases the enzyme affinity for Ca^{++}, the Ca^{++}-dependent ADP-ATP exchange rate, and the maximal rate of the pump (19). The affinity for ATP at the low-affinity site, which may be important in regulation, is also increased. It is postulated that there is a 9-kD protein sequence at the C-terminus of the pump, which, in the absence of calmodulin, inhibits ATPase activity by interfering with a high-affinity Ca^{++}-binding site (58–60). An elevation in cytoplasmic Ca^{++} concentration, however, results in more Ca^{++}-calmodulin binding to this 9-kD segment, thus activating the PM Ca^{++}-pump by disrupting interaction of this segment with the Ca^{++} binding site. This interaction can also be disrupted by limited proteolysis, accounting for the increases in V_{max} and Ca^{++} affinity observed in previous studies following partial digestion of the pump protein (60, 61).

The V_{max} and Ca^{++} affinity of the PM Ca^{++}-pump is also increased by acidic phospholipids such as phosphatidylinositol and phosphatidylserine (62). Self-association of the enzyme also increases V_{max} and Ca^{++} affinity (63). Target inactivation, chemical cross-linking, and electron microscopy studies indicate that ATPase molecules may interact under normal conditions with the dominant oligomeric form being either the dimer or tetramer (64).

The pump is also activated by long-chain polyunsaturated fatty acids, organic solvents (i.e., dimethyl sulfoxide), and phospholipase A2 (4, 65). Carbachol at extremely high concentrations, N', N'-dicyclohexylcarbodiimide, and AlF_4^- inhibit the pump (35). Finally, hormones such as the thyroid hormone have been reported to activate or inhibit the pump in erythrocytes depending on the nutritional status of the animals (4).

Smooth Muscle

Internal Ca^{++}-Pump Structure and Localization.   Phosphorylation experiments provided early evidence that the subunit molecular weight of the internal

Table 1. Summary of calcium-pump proteins identified to date (based on cDNA sequences).

Plasma Membrane	
3 genes × 4 splices	127–135 kD
Internal Membrane	
Slow-twitch/cardiac gene	
I_c	110 kD
I_s	115 kD
HKS gene	109 kD
Fast-twitch skeletal gene	
Adult	110 kD
Neonatal	111 kD

Ca^{++}-pump in SM ER-enriched fractions was about 100 kD (40, 66). Ca^{++} uptake by the ER-enriched vesicles was stimulated by oxalate. This stimulation somewhat paralleled the distribution of the ER markers NADPH:cytochrome-c-reductase and rotenone-insensitive NADH:cytochrome-c-reductase even though the recovery of the oxalate-stimulated uptake decreased on fractionation (67). Examination of tryptic digestion patterns confirmed that this pump was not a proteolytic digestion product of the PM Ca^{++}-pump (57). Antibodies against the heart but not the skeletal muscle SR Ca^{++}-pump reacted with the ER pump in stomach SM (40–42). Transcripts for three different isoforms of the internal Ca^{++}-pump have been reported, although it is not established whether they are all present in SM. Very low levels of transcripts for the cardiac/slow-twitch Ca^{++}-ATPase (I_c) are present in some SM. It is most abundant in soleus and cardiac tissue (68–70). The second isoform, the SM/nonmuscle Ca^{++}-ATPase (I_s), differs in that the terminal 4 amino acids are replaced by 49 amino acids due to the recognition of a cryptic splice site (54, 72, 73). This is the most abundant isoform found in SM and nonmuscle tissue. Hybridization and nuclease protection studies have revealed that the uterus, stomach, trachea, large and small intestines, as well as the liver, kidney, and spleen, all contain transcripts for I_s almost exclusively (i.e., 85%–100%) (69). Esophagus, testis, aorta, urinary bladder, and brain contain varying amounts of mRNA for both I_c and I_s (68).

Recently a gene encoding the third intracellular Ca^{++}-pump isoform in SM has been identified in rat kidney (I_k) (74). It exhibits 75%–77% amino acid identity with the slow-twitch/cardiac and fast-twitch isoforms of the SR Ca^{++}-ATPase. Very low levels of mRNA coding for I_k are expressed in the uterus, lung, testes, and large and small intestines, as well as the pancreas, brain, liver, kidney, heart, and skeletal muscle. In rabbit stomach SM, however, we have observed transcripts and protein products only for I_s (75).

Regulation of the tissue-specific expression of the three isoforms remains unknown. We have proposed that the alternate splicing may serve to control both the type and level of the isoforms produced in a tissue-specific manner (75). Another question is where these different isoforms are located within the cell and how they differ in their function. Most researchers have only addressed the question of whether the mRNA for these isoforms is present in different tissues; they have not studied cellular localization of the protein at all. In some studies, whole organs were used, and thus reports of a particular isoform being expressed in specified tissues may also be unreliable. Therefore, when addressing these and other questions, it is very important that the cell type be as homogeneous as possible.

Internal Ca++-Pump Regulation. In SM the internal membrane Ca^{++}-pump is regulated by phospholamban in the same manner as it is in the cardiac and slow-twitch skeletal muscles. Beta-adrenergic receptor activation is therefore postulated to induce SM relaxation by increasing intracellular cAMP or cGMP levels, resulting in the activation of protein kinases and the resulting phosphorylation of phospholamban (1). The SM internal Ca^{++}-pump is also subjected to other forms of regulation as has been described previously for other internal pumps.

PM Ca++-Pump Structure. Immunologically, this pump is similar to the erythro-cyte PM Ca^{++}-pump (76, 77). Both the pumps are stimulated by calmodulin, and this stimulation parallels the subcellular distribution of PM markers (i.e., 5' nucleotidase activity). Acid-stable acylphosphate-enzyme studies have confirmed this similarity. The acylphosphate intermediate of both the pumps is stabilized by La^{+++} and has a subunit molecular weight of 135 ± 5 kD (66). The PM Ca^{++}-pumps present in SM or erythrocytes, however, have not been cloned, and thus their structural similarity has not been confirmed. Northern blot analysis has revealed that the SM PM Ca^{++}-pump may also be similar to one isoform cloned from rat brain (78).

The rat brain contains cDNA coding for three distinct isoforms of the PM Ca^{++}-pump. These include $PMCA_1$ ($M_r = 129,500$), $PMCA_2$ ($M_r = 132,605$) and $PMCA_3$ ($M_r = 127,000$) (78). $PMCA_1$ and $PMCA_2$ exhibit 82% amino acid identity, and $PMCA_3$ had 81% and 85% amino acid identity with $PMCA_1$ and $PMCA_2$, respectively. All have been proposed to be encoded by different genes. An interest-ing observation is that the 3^1-coding untranslated sequence of $PMCA_1$ contains a 154-nucleotide sequence, which, if excised, would result in a C-terminus like that of $PMCA_2$ (79). This was the first suggestion of an alternate processing event that may contribute to additional diversity in the PM Ca^{++}-pump proteins. Thus $PMCA_1$ and $PMCA_2$ differ in their potential for regulation by cAMP-dependent kinases and calmodulin. In human fetal skeletal muscle alternate splicing of this 154-bp exon in PMCA resulted in four different mRNA transcripts arising from a single gene as predicted (79).

Northern blot analysis using probes from the cDNA corresponding to the 5' end and 3' untranslated region of $PMCA_1$ revealed that $PMCA_1$ or a pump similar to it is expressed in a wide range of tissues including SM (74). These smooth muscles include the uterus, lung, testes, stomach, and large and small intestines. Northern blot analysis also revealed the appearance of different sizes of transcripts for each of the three PMCA isoforms (71).

PM Ca⁺⁺-Pump Regulation. The SM PM Ca⁺⁺-pump is stimulated by the binding of calmodulin, negatively charged phospholipids, and in some instances by small increases in pH within the physiological range (6.9–7.4) (62, 80). The pH elevation may increase the affinity of the pump for Ca⁺⁺ (80). Oxytocin inhibits the pump in rat myometrial PM by reducing the affinity of the pump for Ca⁺⁺ (81). This inhibition depends, however, on the hormonal status of the rat, because the administration of progesterone together with diethylstilbestrol abolishes this inhibitory action. The pump in some studies has also been reported to be 10 times more sensitive to inhibition by vanadate than the SM internal Ca⁺⁺-pump (1). Finally, in some instances cGMP-dependent protein kinase stimulates the PM Ca⁺⁺-pump, as predicted from the alternate splicing event outlined previously.

FUTURE DIRECTIONS

Future research efforts are needed to understand the structural and functional significance of the differences that exist between the many internal membrane and PM Ca⁺⁺-pump isoforms. Studies using chimeric enzymes or monoclonal antibodies to these divergent regions may be particularly useful in answering whether these differences play an important physiological role in pump regulation and tissue targeting or have some developmental importance.

Another unknown is the identity of the factors that regulate these alternate splicing events resulting in the formation of different isoforms. What determines the relative abundance of the isoforms in different tissues? One possibility might be that the mRNA of different isoforms have different translation efficiencies due to different mRNA secondary structures. The stability of mRNA or Ca⁺⁺-pump proteins may also influence their relative abundance. Possibly answers will be obtained by studying the expression of these isoforms in model systems in in vivo and in vitro. This will help to better understand the molecular mechanisms regulating $[Ca^{++}]_i$ in health and disease.

REFERENCES

1. Daniel E, Grover A, Kwan C. Calcium. In: Stephens NL, ed. Biochemistry of smooth muscle, vol 3. Boca Raton, FL: CRC Press, 1983:1-72.
2. Somlyo A, Himpens B. Cell calcium and its regulation in smooth muscle. FASEB J 1989;3:2266-76.
3. Villereal M, Palfrey H. Intracellular calcium and cell function. Annu Rev Nutr 1989;9:347-76.
4. Carafoli, E. Intracellular calcium homeostasis. Annu Rev Biochem 1987;56:395-433.
5. Ehara T, Noma A, Ono K. Calcium-activated non-selective cation channel in ventricular cells isolated from adult guinea-pig hearts. J Physiol 1988;403:117-133.
6. Zaloga G. Calcium homeostasis in the critically ill patient. Magnesium 1989;8: 190-200.
7. Grover A. Calcium transport and ATPases in smooth muscle PM. In: Kidwai AM, ed. CRC sarcolemmal biochemistry, vol 1. Boca Raton, FL: CRC Press, 1987:99-116.
8. Kirber M, Walsh J, Singer J. Stretch-activated ion channels in smooth muscle: a

mechanism for the initiation of stretch-induced contraction. Pflügers Arch 1988;412:339-45.

9. Van Breemen C. Cellular mechanisms regulating $[Ca^{++}]_i$ smooth muscle. Annu Rev Physiol 1989;51:315-29.

10. Gurney A, Charnet P, Pye J, et al. Augmentation of cardiac calcium current by flash photolysis of intracellular caged-Ca molecules. Nature 1989;341:65-8.

11. Benham C, Tsien R. A novel receptor-operated Ca-permeable channel activated by ATP in smooth muscle. Nature 1987;328:275-8.

12. Fleischer S, Inui M. Biochemistry and biophysics of excitation-contraction coupling. Annu Rev Biophys Chem 1989;18:333-64.

13. Rooney T, Sass E, Thomas A. Characterization of cytosolic calcium oscillations induced by phenylephrine and vasopressin in single fura-2-loaded hepatocytes. J Biol Chem 1989;264:17131-41.

14. Walker J, Somlyo A, Goldman Y, et al. Kinetics of smooth and skeletal muscle activation by laser pulse photolysis of caged inositol 1,4,5-triphosphate. Nature 1987;327:249-52.

15. Lai F, Misra M, Xu L, et al. The ryanodine receptor-Ca release channel complex of skeletal muscle SR. J Biol Chem 1989;264:16776-85.

16. Anderson K, Lai F, Liu Q, et al. Structural and functional characterization of the purified cardiac ryanodine receptor-Ca^{++} release channel complex. J Biol Chem 1989;264:1329-35.

17. Palade P, Dettbarn C, Volpe P, et al. Direct inhibition of inositol-1,4,5-trisphosphate-induced Ca release from brain microsomes by K^+ channel blockers. Mol Pharmacol 1989;36:673-80.

18. Palade P, Dettbarn C, Alderson B, et al. Pharmacologic differentiation between inositol-1,4,5-triphosphate-induced Ca release and Ca- or caffeine-induced Ca release from intracellular membrane systems. Mol Pharmacol 1989;36:673-80.

19. Volpe P, Krause K, Hashimoto S, et al. "Calciosome," a cytoplasmic organelle: the inositol 1, 4, 5-triphosphate-sensitive Ca store of nonmuscle cells? Proc Natl Acad Sci USA 1988;85:1091-5.

20. Alderson B, Volpe P. Distribution of ER and calciosome markers in membrane fractions isolated from different regions of the canine brain. Arch Biochem Biophys 1989;272:162-74.

21. Wuytack F, Raeymaekers L, Verbist J, et al. Evidence for the presence in smooth muscle of two types of Ca-transport ATPase. Biochem J 1984;224:445-51.

22. Philipson K. Sodium-calcium exchange in PM vesicles. Annu Rev Physiol 1985;47:561-71.

23. Schatzmann H. The calcium pump of the surface membrane and of the SR. Annu Rev Physiol 1989;51:473-85.

24. Inesi G. Mechanism of calcium transport. Annu Rev Physiol 1985;47:573-601.

25. Jencks WP. How does a calcium pump pump calcium? J Biol Chem 1989;264:18855-8.

26. Jorgensen P, Anderson J. Structural basis for E_1-E_2 conformational transitions in Na, K-pump and Ca-pump proteins. J Membrane Biol 1988;103:95-120.

27. Clarke DM, Loo TW, Inesi G, MacLennan DH. Location of high affinity Ca-binding sites within the predicted transmembrane domain of the sarcoplasmic reticulum Ca-ATPase. Nature 1989;339:476-8.

28. Clarke D, Maruyama K, Loo T, et al. Functional consequences of glutamate, aspar-

tate, glutamine, and asparagine mutations in the stalk sector of the Ca-ATPase of sarcoplasmic reticulum. J Biol Chem 1989;264:11246-51.

29. Vilsen B, Andersen J, Clarke D, et al. Functional consequences of proline mutations in the cytoplasmic and transmembrane sectors of the Ca-ATPase of SR. J Biol Chem 1989;264:21024-30.

30. Maruyama K, Clarke D, Fujii J, et al. Function consequences of alterations to amino acids located in the catalytic centre (isoleucine 348 to threonine 357) and nucleotide-binding domain of the Ca-ATPase of sarcoplasmic reticulum. J Biol Chem 1989;264:13038-42.

31. Heilmann C, Spamer C, Gerok W. Mechanisms of the calcium pump in the ER of liver: phosphoproteins as reaction intermediates. Cell Calcium 1989;10:275-87.

32. Chipman D, Jencks W. Specificity of the SR calcium ATPase at the hydrolysis step. Biochemistry 1988;27:5707-12.

33. Briggs F, Cable M, Geisow M, et al. Primary structure of the nucleotide binding domain of the Ca, Mg-ATPase from cardiac SR. Biochem Biophys Res Comm 1986;135:864-9.

34. Maruyama K, MacLennan D. Mutation of aspartic acid-351, lysine-352, and lysine-515 alters the Ca-transport activity of the Ca-ATPase expressed. Proc Natl Acad Sci USA 1988;85:3314-8.

35. Breier A, Turi-Nagy L, Ziegelhoffer A, et al. Hypothetical structure of the ATP-binding site of $(Na^+ + K^+)$-ATPase. Gen Physiol Biophys 1989;8:283-6.

36. Andersen J, Vilsen B, Leberer E, et al. Functional consequences of mutations in the B-strand of the Ca-ATPase of SR. J Biol Chem 1989;264:21018-23.

37. Suzuki S, Kawato S, Kouyama T, et al. Independent flexible motion of submolecular domains of the Ca^{2+}, Mg^{2+}-ATPase of SR measured by time resolved fluorescence depolarization of site-specifically attached probes. Biochem 1989;28:7734-40.

38. MacLennan D, Brandl C, Korczak B, et al. Amino-acid sequence of a $Ca^{2+} + Mg^{2+}$-dependent ATPase from rabbit muscle SR, deduced from its complementary DNA sequence. Nature 1985;316:696-700.

39. Caride A, Gorski J, Penniston J. Topology of the erythrocyte Ca^{2+} pump. Biochem J 1989;255:663-70.

40. DeFoor P, Levitsky D, Biryukova T, et al. Immunological dissimilarity of the calcium pump protein skeletal and cardiac muscle SR. Arch Biochem Biophys 1990;200:196-205.

41. Damiani E, Betto R, Salvatori S, et al. Polymorphism of SR adenosine triphosphatase of rabbit skeletal muscle. Biochem J 1981;197:245-8.

42. Eggermont J, Vrolix M, Wuytack F, et al. The (Ca-Mg)-ATPase of the PM and of the ER in SM cells and their regulation. J Card Pharmacol 1988;12:S51-5.

43. Brandl J, Green N, Korczak B, et al. Two Ca ATPase genes: homologies and mechanistic implications of deduced amino acid sequences. Cell 1986;44:597-607.

44. MacLennan D, Brandl C, Chanpaneria S, et al. Fast-twitch and slow-twitch/cardiac Ca ATPase genes map to human chromosomes 16 and 12. Somatic Cell Mol Gen 1987;13:341-6.

45. Brandl C, deLeon S, Martin D, et al. Adult forms of the Ca-ATPase of SR. J Biol Chem 1987;262:3768-74.

46. Korczak B, Zarain-Herzberg A, Brandl C, et al. Structure of the rabbit fast-twitch skeletal muscle Ca-ATPase gene. J Biol Chem 1988;263:4813-9.

47. Raeymaekers L, Hofmann F, Casteels R. Cyclic GMP-dependent protein kinase phosphorylates phospholamban in isolated SR from cardiac and smooth muscle. Biochem J 1988;252:269-73.
48. James P, Inui M, Tada M, et al. Nature and site of phospholamban regulation of the Ca pump of SR. Nature 1989;342:90-2.
49. Peuch C, DeMaille J. Covalent regulation of the cardiac SR calcium pump. Cell Calcium 1989;10:397-400.
50. Knowles A, Eytan E, Racker E. Phospholipid-protein interactions in the Ca^{2+}-adenosine triphosphatase of SR. J Biol Chem 1976;251:5161-5.
51. Petretski J, Wolosker H, de Meis L. Activation of Ca^{2+} uptake and inhibition of reversal of the SR Ca pump by aromatic compounds. J Biol Chem 1989;264:20339-43.
52. Missiaen L, Wuytack F, De Smedt H, et al. AlF_4-induced inhibition of the ATPase activity, the Ca-transport activity and the phosphoprotein-intermediate formation of PM and ER(SR) Ca-transport ATPases in different tissues. Biochem J 1989;261:655-60.
53. Seidler N, Jona I, Vegh M, et al. Cyclopiazonic acid is a specific inhibitor of the Ca-ATPase of SR. J Biol Chem 1989;264:17816-23.
54. Lytton J, MacLennan D. Molecular cloning of cDNAs from human kidney coding for two alternatively spliced products of the cardiac Ca-ATPase gene. J Biol Chem 1988;263:15024-31.
55. Verma A, Filoteo A, Stanford D, et al. Complete primary structure of a human plasma membrane Ca pump. J Biol Chem 1988;263:14152-9.
56. Papp B, Sarkadi B, Enyedi A, et al. Functional domains of the in situ red cell membrane calcium pump revealed by proteolysis and monoclonal antibodies. J Biol Chem 1989;264:4577-82.
57. Zurini M, Krebs J, Penniston J, et al. Controlled proteolysis of the purified Ca-ATPase of the erythrocyte membrane. J Biol Chem 1984;259:618-27.
58. Benaim G, Clark A, Carafoli E. ATPase activity and Ca transport by reconstituted tryptic fragments of the Ca pump of the erythrocyte PM. Cell Calcium 1986;7:175-86.
59. Brandt P, Zurini M, Neve R, et al. A C-terminal calmodulin-like regulatory domain from the PM Ca-pumping ATPase. Proc Natl Acad Sci USA 1988;85:2914-8.
60. Enyedi A, Vorherr T, James P, et al. The calmodulin binding domain of the PM Ca pump interacts both with calmodulin and with another part of the pump. J Biol Chem 1989;264:12313-21.
61. Wuytack F, Raeymaekers L, Droogmans G, et al. The Ca^{2+}-transport ATPases in smooth muscle. Biochem J 1989;264:609-12.
62. Missiaen L, Raeymaekers L, Droogmans G, et al. Role of arginine residues in the stimulation of the smooth muscle PM Ca pump by negatively charged phospholipids. Biochem J 1989;264:609-12.
63. Kosk-Kosicka D, Bzdega T. Activation of the erythrocyte Ca-ATPase by either self-association or interaction with calmodulin. J Biol Chem 1989;263:18184-9.
64. Keresztes T, Jona I, Pikula S, et al. Effect of calcium on the interactions between Ca-ATPase molecules in SR. Biochim Biophys Acta 1989;984:326-38.
65. Benaim G, de Meis L. Activation of the purified erythrocyte PM Ca-ATPase by organic solvents. FEBS Lett 1989;2:484-6.
66. Wuytack F, Raeymaekers L, De Schutter G, et al. Demonstration of the phosphorylated intermediates of the Ca-transport ATPase in a microsomal fraction and in a

(Ca^{2+} + Mg^{2+})-ATPase purified from smooth muscle by means of calmodulin affinity chromatography. Biochim Biophys Acta 1982;693:45-52.

67. Grover A, Boonstra I, Garfield R, et al. Ca pumps in rabbit stomach smooth muscle PM and ER. Biochem Arch 1988;4:169-79.

68. Lytton J, Zarain-Herzberg A, Periasamy M, et al. Molecular cloning of the mammalian smooth muscle SR (ER) Ca-ATPase. J Biol Chem 1989;264:7059-65.

69. Lompre A, de la Bastie D, Boheler K, et al. Characterization and expression of the rat heart SR Ca-ATPase mRNA. FEBS Lett 1989;249:35-41.

70. Greeb J, Shull G. Molecular cloning of a third isoform of the calmodulin-sensitive PM Ca-transporting ATPase that is expressed predominantly in brain and skeletal muscle. J Biol Chem 1989;264:18569-76.

71. Eggermont J, Wuytack F, De Jaegere S, et al. Evidence for two isoforms of the ER Ca pump in pig smooth muscle. Biochem J 1989;260;757-61.

72. de la Bastie D, Wisnewsky C, Schwartz K, et al. (Ca^{2+} + Mg^{2+})-dependent ATPase mRNA from smooth muscle SR differs from that in cardiac and fast skeletal muscles. FEBS Lett 1988;229:45-8.

73. Gunteski-Hamblin A, Greeb J, Shull G. A novel Ca pump expressed in brain, kidney, and stomach I_s encoded by an alternative transcript of the slow-twitch muscle SR Ca-ATPase gene. J Biol Chem 1988;263:15032-40.

74. Burk S, Lytton J, MacLennan D, et al. cDNA cloning, functional expression, and mRNA tissue distribution of a third organellar Ca pump. J Biol Chem 1989;264:18561-8.

75. Khan I, Spencer G, Samson S, et al. Abundance of SR calcium pump isoforms in stomach and cardiac muscles. Biochem J 1990;264:18561-8.

76. Verbist J, Wuytack F, Raeymaekers L, et al. A monoclonal antibody to the calmodulin-binding (Ca^{2+} + Mg^{2+})-dependent ATPase from pig stomach smooth muscle inhibits plasmalemmal (Ca^{2+} + Mg^{2+})-dependent ATPase activity. Biochem J 1986;240:633-40.

77. Verbist J, Wuytack F. Raeymaekers L, et al. Inhibitory antibodies to plasmalemmal Ca^{2+}-transporting ATPases. Biochem J 1985;231:737-42.

78. Shull G, Greeb J. Molecular cloning of two isoforms of the PM Ca-transporting ATPase from rat brain. J Biol Chem 1988;263:8646-57.

79. Strehler E, Strehler-Page M, Vogel G, et al. mRNAs for PM calcium pump isoforms differing in their regulatory domain are generated by alternative splicing that involves two internal donor sites in a single exon. Proc Natl Acad Sci USA 1989;86:6908-12.

80. Missiaen L, Droogmans G, De Smedt H, et al. Alkalinization stimulates the purified PM Ca pump by increasing its Ca affinity. Biochem J 1989;262:361-4.

81. Enyedi A, Brandt J. Minami J, et al. Oxytocin regulates the PM Ca-transport in rat myometrium. Biochem J 1989;261:23-8.

82. Vrolix M, Raeymaekers L, Wuytack F, et al. Cyclic GMP-dependent protein kinase stimulates the plasmalemmal Ca pump of smooth muscle via phosphorylation of phosphatidylinositol. Biochem J 1988;255:855-63.

6

Hormonal Regulation of Myometrial Intracellular Calcium

Barbara M. Sanborn and Khursheed Anwer

Department of Biochemistry and Molecular Biology, University of Texas Medical School at Houston

A s described in detail in Chapter 4, the phosphorylation of myosin 20-kD light chains (MLC) by myosin light-chain kinase (MLCK) accompanies initiation of contraction and parallels the rise in intracellular calcium ($[Ca]_i$) (1, 2). In myometrium, such an increase in myosin phosphorylation accompanies spontaneous and hormone-induced contractions (3–8). Myometrial MLCK is a calcium-calmodulin-dependent enzyme (1, 5). Hence an increase in $[Ca]_i$ can influence the contractile apparatus by increasing MLCK activity and, in turn, MLC phosphorylation. Other calcium-dependent regulatory mechanisms may also exist. However, there does not appear to be much evidence in favor of a major contribution of the latch state (persistent tension in the face of decreasing MLC phosphorylation) in uterus; phosphorylation levels persist at relatively high levels following contraction (5, 9, 10).

Mechanisms for myometrial relaxation are less clearly delineated. In contracting myometrium, spontaneous and agonist-induced relaxation is accompanied by a decrease in MLC phosphorylation (3–6). The decrease in MLC phosphorylation could result from a decrease in MLCK activity as a result of decreased $[Ca]_i$ (1), decreased MLCK affinity for calcium-calmodulin as a result of phosphorylation (5, 11), increased myosin phosphatase activity, or a combination of these effects.

From the preceding discussion, it is clear that control of $[Ca]_i$ by contractants and relaxants is important in the regulation of uterine contractile activity. Figure 1 illustrates possible points of control, some of which have not yet been explored in the myometrium.

The extracellular environment serves as a major source of $[Ca]_i$ in many smooth muscles, including myometrium. At the level of the plasma membrane, receptor-operated (ROC), voltage-operated (VOC), second-messenger-operated

Acknowledgments: The research reported here was supported by NIH grant HD-09618.

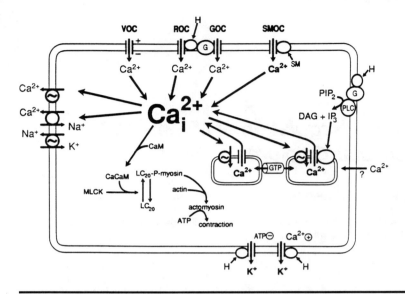

Fig. 1. Potential mechanisms for control of intracellular calcium as defined and described in text.

(SMOC), and GTP-binding protein (G-protein), and gated (GOC) ion channels control the influx of Ca (12). Other ion channels influence VOC indirectly by altering membrane potential. For example, activation of Ca-activated K-channels and ATP-sensitive K-channels, resulting in membrane repolarization, is thought to be involved in the termination of the Ca signal in smooth muscle (13, 14). In the plasma membrane, the Na–Ca exchanger and calmodulin-dependent Ca-ATPase function in calcium extrusion, each in different Ca ranges (15). Furthermore, the membrane contains phosphoinositides and phospholipase C (PLC) activity. Receptor-operated activation of PLC, often coupled through a G-protein, results in the release of inositol trisphosphate (IP_3) and diacylglycerol (16). IP_3 releases calcium from intracellular stores, and diacylglycerol activates protein kinase C (PKC) (17).

Other potentially significant sources of $[Ca]_i$ for contraction are nonmitochondrial compartments described variously as the endoplasmic reticulum and other pools (17, 18). IP_3, acting via a specific receptor, increases release of Ca into the cytoplasmic compartment from one such pool (17, 18). This pool apparently refills from extracellular sources by mechanisms not well understood. An IP_3-insensitive intracellular calcium pool has also been described; it responds to increased $[Ca]_i$ with Ca release (17, 18). Active pumps move Ca into these compartments (15, 18).

It is the purpose of this discussion to explore the acute effects of hormones promoting uterine contraction and relaxation on a number of the biochemical activities just described. Long-term effects, such as hormonal regulation of the expression of components of these systems, are beyond the scope of this chapter but are discussed elsewhere in this book.

UTERINE CONTRACTANTS

Increase of Myometrial Intracellular Calcium by Increasing Influx from the Extracellular Environment

A number of uterine contractants have been postulated to increase $[Ca]_i$ by increasing influx of ^{45}Ca across the plasma membrane (19, 20). However, uptake data in themselves do not provide direct evidence of an increase in $[Ca]_i$.

We have directly observed an increase in $[Ca]_i$ following addition of oxytocin, norepinephrine, and carbachol to myometrial cells isolated from estrogen-primed rats (21). The effects are dose-dependent and partially decreased by the removal of extracellular Ca (Fig. 2). These data suggest that at least part of the increase in $[Ca]_i$ can be attributed to enhanced influx of Ca into the cells. The effect of oxytocin is not affected by 30-µM D600 (21) or 1-µM nifedipine (Singh, Anwer, and Sanborn, unpublished data), suggesting that receptor-operated (or second messenger-operated) rather than voltage-operated channels are involved.

At first glance these data seem to contradict observations that Ca channel blockers progressively inhibit oxytocin-, carbachol-, and acetylcholine-induced uterine contractions, although with less sensitivity than to K-induced contraction (22, 23). The blockage of contractions may reflect the interaction of the contributions of ROC and VOC in intact tissue responses of a secondary activation of VOC by contractants or actions of Ca channel blockers at additional sites. The release of intracellular bound Ca may account for the blocker-insensitive contraction. Alternatively, VOC and ROC may simply represent different conformations of the same channel (22, 24), and channel blockers may alter hormonal access (12). More work is needed to elucidate the mechanisms involved.

Stimulation of Phosphoinositide Turnover and Release of Calcium from Intracellular Stores

The effect of oxytocin on myometrial $[Ca]_i$, in addition to being partially reduced by removing extracellular Ca, is also partially inhibited by pertussis-toxin treatment (21). Figure 3 shows that the inhibition is additive with the effect of removing extracellular Ca. This suggests an additional effect of oxytocin: mobilization of Ca from intracellular stores, perhaps via generation of IP_3. Oxytocin does increase $[^3H]$-IP_3 formation by a process independent of the presence of extracellular Ca and inhibited by pertussis-toxin treatment (25) (Fig. 3). These data suggest a hormonal activation of PLC, mediated through a pertussis-toxin-sensitive G-protein in the rat. Similar results have been obtained using carbachol (26). Norepinephrine also increases turnover of phosphoinositide (27). However, in guinea pig myometrium, pertussis-toxin treatment does not inhibit the effect of carbachol or oxytocin (28), suggesting some species variability in the nature of the G-protein involved.

Reports of contractions elicited in Ca-free media and with skinned

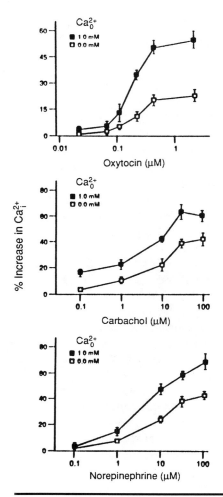

Fig. 2. Effect of contractants on myometrial cell intracellular calcium as mea-sured by fura-2 fluorescence in the absence and presence of 1-mM extracellular Ca. (From Anwer K, Sanborn BM, Changes in intracellular free calcium in isolated myometrial cells: role of extracellular and intracellular calcium and possible involvement of guanine nucleotide-sensitive proteins, Endocrinology 1989;124:17–23, with permission.)

myometrial fibers have provided indirect evidence for agonist-stimulated release of Ca from uterine microsomes (23, 29–33). However, Ca-independent contraction may also occur (34). IP_3 has been shown to release calcium from uterine micro-somes (35–37). Furthermore, measurements of ^{45}Ca efflux from intact and permeabilized cells have been interpreted as indicating increased intracellular Ca release in response to oxytocin (19, 36). These data are consistent with a role for agonist-generated IP_3 in intracellular Ca release in myometrium.

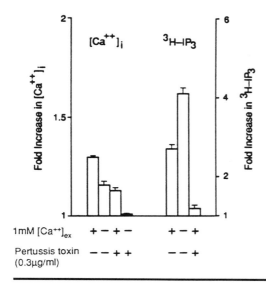

Fig. 3. Effect of pertussis-toxin treatment and removal of extracellular Ca on the oxytocin-stimulated increase in myometrial $[Ca]_i$ (see reference 21), and effect of pertussis-toxin treatment and removal of extracellular Ca on the oxytocin-stimulated increase in myometrial $[^3H]$-IP_3 formation (see reference 25).

UTERINE RELAXANTS

Inhibition of Oxytocin-Induced Calcium Rises and Phosphoinositide Turnover

Isoproterenol and porcine relaxin inhibit both spontaneous and oxytocin- or prostaglandin $F_{2\alpha}$-induced contractions of uterine strips from estrogen-primed rats and oxytocin-induced shape changes in myometrial cells in culture (5, 7, 38). Isoproterenol and relaxin have little detectable effect on resting $[Ca]_i$ but inhibit the oxytocin-induced rise in $[Ca]_i$ (25). The inhibitory activity is not abolished by removal of extracellular Ca or pretreatment with pertussis toxin, suggesting that these relaxants affect actions of oxytocin on both Ca influx and release. Figure 4 illustrates the effect of relaxin. Isoproterenol and relaxin also inhibit the oxytocin-induced increase in phosphoinositide turnover (25). Forskolin and CPT-cAMP attenuate the effect of oxytocin on $[Ca]_i$ and on phosphoinositide turnover as well (25). These data are consistent with a role for cAMP in this process. In contrast, in the guinea pig, the stimulation of phosphoinositide turnover by carbachol, but not oxytocin, was inhibited by forskolin (28).

Effect of Ion Flux in Myometrium

Both isoproterenol and relaxin increase ^{45}Ca efflux from myometrial tissue (39, 40) and cells (41, 42). This is apparently not due to increased Na–Ca exchange coupled

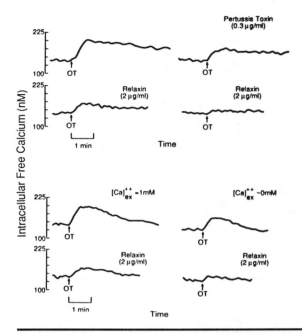

Fig. 4. Ability of relaxin to attenuate the oxytocin-stimulated increase in intracellular Ca in the presence and absence of extracellular Ca and after pertussistoxin treatment. (From Anwer K, Sanborn BM, Changes in intracellular free calcium in isolated myometrial cells: role of extracellular and intracellular calcium and possible involvement of guanine nucleotide-sensitive proteins, Endocrinology 1989;124:17–23, with permission.)

to indirect stimulation of Na-K-ATPase activity. The ^{86}Rb uptake is not affected by isoproterenol or relaxin (43).

The presence and characteristics of ion channel activities in myometrium are discussed in detail elsewhere in this book. Studies of hormonal effects on ion channels and the relationship of channel activity to [Ca]$_i$ and contractile activity are important to a total understanding of hormone-regulated events in the myometrium. To date, there has been no demonstration of an acute effect of a hormone on uterine Ca channels. Studies on hormonal regulation of uterine K-channels are also incomplete. Norepinephrine has been shown to potentiate fast and reduce intermediate K-channels (44). Forskolin has been reported to hyperpolarize rat myometrial membranes, but mechanisms have not been defined (45). GABA-regulated Cl channels, which function to inhibit contractile activity, may be activated by tetrahydroprogesterone and other steroids (46).

Mechanisms of Action

The role of cyclic nucleotides in smooth-muscle contraction and relaxation has been controversial. Clearly, an elevation in cAMP is not a requirement for relaxation (47). In addition, some agents, notably prostaglandins, elevate cAMP but contract the uterus (47, 48). Isoproterenol increases cAMP in rat uterine strips (7, 47) and in myometrial cells (49). The effect is rapid and is accompanied by an increase in the activity of cAMP-dependent protein kinase A (PKA) (50). However, actions of isoproterenol unrelated to cAMP elevation have been reported in uterus (48, 51), thus calling into question the exclusive role of PKA in the relaxant action of isoproterenol. Relaxin, on the other hand, elevates uterine and myometrial cAMP with a slower time-course than that seen for physical effects, and a slower activation of PKA (7, 49, 52). Consequently, it was not at all obvious that cAMP would play an obligatory role in the mechanism of action of relaxin or isoproterenol.

To study the possible role of PKA in the action of isoproterenol and relaxin, we have made use of the PKA inhibitor H-8 (53). In work described in detail in reference 54, we demonstrate that at 100 μM, H-8 is more potent than the PKC inhibitor H-7 at inhibiting the effect of CPT-cAMP on the oxytocin-induced increase in myometrial [Ca]$_i$ and phosphoinositide turnover. H-8 reverses the inhibitory effects of isoproterenol on oxytocin-induced uterine contractions (Fig. 5). H-8 also reverses the effects of isoproterenol on the oxytocin-induced rise in [Ca]$_i$, including those seen in the absence of extracellular Ca, and on phosphoinositide turnover (Fig. 5). Similar results were observed with relaxin, including reversal of relaxant effects retained after pertussis toxin treatment (54).

A number of other actions of isoproterenol and relaxin in myometrium have been attributed to PKA indirectly. Isoproterenol increases phosphorylation of uter-

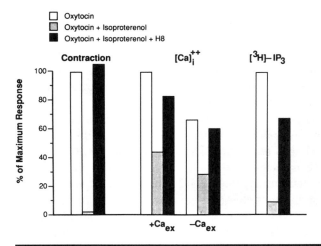

Fig. 5. Ability of 100-μM H-8 pretreatment for 1 h to reverse the inhibition by isoproterenol of the oxytocin-stimulated increases in contractile activity, [Ca]$_i$, and [³H]-IP$_3$ formation, measured as described in references 21 and 25.

ine microsomal proteins and ^{45}Ca uptake into microsomes, as does cAMP treatment (7, 47). The effect of relaxin on the latter is markedly dependent on hormonal state and does not correlate with physiological effectiveness (7). Relaxin treatment decreases the affinity for calmodulin of MLCK extracted subsequently from myometrial strips or myometrial cells (5, 55). This change in affinity is mimicked by phosphorylation of purified enzyme in vitro with cAMP-dependent protein kinase (7). However, direct evidence of hormonally stimulated phosphorylation has yet to be produced.

Thus, despite some evidence to the contrary, it appears that the relaxant activities of isoproterenol and relaxin versus oxytocin in the estrogen-primed rat uterus can be explained by actions of PKA. This implicates cAMP in the mechanism of action of these relaxants on contraction, Ca_i mobilization from extracellular and intracellular sources, and phosphoinositide turnover.

Agents that elevate cGMP also relax the uterus (47). Recent studies implicate an increase in Ca-ATPase activity, which may be indirect (56, 57) and an inhibition of PLC via an effect on the associated G-protein (58) in its mechanism of action. Accordingly, there are multiple pathways to achieving similar physical effects.

The fact that the PKC inhibitor H-7 and acute administration of 0.1–1.0 μM phorbol ester have no effect on basal or agonist-stimulated $[Ca]_i$ or phosphoinositide turnover (54) suggests that PKC has little effect on these parameters in the estrogen-dominated rat uterus. Others have found no effects (59) or inhibitory effects (60) of phorbol esters on nonpregnant myometrium.

POTENTIAL MECHANISMS FOR THE HORMONAL CONTROL OF UTERINE INTRACELLULAR CALCIUM

At the level of the plasma membrane, the nature of the Ca channel stimulated by oxytocin, including the possible involvement of a G-protein, is yet to be described. The inhibitory action of relaxants on Ca influx could reflect a direct effect of PKA on hormone-stimulated Ca channels or alteration of a channel-associated G protein. Although oxytocin and carbachol have been shown to slightly depolarize myometrial plasma membrane (61, 62), the mechanisms of these effects and their relationship to VOC are not well understood.

A more detailed understanding of the effects of contractants and relaxants on the activity of K-channels is also crucial to an understanding of ion dynamics. Ca-activated K-channels are stimulated by β-adrenergic agents and inhibited by acetylcholine in smooth muscle (63, 64). On the other hand, vasodilators (14, 65) have been reported to activate ATP-sensitive K-channels. It will be important to determine the effects of different classes of relaxants on activation of K-channels in myometrial cells. Also, the regulation of Cl channels by steroids, GABA, and other agents holds potential for understanding ionic mechanisms in the uterus.

Although sporadic reports of inhibition by contractants of myometrial plasma membrane Ca-ATPase have appeared (66–68), it is not clear that these relate directly to Ca-pump activity (69). The pump itself is inhibited under certain conditions by oxytocin (70, 71), but mechanisms have not been explored. Furthermore, no effects of relaxants on this activity have been described. In liver, a cholera-toxin-sensitive G-protein regulates plasma membrane Ca-ATPase (72), suggesting one possible link to receptor-mediated events.

Although guinea pig uterine phosphatidyl inositol-specific PLC-I has been purified (73), little is known to date about how it associates with plasma membrane or the nature of its interaction with G-proteins. The cAMP-dependent phosphorylation of PLC from two cell lines has been demonstrated but does not affect enzyme activity, prompting the suggestion that association with key components in the membrane has been altered (73, 74). Such studies are currently underway in myometrium. The mechanism of regulation by cGMP of G-proteins coupled to PLC activation may provide additional insight into this system.

Regarding the mobilization of Ca from intracellular stores, the relative importance of IP_3-mediated and Ca-activated Ca release in uterus has yet to be addressed. The IP_3 receptor has been isolated from several tissues, but not rat myometrium. The receptor is apparently also associated with G-proteins and can be phosphorylated by cAMP-dependent protein kinase in the brain (75). This phosphorylation causes no change in binding characteristics but decreases the releasing capability of IP_3. However, enhancement of IP_3-mediated Ca release was observed after treating permeabilized aortic smooth-muscle cells with cAMP (76). The effect of uterine relaxants on the IP_3 receptor and on IP_3- and Ca-mediated $[Ca]_i$ release needs more study. Communication between IP_3-sensitive and Ca-insensitive stores, thought to be regulated by GTP (18), has yet to be addressed in the uterus.

Uterine microsomal Ca-pumps have been cloned, as described in detail in Chapter 5. Specific localization relative to IP_3-sensitive and -insensitive stores has yet to be delineated. Relaxants, in general, stimulate while contractants inhibit $[Ca]_i$ uptake (7, 36, 37), but these effects are yet to be defined mechanistically. Microsomal proteins phosphorylated by PKA are too small to be the Ca pump, and the relationship of these phosphorylated proteins to pump activity remains to be defined. Also, the relative importance of stimulation by relaxants of sequestration versus inhibition of release of intracellular Ca in the uterus is yet to be determined.

Although relaxant-induced changes in uterine MLCK have been demonstrated (5, 55), direct phosphorylation of uterine MLCK in response to stimulation by agents that elevate cAMP has yet to be demonstrated. Evidence for a change in MLCK activity has been lacking in trachaeal smooth muscle (1), but there is a decrease in MLC phosphorylation with no change in $[Ca]_i$, suggesting that a role may exist for MLCK (2). Alternative Ca-mediated mechanisms controlling the contractile apparatus in uterus and the importance of latch states during tonic and phasic contractions are unresolved questions. Furthermore, there are a number of reports of indirect effects of cAMP on the contractile apparatus itself (29, 77).

Conclusion

We now know a considerable amount about the mechanisms by which uterine contractants and relaxants achieve their effects. Direct influx of Ca through receptor-operated channels increase [Ca]$_i$, triggering Ca-mediated myosin light-chain phosphorylation, which activates the contractile apparatus. Contractants also increase IP$_3$ formation, which releases Ca from intracellular stores. Some relaxants, at least, inhibit these actions via mechanisms involving PKA. They also increase efflux of Ca and promote its resequestration in intracellular stores. Nonetheless, many questions remain. For example, only certain classes of contractants and relaxants have been studied in detail. Species differences may illuminate central control points and variations on the general theme. The differences in responses in different hormonal states and at different stages of pregnancy may reveal the importance of other factors in controlling the relative predominance of one mechanism over the other. Such studies should greatly increase our understanding of the regulation of uterine contractility.

REFERENCES

1. Kamm KE, Stull JE. The function of myosin and myosin light chain kinase phosphorylation in smooth muscle. Annu Rev Pharmacol Toxicol 1985;25:593-620.
2. Taylor DA, Bowman BF, Stull JT. Cytoplasmic Ca^{2+} is a primary determinant for myosin phosphorylation in smooth muscle cells. J Biol Chem 1989;264:6207-13.
3. Janis RA, Moats-Staats BM, Gualtier RT. Protein phosphorylation during spontaneous contraction of smooth muscle. Biochem Biophys Res Commun 1980;96:265-70.
4. Janis RA, Barany K, Barany M, Sarmiento JG. Association between myosin light chain phosphorylation and contraction of rat uterine smooth muscle. Mol Physiol 1981;1:3-11.
5. Nishikori K, Weisbrodt NW, Sherwood OD, Sanborn BM. Effects of relaxin on rat uterine myosin light chain kinase activity and myosin light chain phosphorylation. J Biol Chem 1983;258:2468-74.
6. Dokhac L, D'Albis A, Janmot C, Harbon S. Myosin light chain phosphorylation in intact rat uterine smooth muscle. Role of calcium and cyclic AMP. J Musc Res Cell Mot 1986;7:259-68.
7. Sanborn BM. The role of relaxin in uterine function. In: Huszar G, ed. The physiology and biochemistry of the uterus in pregnancy and labor. Boca Raton, FL: CRC Press, 1986:225-38.
8. MacKenzie LW, Word RA, Casey ML, Stull JT. Myosin light chain phosphorylation in human myometrial smooth muscle cells. Am J Physiol 1990;258:C92-8.
9. Csabina S, Barany M, Barany K. Comparison of mysoin light chain phosphorylation in uterine and arterial smooth muscles. Comp Biochem Physiol 1987;87B:271-7.
10. Haeberle JR, Hathaway DR, DePaoli-Roach AA. Dephosphorylation of myosin by the catalytic subunit of a type-2 phosphatase produces relaxation of chemically skinned uterine smooth muscle. J Biol Chem 1985;260:9965-8.
11. DeLanerolle P, Nishikawa M, Yost DA, Adelstein RS. Increased phosphorylation of myosin light chain kinase after an increase in cyclic AMP in intact smooth muscle. Science 1984;223:1415-7.
12. Rosenthall W, Hescheler J, Trautwein W, Schultz G. Receptor- and G-protein-mediated modulations of voltage-dependent calcium channels. Cold Spring Harbor Symp Quant Biol 1988;53:247-54.
13. Singer JJ, Walsh Jr JV. Characterization of calcium-activated potassium channels in

single smooth muscle cells using the patch-clamp technique. Pflügers Arch 1987;408:98-111.

14. Standen NB, Quayle JM, Davies NW. Brayden JE, Huang Y, Nelson MT. Hyperpolarizing vasodilators activate ATP-sensitive K^+ channels in arterial smooth muscle. Science 1989;245:179-80.

15. Grover AK. Role of cellular organelles in calcium-mobilization of uterine smooth muscle. In: Huszar G, ed. The physiology and biochemistry of the uterus in pregnancy and labor. Boca Raton, FL: CRC Press, 1986:93-106.

16. Berridge MJ, Irvine RF. Inositol phosphates and cell signaling. Nature 189;341:197-205.

17. Putney JW Jr, Takemura H, Hughes AR, Horstman DA, Thastrup O. How do inositol phosphates regulate calcium signaling? FASEB J 1989;3:1899-905.

18. Schulz I, Thevenod F, Dehlinger-Kremer M. Modulation of intracellular free Ca^{2+} concentration by IP_3-sensitive and IP_3-insensitive nonmitochondrial Ca^{2+} pools. Cell Calcium 1989;10:325-36.

19. Batra S. Effect of oxytocin on calcium influx and efflux in the rat myometrium. Eur J Pharmacol 1986;120;57-61.

20. Urono T, Sekiguchi T, Sunagane N, Matsuoka Y, Kubota K. Effects of high potassium depolarization, carbachol and oxytocin on the lanthanum-resistant ^{45}Ca fraction in rat myometrium. Jpn J Pharmacol 1983;183;33:1-8.

21. Anwer K, Sanborn BM. Changes in intracellular free calcium in isolated myometrial cells: role of extracellular and intracellular calcium and possible involvement of guanine nucleotide-sensitive proteins. Endocrinology 1989;124:17-23.

22. Janis RA, Triggle DJ. Effects of calcium channel antagonists on the myometrium. In: Huszar G, ed. The physiology and biochemistry of the uterus in pregnancy in labor. Boca Raton, FL: CRC Press, 1986:201-23.

23. Kyozuka M, Crankshaw J, Berezin I, Collins SM, Daniel EE. Calcium and contractions of isolated smooth muscle cells from rat myometrium. Can J Physiol Pharmacol 1987;65:1966-75.

24. Van Breeman C, Saida K. Cellular mechanisms regulating $[Ca^{2+}]$ in smooth muscle. Annu Rev Physiol 1989;51:315-29.

25. Anwer K, Hovington JA, Sanborn BM. Antagonism of contractants and relaxants at the level of intracellular calcium and phosphoinositide turnover in the rat uterus. Endocrinology 1989;124:2295-3002.

26. Ruzycky AL, Crankshaw DJ. Role of inositol phospholipid hydrolysis in the initiation of agonist-induced contractions of rat uterus: effects of domination by 17β-estradiol and progesterone. Can J Physiol Pharmacol 1988;66:10-7.

27. Riemer RK, Goldfien A, Roberts JM. Estrogen increases adrenergic but not cholinergic-mediated production of inositol phosphates in rabbit uterus. Mol Pharmacol 1987;32:663-8.

28. Marc S, Leiber D, Harbon S. Fluoroaluminates mimic muscarinic- and oxytocin-receptor-mediated generation of inositol phosphates and contraction in the intact guinea-pig myometrium. Biochem J 1988;255:705-13.

29. Savineau JP, Mironneau J, Mironneau C. Contractile properties of chemically skinned fibers from pregnant rat myometrium: existence of an internal Ca-store. Pflügers Arch 1988;411:296-303.

30. Missiaen L, Kanmura Y, Wuytack F, Raeymaekers L, Declerk I, Droogmans G, Casteels R. AlF_4- inhibits the accumulation of Ca in the endoplasmic reticulum in

intact myometrial strips, but not in the rabbit ear artery. Pflügers Arch 1989;414: 423-9.

31. Sakai K, Higuchi K, Yamaguchi T, Uchida M. Oxytocin-induced Ca-free contraction of rat uterine smooth muscle: effects of preincubation with EGTA and drugs. Gen Pharmacol 1982;13:393-9.

32. Anselmi E, D'Ocon P, Villar A. A comparison of uterine contraction induced by PGE_1 and oxytocin in Ca-free solution. Prostaglandins 1987;34:351-5.

33. Lalanne C, Mironneau C, Mironneau J, Savineau JP. Contractions of rat uterine smooth muscle induced by acetylcholine and angiotensin II in Ca^{2+}-free medium. Br J Pharmacol 1984;81:317-26.

34. Matsuo K, Gokita T, Karibe H, Uchida MK. Ca^{2+}-independent contraction of uterine smooth muscle. Biochem Biophys Res Commun 1989;165:722-7.

35. Carsten ME, Miller JD. Ca^{2+} release by inositol trisphosphate from Ca^{2+}-transporting microsomes derived from uterine sarcoplasmic reticulum. Biochem Biophys Res Commun 1985;130:1027-31.

36. Molnar M, Asem EK, Hertelendy F. Differential effects of prostaglandin $F_{2\alpha}$ and of prostaglandins E_1 and E_2 on cyclic-3',5'-monophosphate production and intracellular calcium mobilization in avian uterine smooth muscle cells. Biol Reprod 1987;36: 384-91.

37. Carsten ME, Miller JD. A new look at uterine muscle contraction. Am J Obstet Gynecol 1987;157:1303-15.

38. Hsu CJ, Sanborn BM. Relaxin affects the shape of rat myometrial cells in culture. Endocrinology 1986;118:495-8.

39. Kroeger EA, Marshall JM, Bianchi CP. Effect of isoproterenol and D-600 on calcium movements in rat myometrium. J Pharmacol Exp Ther 1975;193:309-16.

40. Ginsburg FW, Rosenberg CR, Schwartz M, Colon JM, Goldsmith LT. The effect of relaxin on calcium fluxes in the rat uterus. Am J Obstet Gynecol 1988;159:1395-401.

41. Fortier M, Chase D, Korenman SG, Krall FJ. β-adrenergic catecholamine dependent properties of rat myometrium primary cultures. Am J Physiol 1983;245:C84-90.

42. Rao MR, Sanborn BM. Relaxin increases calcium efflux from rat myometrial cells in culture. Endocrinology 1986;119:435-7.

43. Sanborn BM. Rat myometrial Na/K ATPase is increased by serum but not by isoproterenol and relaxin. Comp Biochem Physiol 1989;93C:341-4.

44. Toro L, Stefani E, Erulkar S. Potassium and calcium currents in single myometrial cells. Proc Natl Acad Sci USA 1990 (in press).

45. Smith DD, Marshall JM. Forskolin effects on longitudinal myometrial strips from the pregnant rat: relationship with membrane potential and cyclic AMP. Eur J Pharmacol 1986;122:29-35.

46. Majewska MD, Falkay G, Baulieu EE. Modulation of uterine $GABA_A$ receptors during gestation and by tetrahydroprogesterone. Eur J Pharmacol 1989;174:43-7.

47. Sanborn BM, Heindel JJ, Robison GA. The role of cyclic nucleotides in reproductive processes. Annu Rev Physiol 1980;42:37-57.

48. Dokhac L, Mokhtar A, Harbon S. A re-evaluated role for cyclic AMP in uterine relaxation. Differential effect of isoproterenol and forskolin. J Pharmacol Exp Ther 1986;239:236-42.

49. Hsu CJ, McCormack S, Sanborn BM. The effect of relaxin on cyclic AMP concentrations in rat myometrial cells in culture. Endocrinology 1985;116:2029-35.

50. Korenman SG, Bhalla RC, Sanborn BM, Stevens RG. Protein kinase translocation as an early event in the hormonal control of uterine contraction. Science 1974;183:430-2.
51. Overweg NIA, Schiff JD. Two mechanisms of isoproterenol inhibition of smooth muscle. Eur J Pharmacol 1978;47:231-3.
52. Sanborn BM, Sherwood OD. Effect of relaxin on bound cAMP in rat uterus. Endocr Res Commun 1981;8:179-92.
53. Hagiwara M, Inagaki M, Hidaka H. Specific binding of a novel compound, N-[2-(methylamino)ethyl]-5-isoquinoline-sulfonamide (H-8) to the active site of cAMP-dependent protein kinase. Mol Pharmacol 1987;31:523-8.
54. Anwer K, Hovington JA, Sanborn BM. Involvement of protein kinase A in the inhibition of the oxytocin-stimulated increase in intracellular free calcium and phosphoinositide turnover by uterine relaxants. Endocrinology, 1990 (submitted).
55. Hsu CJ, Sanborn, BM. Relaxin treatment alters the kinetic properties of myosin light chain kinase activity in rat myometrial cells in culture. Endocrinology 1986;118:499-505.
56. Rashatwar SS, Cornwall TL, Lincoln TM. Effects of 8-bromo-cGMP on Ca^{2+} levels in vascular smooth muscle cells: possible regulation of Ca^{2+}-ATPase by cGMP-dependent protein kinase. Proc Natl Acad Sci USA 1987;84:5685-9.
57. Vrolix M, Raeymaekers L, Wuytack F, Hofmann F, Casteels R. Cyclic GMP-dependent protein kinase stimulates the plasmalemmal Ca^{2+} pump of smooth muscle via phosphorylation of phosphatidylinositol. Biochem J 1988;255:855-63.
58 Hirata M, Kohse KP, Chang CH, Ikebe T, Murad F. Mechanism of cyclic GMP inhibition of inositol phosphate formation in rat aorta segments and cultured bovine aorta smooth muscle cells. J Biol Chem 1990;265:1268-73.
59. Missiaen L, Kamura Y, Eggermont JA, Casteels R. TPA- and agonist-induced force development in myometrium from pregnant and nonpregnant rats. Biochem Biophys Res Commum 1989;158:302-6.
60. Baraban JM, Gould RJ, Peroutka ST, Snyder SH. Phorbol ester effects on neuro-transmission: interaction with neurotransmitters and calcium in smooth muscle. Proc Natl Acad Sci USA 1985;82:604-7.
61. Mironneau C, Mironneau J, Savineau JP. Maintained contractions of rat uterine smooth muscle incubated in a Ca^{2+}-free solution. Br J Pharmacol 1984;82:735-43.
62. Garfield RE, Beier S. Increased myometrial responsiveness to oxytocin during term and preterm labor. Am J Obstet Gynecol 1989;161:454-61.
63. Kume H, Takai A, Tokuno H, Tomita T. Regulation of Ca^{2+}-dependent K^+-channel activity in tracheal myocytes by phosphorylation. Nature 1989;341:152-4.
64. Cole CW, Carl A, Sanders KM. Muscarinic suppression of Ca^{2+}-dependent K current in colonic smooth muscle. Am J Physiol 1989;257:C481-7.
65. McPherson GM, Angus JA. Phentolamine and structurally related compounds selectively antagonize the vascular actions of the K^+ channel opener, cromakalim. Br J Pharmacol 1989;97:941-9.
66. Soloff MS, Sweet P. Oxytocin inhibition of $(Ca^{2+} + Mg^{2+})$-ATPase activity in rat myometrial plasma membranes. J Biol Chem 1982;257:10687-93.
67. Wuytack F, Casteels R. Demonstration of a $(Ca^{2+} + Mg^{2+})$-ATPase activity probably related to Ca^{2+} transport in the microsomal fraction of porcine coronary artery smooth muscle. Biochim Biophys Acta 1980;595:257-63.
68. Deliconstantinos G, Fotiou S. Effect of prostaglandins E_2 and $F_{2\alpha}$ on membrane

calcium binding, Ca^{2+}/Mg^{2+}-ATPase activity and membrane fluidity in rat myometrial plasma membranes. J Endocrinol 1986;110:395-404.

69. Enyedi A, Minami J, Caride AJ, Penniston JT. Characteristics of the Ca^{2+} pump and Ca^{2+} "ATPase" in the plasma membrane of rat myometrium. Biochem J 1988;252: 215-220.

70. Missiaen L, Kanmura Y, Wuytack F, Casteels R. Carbachol partially inhibits the plasma membrane Ca^{2+}-pump in microsomes from pig stomach smooth muscle. Biochem Biophys Res Commun 1988;150:681-6.

71. Enyedi A, Brandt J, Minami J, Penniston JT. Oxytocin regulates the plasma membrane Ca^{2+} transport in rat myometrium. Biochem J 1989;261:23-8.

72. Lotersztajn S, Pavione C, Mallat A, Stengel D, Insel PA, Pecker F. Cholera toxin blocks glucagon-mediated inhibition of the plasma membrane $(Ca^{2+} + Mg^{2+})$-ATPase. J Biol Chem 1987;262:3114-7.

73. Bennett CF, Crooke ST. Purification and characterization of a phosphoinositide-specific phospholipase C from guinea pig uterus. J Biol Chem 1987;262:13789-97.

74. Kim UH, Kim JW, Rhee SG. Phosphorylation of phospholipase C-γ by cAMP-dependent protein kinase. J Biol Chem 1989;264:20167-70.

75. Suppattapone S, Danoff SK, Theibert A, Joseph SK, Steiner J, Synder SH. Cyclic-AMP-dependent phosphorylation of a brain inositol trisphosphate receptor decreases its release of calcium. Proc Natl Acad Sci USA 1988;85:8747-50.

76. Tawada Y, Furukawa KI, Shigekawa M. Cyclic AMP enhances inositol trisphosphate-induced mobilization of intracellular Ca^{2+} in cultured aortic smooth muscle cells. J Biochem 1988;104:795-800.

77. Nishimura J, Van Breeman C. Direct regulation of smooth muscle contractile elements by second messengers. Biochem Biophys Res Commun 1989;163:929-35.

MECHANISMS OF ACTION OF AGENTS ALTERING UTERINE CONTRACTILITY

7

Myometrial Contractility In Vitro: Its Role in an Understanding of the Mechanisms Controlling Uterine Activity

D. J. Crankshaw

Department of Obstetrics and Gynecology and Division of Physiology and Pharmacology, Department of Biomedical Sciences, McMaster University, Hamilton, Ontario, Canada

A bnormalities in uterine contractility are thought to contribute, to some extent, to such clinical problems as preterm labor, delayed onset of labor, and dysmenorrhea. It seems valid, therefore, to speculate that a deeper understanding of the mechanisms controlling uterine activity will lead to the formulation of more appropriate and effective management practices than those currently in use. In this chapter I will attempt to make a case for the more extensive use of the study of myometrial contractility in vitro as a simple tool for elucidating the mechanisms controlling uterine activity. I outline the advantages and drawbacks of this technique, and I describe in some detail one method that is currently in use in my laboratory, by which in vitro contractility can be quantified. I stress the importance of quantification and point out the dangers of empiricism. I examine one instance where studies of in vitro contractility have led to some controversy about the mechanisms controlling uterine activity. An attempt to understand what happens to the uterus during normal parturition seems an appropriate place to start.

Perhaps the major function of the myometrium is to contract during parturition and help to expel the conceptus. At earlier stages of pregnancy it should be relatively quiescent to ensure adequate fetal-maternal exchanges, thus providing the fetus with optimal conditions for growth. The question of what mediates the change from quiescence to expulsive contractions is of considerable importance, since an answer will give insight into the clinical problems referred to above.

That the excitability of the myometrium changes during pregnancy, becoming maximal at the time of parturition, was clearly demonstrated by Csapo (1). As a result of this work, we now realize that the myometrium must go through some "priming process" (others have referred to it as a "preparatory phase of labor" [2]), before it can respond to uterotonic agents in a manner likely to lead to efficient expulsion of the conceptus. The task is to discover this priming process.

One hypothesis suggests the occurrence of a "membrane block" that serves to stabilize a pool of activator Ca so that it cannot be released by uterotonic agents (1). As parturition approaches, the membrane block is lifted, and the myometrium becomes excitable. Activator Ca may come from a number of different sources by a number of different mechanisms (3).

A second hypothesis is concerned with the formation of gap junctions between myometrial cells (4). In several species, the number of these specialized contacts is low or nonexistent during early pregnancy, their numbers increase dramatically during parturition, and they decrease again postpartum. The presence of gap junctions in the myometrium has been suggested to contribute to the successful termination of pregnancy by allowing electrical propagation through the myometrium, resulting in synchronous activity. The formation of gap junctions thus ought to increase excitability.

A third hypothesis is concerned with regulation of receptors for uterotonic agents (5). The concept that receptors themselves are dynamic entities whose numbers and perhaps affinities for target ligands might vary with changing physiological or pathological conditions (6) has changed current thinking about regulatory mechanisms. This is an important concept for the myometrium and its regulation because if, for instance, the number of receptors for a uterotonic agent can be regulated, then the excitability of the myometrium to that agent can also be regulated (5). In other words, the priming process mentioned above might represent the appearance of functional receptors.

The three hypotheses presented are not mutually exclusive, and it is possible that all contribute in some way. If the membrane block or gap-junction mechanisms are operative, nonspecific effects will most likely be produced such that all uterotonic agents are affected in the same way. Receptor regulation by its very nature should be agonist specific.

THE CASE FOR STUDYING MYOMETRIAL CONTRACTILITY IN VITRO

The most appropriate technique to assess whether changes in excitability are agonist specific or nonspecific, to determine the temporal characteristics of these changes, and therefore to provide clues as to what the overall controlling mechanisms might be is the study of the response of isolated strips of myometrium, taken at different stages of pregnancy to challenge with appropriate agonists (7–11)—in other words, the study of myometrial contractility in vitro. Furthermore, this is the first-line technique for determination of the effectiveness of putative mediators (12, 13) since, contrary to some opinions, results of radioimmune assays showing high concentrations of substance X in amniotic fluid at term do not prove the hypothesis that substance X plays an important role in mediating uterine contractions. In addition, a demonstration of effects on myometrial contractility in vitro is a prerequisite for development of therapeutic agents for control of disorders of uterine activity (14–17).

Of course, the animal uterus in vitro has been used extensively for many years, not only for the purposes mentioned above, but also as a bioassay tool (18), as an aid to an understanding of the relationship between structure and activity in peptide series (19), to help with the characterization of drug receptors and the understanding of receptor mechanisms in the uterus (20, 21), and for numerous other purposes. Unfortunately, the vast body of evidence that has accumulated has not been summarized and critically appraised recently. This latter statement is also true for the existing literature on the human uterus in vitro, and while this chapter is not the place to rectify this deficit, one observation must be made: Namely, there are major gaps in our knowledge that are readily and easily rectifiable. For instance, although prostanoids have been implicated as mediators of uterine contractions of parturition (32) and of dysmenorrhea (23) for some time, we still do not have a clear picture of dose-response relationships for individual agents, parts of the uterus affected (e.g., longitudinal versus circular muscle, lower segment versus body), the influence of hormonal status and even in some cases whether the response is excitatory or inhibitory (17). Although some work has explored the action of β-adrenoceptor agonists in vitro, particularly with an aim at understanding the development of tolerance (24, 25), we have virtually no evidence about the relative abilities of these agents to inhibit contractions driven by different agonists. Surely such evidence would be useful in further refining the conditions under which these agents can be expected to be therapeutically useful. The list could go on, but we need to ask the question: Why do these gaps remain?

Certainly studies of myometrial contractility in vitro do present some technical difficulties, more in their interpretation than in their execution, but these are minor and ought not to deter the inquisitive investigator. Such studies are unpopular, I believe, for two major reasons. First, there is a widely held myth, which I hope the foregoing has helped to dispel, that we have all the answers. Second, in vitro contractility is out of vogue; as an attractant to funding agencies, it lacks the power of such terms as patch clamp, cDNA, or even RIA. Everyone old enough remembers frightful undergraduate days huddled around a smoked drum, when curses and incantations seemed more likely to produce meaningful results than any attempt at application of the scientific method. And those not old enough have heard the stories. Consequently, few have faith in the value of in vitro contractility when compared to those other, more glamorous techniques.

ADVANTAGES OF THE STUDY OF MYOMETRIAL CONTRACTILITY IN VITRO

Technically, the study of myometrial contractility in vitro is relatively simple (see later), and although the equipment used to collect and analyze data can be at any of several levels of complexity, even the most complex is relatively inexpensive.

If the process of uterine activity itself is to be studied, then in vitro techniques present far fewer difficulties than in vivo techniques. Besides the obvious additional responsibility of attending to the welfare of an intact animal (or even more so, a patient), in vivo contractility presents a number of interpretational problems that make it useful as an empirical method at best. One has to decide whether to monitor activity through the medium of intrauterine pressure, external tocodynamometer, or strain gauges attached to the uterine surface. For obvious reasons, this latter can be ruled out for the study of human subjects. For intra-uterine pressure recording, one then must debate the relative merits of open-ended catheters, balloons, and so on, all of which is somewhat academic since the rela-tionship between intrauterine pressure and activity of the myometrium is ex-tremely complex (e.g., shortening at some sites, relaxation at others) and, in fact, defies interpretation except in the most extreme of circumstances. But most im-portantly, if we are to learn anything about changes in contractility of the myometrium that will lead to an understanding of the process of parturition, for instance, then we must have an accurate measure of the sensitivity of the myometrium and the maximal response of the myometrium to a given agent at a given time. Such information can be obtained with reliable accuracy only from properly conducted dose-response experiments. Properly conducted dose-response experiments are barely possible in vivo for many reasons, including the complica-tion of crossover effects of the drug under study on systems other than the myometrium, the difficulty in reaching a maximum response, and the extreme difficulty (if not impossibility) of comparing the magnitude of the effect from one subject to another. In this area, in vitro studies are clearly superior because they have none of these disadvantages.

Many of the ethical considerations that impinge upon the use of intact animals or the study of human subjects disappear when studies are performed in vitro, which is not to suggest that there are not important ethical considerations in both these cases. In the case of humans, small pieces of tissue, sufficient to produce material for up to 8 muscle bath strips can be taken from the upper margin of a lower uterine segment incision at the time of cesarean section without danger to mother or fetus. Institutional review boards have little difficulty approving re-quests to obtain such tissue through informed consent from appropriate patients who will be properly safeguarded. In our experience (13, 17), a large percentage of patients are willing to give such consent. Perhaps the biggest impediment to the study of pregnant human myometrium in vitro is the poor compliance of surgeons and operating room staff in actually collecting tissue once consent has been ob-tained.

Interpretation of in vitro experiments is relatively simple since measure-ments are unidirectional. In fact, only as a result of in vitro studies that compared the activity of isolated strips of circular muscle with that of isolated strips of longitudinal muscle (8, 26) or longitudinally oriented strips with circularly oriented strips (7), do we realize that the two muscle layers can behave quite differently in response to the same agonist. Only in vitro can the responses of the two layers be studied separately, with the potential to yield more information about overall control mechanisms. Similarly, only in vitro studies can accurately determine the

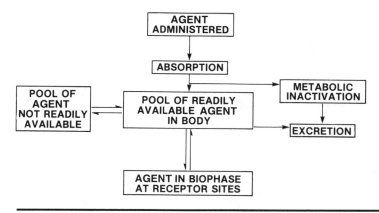

Fig. 1. The pharmacokinetic influences on a biologically active agent.

role of the endometrium in modulating the myometrium, through studies of the contractility of strips both including and lacking this layer. Indeed, this area has the potential to yield some exciting findings concerning the regulation of uterine activity if the interactions between endothelium (27) or epithelium (28) and underlying smooth muscles, which have recently been described, turn out to be general phenomena. The interaction between oxytocin, endometrium, prostanoids, and myometrium is already well documented (29–31).

Another important advantage of in vitro methods is the elimination, to a large extent, of pharmacokinetic variables. The response to an agonist is proportional to the concentration of that agonist at its receptor sites. Unfortunately for the investigator, in intact animals, this concentration is determined by many other factors besides the dose of the agent administered (see Fig. 1). Thus, a change in the response to a fixed dose might be brought about, not because the target organ has become more or less sensitive, but because a different concentration of the agent is reaching the receptor sites as a result of changes in pharmacokinetics. Although changes of a pharmacokinetic nature can still occur in vitro, the number of variables is considerably reduced and interpretations are more straightforward.

DISADVANTAGES OF THE STUDY OF MYOMETRIAL CONTRACTILITY IN VITRO

The use of isolated tissues is at least as old as the discipline of experimental pharmacology, and consequently, there is a large literature on this general topic. I will not attempt to summarize this general literature with regard to the drawbacks of the technique and the many precautions that should be taken, particularly since Kenakin (32) has done this thoroughly. Instead, I will outline a few of the problems which I feel should be of special concern to those of us who study the myometrium.

While removal of the tissue from its natural environment through elimination of the number of complex interactions described above can be of great benefit to an understanding of underlying mechanisms, it is also a potentially serious impediment to an understanding of the overall picture of the control of uterine activity. There are three areas where this is particularly important: interactions, the hormonal milieu, and dose-response relationships.

Interactions.   The area of interactions can be divided into two separate sections. First of all, there is the importance of interactions within the uterus itself. The ways in which longitudinal and circular muscle layers interact with each other and with the endometrium are indubitably very complex. A simple technique like the measurement of in vitro contractility is incapable of modeling precisely the forces that result from these interactions and that consequently impinge upon the fetus, for example.

   The physiological or pharmacological significance of the interaction of drugs or endogenous mediators with extra-uterine sites obviously should not be discounted and may be of particular relevance. Prostanoids, for instance, have myriad effects (33), and it is not beyond the bounds of possibility that when these compounds are produced in vitro, effects that they might have on blood flow (34) or steroid hormone production (35) could indirectly affect uterine contractility. Such properties will not manifest themselves when the effects of prostanoids on myometrial contractility are studied in vitro, and inappropriate conclusions about the role of these agents might be drawn. Therefore, discrepancies between in vitro and in vivo effects may be of considerable importance.

Hormonal Milieu.   The contractile activity of the myometrium, much more than any other smooth muscle, has been shown to be dependent upon the steroid hormonal milieu, particularly the relative dominance of estrogens to progestagens (36). When tissues are removed from their natural milieu and placed in tissue baths, control by steroid hormones may be lost. There is a general tendency to believe that effects of steroid hormones on contractility are rather long-lasting and, thus, that steroid hormone wash-out is of no consequence to the study of myometrial contractility in vitro. This is, in fact, only partially supported by experimental evidence, which shows a relatively slow but nevertheless significant rate of loss of progesterone's effect on rabbit myometrial contractility in vitro (37) and the development of gap junctions (which presumably affect contractility) when myometrium is incubated in vitro (38). These studies should at least place an upper time limit on the ability of in vitro studies to reflect the behavior of tissues in the environment from which they are recently removed. Unfortunately, we know very little indeed about quickly reversible forms of control of uterine activity. When myometrial tissues are incubated in vitro, they almost always develop spontaneous contractions (see Fig. 2). There is little evidence to suggest that such contractions are always present in vivo. One explanation might be that in vivo the uterus is, in most physiological circumstances, under constant tonic inhibition and that this inhibition is rapidly released in vitro. If so, the effect of agonists in vitro on a disinhibited tissue might be quite different from their effects in vivo. The possibility that relaxin acts to provide this kind of tonic inhibition of uterine activity in some species during late pregnancy (39) is an example of this problem. In a much more general sense, a

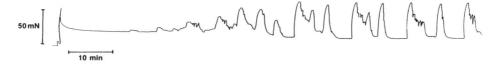

Fig. 2. Development of spontaneous contractile activity in a piece of human lower uterine segment tissue incubated in vitro.

developing body of evidence suggests tissues change more fundamentally than had been previously suspected when incubated in vitro. Thus, in at least one case, the development of responses to agonists during in vitro incubation, which is often referred to as "equilibration," has been shown to be dependent upon protein synthesis and perhaps to involved de novo synthesis of receptors (40, 41).

Even though the importance of a precise determination of the relationship between dose and response (or concentration and effect) cannot be overstated, this does not imply that knowledge of this relationship can necessarily be translated into a full understanding of myometrial physiology. In situations where changes in milieu can be disregarded, there are still problems of interpretation. Perhaps of foremost importance is the fact that we do not understand the relationship between the magnitude of a response in vitro and the physiological significance of the matching response in vivo. It is probable, but not proven, that even those contractions of the myometrium responsible for the expulsive contractions of parturition occur at the lower part of the dose-response curve. A relationship like this has been suggested to exist between in vitro responses of airway smooth muscle and airway narrowing in vivo (42). Another factor that makes interpretation of the significance of dose-response data difficult is a lack of understanding of the relationship between plasma concentrations of agents and their concentration at receptor sites, this is a particularly important problem for compounds that act in a paracrine manner and have a high rate of biotransformation in the target tissue. This is not an excuse to neglect collecting dose-response data. Even the relationship between tissue bath concentration and receptor site concentration is not always clear (32), and some additional problems that may be relevant to prostanoids have recently been pointed out (43).

All this being stated, I still firmly believe that the major problem associated with dose-response experiments appears when they are not done, when conclusion about the effects of agonists on myometrial contractility are made using the methods of empiricism, which have been described as follows:

> First, experience is identified as that part of a newly conceived hypothesis that can most readily be illustrated by simple and eye-catching procedures. Secondly, the experience so defined is made solid by the success (which may have been brought about with the help of ad hoc assumptions) of the hypothesis it illustrates as well as the vividness of the illustrating examples. Thirdly, it is given the appearance of stability through a method of

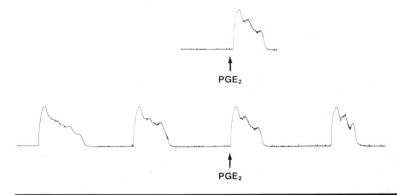

Fig. 3. Empiricism in action. The upper panel shows a clear effect of PGE_2 on human myometrial contractility. In the lower panel, the effect is not so clear.

interpretation that aims at, and succeeds in, concealing all change. The aim is reached by concentrating on the illustrations themselves rather than on the role they play in a particular theory (the same picture, after all, can illustrate very different things). [44]

Far too many times one finds proof that a newly discovered mediator is uterotonic based upon evidence similar to that shown in the upper part of Figure 3: no indication of dose, no indication of reproducibility, no indication of controls. In many cases, one is forced to conclude that if the entire tracing were displayed it would look like the lower part of Figure 3. An exaggeration perhaps? Perhaps not. Those who care to review the evidence concerning the direct effect of prostanoids on myometrial contractility in vitro, as we did for a number of our studies (13, 17, 45), will be surprised to find on what tenuous ground some current beliefs are based. Such a lack of rigor is unthinkable in other disciplines and should not be tolerated here. Well-controlled, reproducible dose-response experiments must be performed before any credence is given to claims for a new mediator.

A METHOD TO ANALYZE MYOMETRIAL CONTRACTILITY IN VITRO

For reasons that I hope have been made obvious by the preceding section, I will here describe in detail one method to analyze myometrial contractility in vitro.

The one property that sets isolated myometrium apart from most other smooth muscles studied in vitro is the development of high levels of spontaneous activity (Fig. 2). Spontaneous activity presents such a serious problem to the analysis of the effects of spasmogens that investigators in the past have taken rather bold steps to eliminate it, these include reducing the temperature of the tissue bath, reducing the Ca^{++} concentration of the bathing medium, and reducing the Mg^{++} concentration of the bathing medium. All of these ploys are to some extent effective and allow some form of analysis to be made, but how are such analyses to be interpreted? Will not measures that interfere with spontaneous contractility also interfere with agonist-induced contractility? Such manipulations would seem to be particularly dangerous when we seek to compare the effects of different agonists under similar conditions or the same agonist at different times during pregnancy, for example.

What if postreceptor mechanisms involved in the response to one agonist are more temperature-dependent than those to another? There is good evidence to suggest that different agonists utilize different Ca^{++} pools to produce excitation (46); thus they might be affected differently if external Ca^{++} is reduced. Similarly, oxytocin responses, which are sensitive to Mg^{++} (47), would be attenuated when this ion is reduced as compared to responses to Mg^{++}-insensitive agonists. For these reasons, I prefer a method by which tissues are incubated under "normal" conditions, spontaneous activity is allowed to develop, and the spontaneous activity is filtered out to reveal the agonist-induced activity. Given appropriate recording devices such filtering can be done manually (48), but the tedium is indescribable. The age of the microcomputer has made our work much easier.

The method currently in use in my laboratory has evolved from a number of our studies (7, 11, 13, 17, 45). Strips of myometrium approximately 20 mm in length and 2–3 mm in thickness are tied at each end with silk thread and suspended vertically in a tissue bath that is maintained at 37°C and contains a physiological salt solution that is continuously bubbled with a gas mixture containing 95% O_2 and 5% CO_2. The physiological salt solution contains the following salts: potassium chloride, 4.6 mmol/l; magnesium sulfate, 1.16 mmol/l; sodium dihydrogen phosphate, 1.16 mmol/l; calcium chloride, 1.8 mmol/l; sodium chloride, 115.5 mmol/l; sodium bicarbonate, 21.9 mmol/l; and glucose, 11.1 mmol/l. Indomethacin at a final concentration of 10 μmol/l may also be added if necessary. Like numerous other investigators of smooth muscle, we used a calcium chloride concentration of 2.5 mmol/l in our earlier studies (7, 45). This is not appropriate because it represents the total rather than the free concentration of Ca^{++} in the plasma.

One end of the myometrial strip is fixed to the bath and the other is tied to a Grass Instruments FTO3C transducer. A resting force is applied to each tissue and is readjusted as necessary until stable. The resting force chosen is that at which actively developed force (induced by agonists) is maximal. This optimal resting force is 25 mN for term pregnant human lower uterine segment (13, 17), for example. Tissues are rested for 30 min, then challenged with potassium chloride (90 mmol/l); those that do not respond with a contraction are discarded. The potassium chloride is washed from the bath, and tissues are rested for a further 30 min, during which time spontaneous activity, if not already present, usually develops. The experiment proper is now begun.

Activity of the tissue is measured by recording changes in developed force at a fixed length (i.e., isometrically). The signal flow and processing steps are shown schematically in Figure 4. The output of the transducer is amplified (Grass model 7P122), and the amplified signal is used in two ways. In one instance, it is used to drive a writing oscillograph (Grass 7D polygraph) and provide an analog record of

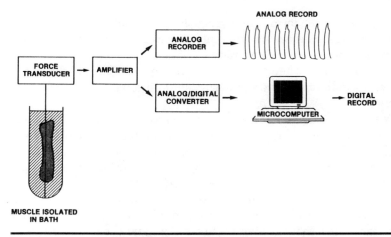

Fig. 4.   Signal flow in the analysis of myometrial contractility in vitro.

events. In the second instance, it is simultaneously sampled, digitized, and stored by the microcomputer to provide a digital record of events. Most often digitized samples are taken at a frequency of 2Hz and stored in epochs of 10 min duration. Usually there is a 2-min gap between the end of one epoch and the beginning of the next. For each epoch, the following parameters are of particular interest: the maximum force, the minimum force, and the mean force (i.e., the sum of all samples taken during that epoch divided by the number of samples). Because of the nature of drug-induced responses under these conditions (7, 45), we have found the mean force to be the most useful index of contractile activity.

When mean force is recorded continuously under these conditions for up to 2 h, an interesting pattern emerges. Rather than the erratic behavior we expect, contractile activity within a single muscle strip is in fact remarkably consistent (11, 13, 45). This observation then makes it possible to design a relatively simple protocol. The first epoch recorded after potassium chloride washout is a control: subsequent increases or decreases from this value will be taken as drug-induced effects provided that a longitudinal control (i.e., one tissue is selected at random from those being studied and remains untreated for the duration of the experiment) does not show significant change in activity for the duration of that experiment.

Drugs under test are added to the bath in small volumes (no greater than 30 μl is optimal) 1 min before the beginning of the next collection epoch. Drugs are added cumulatively (i.e., the bath is not washed out) until further addition produces no further change in activity. Although cumulative additions suit the experimenter quite well, it must be recognized that this method does not always produce the same results as when the bath is washed between additions (32). The control activity is subtracted from the activity in the presence of each cumulative concentration of drug to give the drug-induced activity. Activity can be expressed as the mean contractile force (units = Newtons) developed during each epoch. However, in order to be able to compare activity between tissues, it is necessary to normalize to the cross-sectional area of the tissue (Newtons per square centimeter). For this reason the cross section of every tissue is calculated from the length and mass, which are measured at the end of each experiment, and an assumed density of 1.05 g/cm^3 (49). The maximal effect is then calculated, and responses at each concentration of agonist are expressed as a percentage of that maximum. A dose-response curve is then constructed with percentage maximal response (y-axis) plotted against the log of the agonist concentration (x-axis). In the absence of a uniquely applicable model we fit our dose-response data to a third-order polynomial function using least-squares techniques. The concentration of the drug that produces a 50% maximal response (EC$_{50}$) is calculated from the curve by interpolation and taking the antilog. Other relevant parameters, such as slope of the linear portion of the curve, can also be determined (50).

In this way, effects of different agents under similar conditions can be compared by examining EC$_{50}$s and maximal effects (17, 45), and the effects of the same agent under different conditions—for example, at different stages of pregnancy—can also be compared (7, 11) by examining the same parameters. Results from experiments of this type have led to some controversy.

REGULATION OF OXYTOCIN RECEPTORS AND RESPONSES IN RAT MYOMETRIUM: EXAMINATION OF A CONTROVERSY

In the rat uterus, the concentration of binding sites for [^{3}H] oxytocin with a Kd around 1 nmol/l has been shown to increase shortly before term, to remain elevated during parturition, and to fall steeply shortly postpartum; manipulations that produce preterm labor produce premature changes in numbers of binding sites (51). A substantial body of evidence has developed to support the hypothesis that the binding sites for [^{3}H]oxytocin are in fact oxytocin receptors (52). A marked change in the number of oxytocin receptors, leading to an increase in the sensitivity of the uterus to oxytocin would be fully compatible with the observation that the hormone can induce parturition in the rat only 1 day before normal term (53). Thus, a physiological role for oxytocin receptor regulation in parturition has been proposed (5) and actively promulgated (52, 54).

Studies from two different laboratories (7, 8) that have examined the effects of oxytocin on myometrial contractility in vitro throughout pregnancy have produced results that are at odds with the receptor regulation hypothesis. First, rather than behaving in a unitary fashion, longitudinal and circular muscle layers show temporal changes in their responses to oxytocin that are markedly different. Second, the longitudinal muscle layer is sensitive to oxytocin throughout pregnancy and, in particular, at times when oxytocin binding sites are few. Whether there is a change in sensitivity immediately before term is unclear (7, 8). Third, the circular muscle is also responsive to oxytocin early in pregnancy, albeit in an all-or-none rather than a graded fashion, and there is agreement that a change in behavior occurs near term, when response suddenly becomes graded.

Two other studies also show a lack of correlation between oxytocin binding and response. When the total number of oxytocin binding sites in the rat uterus are manipulated either genetically (55) or by steroid hormone treatments (56), the behavior of the uterus in vitro in response to oxytocin remains unchanged.

From the standpoint of the receptor-binding aficionado, the discrepancies are easily explained. Measurements of in vitro contractility are unreliable, and many of the concerns expressed about the method in the preceding section are valid. Obviously, the uterus at the end of a lengthy in vitro experiment is very different from the uterus as first removed from the donor, which normally serves as the basis for binding experiments. In an analogy to cell culture, the uterus in vitro probably "de-differentiates" to a standard type during the course of an experiment. There is also the possibility that the true in vitro response to oxytocin is masked by the artifactual production of other uterotonic substances in vitro as seems to be the case during pregnancy in the rabbit (9). Also, in the rabbit, there is a good correlation between changes in oxytocin binding and changes in response when the steroid hormonal environment is manipulated (57); the problem therefore lies with in vitro contractility.

The observations are easily explained in an alternate manner by adherents of in vitro contractility. The binding sites referred to as oxytocin receptors are in fact no such thing and therefore their regulation is of no consequence for the contractile behavior of the uterus. In support of this view, isolated uterine cells have been shown to possess a binding site for oxytocin with a Kd of around 200 nmol/l, and it is more likely that this is the oxytocin receptor (58) than the approximately 1 nmol/l Kd site normally considered to be the receptor (52). Furthermore these observations are not artifacts of intact cells, since a similar site has been identified on isolated membranes (59). There is no mechanistic or thermodynamic argument in favor of the higher affinity site as the receptor; indeed, in a number of well-documented cases, there is a difference of two orders of magnitude between the EC_{50} and Kd of an agonist (48, 60). In addition, oxytocin has metabolic (61) as well as contractile functions, and the binding sites might represent receptors that mediate the former effects, not the latter.

However, as a dabbler in both receptor binding and in vivo contractility, I would like to believe that the truth lies somewhere between these two extremes. We need to re-examine the basic assumptions underlying each point of view. Only in this way can the full value of each technique be realized and a closer approximation of the true mechanism be attained. One of the first steps should be a re-examination of the model used for oxytocin/receptor interactions.

It is highly unlikely that the relationship between the concentration of oxytocin (OT), its receptor (R), and the response generated can be represented by the simple classical equation

$$OT + R \xrightleftharpoons{K_{1A}} OTR$$

in which the concentration of OTR determines the magnitude of the subsequent response. No matter whether the mechanism of action of oxytocin is through inhibition of a Ca^{++}-ATPase (62), stimulation of inositol phospholipid hydrolysis

(56), a combination of the two, or neither, it is most likely that the relationship is at least as complex as the following.

$$OT + R \overset{K_{1A}}{\rightleftharpoons} OTR + X \overset{K_{2A}}{\rightleftharpoons} OTRX$$

where X is a transducer or effector molecule, and it is the concentration of the ternary complex, OTRX, that determines the magnitude of the subsequent response (63, 64). A number of observations follow from this. Firstly in such as system,

$$EC_{50} = K_{1A}/1 + Rt/K_{2A}$$

where Rt is the total number of receptors (64). Only in cases where Rt/K_{2A} is very small will there be correspondence between EC_{50} and K_{1A} (which represents in our case the Kd for oxytocin), and under these circumstances the coupling efficiency is very low (64).

Knowing the value of EC_{50} from in vitro contractility experiments and of Kd and Rt from binding experiments, we can use the model to predict the value of K_{2A}. But perhaps the most important practical application arises from the observation that the formation of the OTRX complex is dependent not only on the concentrations of OT and R but also on the concentration of X. Thus, X presents another site at which responses to oxytocin can be regulated. In many cases, G-proteins serve the function of X (65). There is practical evidence that in the uterus, G-proteins can be the target of steroid hormone regulation (66), and there is theoretical evidence that in G-protein-modulated systems, changes in GTP concentration affect the apparent potency of agonists (67).

Thus, regulation of the contractile response of the uterus is an extremely complex process involving a large number of pharmacokinetic and pharmacodynamic variables. The study of in vitro contractility is an indispensable tool to help identify and quantify some of these variables.

REFERENCES

1. Csapo AI. The "see-saw" theory of parturition. In: The fetus and birth. Amsterdam: Ciba Foundation Symposium, Elsevier, 1977:159-210.
2. Casey ML, MacDonald PC. Decidual activation: the role of prostaglandins in labor. In: McNellis D, Challis JRG, MacDonald PC, Nathanielsz PW, Roberts JM, eds. The onset of labor: cellular and integrative mechanisms. Ithaca, NY: Perinatology Press, 1988:141-56.
3. Wanner O, Crankshaw DJ, Pliska V. The use of dynamic models to study the role of calcium in the oxytocin-induced contraction of the uterus. Mol Cell Endocrinol 1977;6:281-92.
4. Garfield RE, Sims S, Daniel EE. Gap junctions: their presence and necessity in myometrium during gestation. Science 1977;198:958-60.

5. Soloff MS, Alexandrova M, Fernstrom MJ. Oxytocin receptors: triggers for parturition and lactation? Science 1979;204:1313-5.

6. Catt KJ, Harwood JP, Aguilera G, Dufau ML. Hormonal regulation of peptide receptors and target cell responses. Nature 1979;280:109-16.

7. Crankshaw DJ. The sensitivity of the longitudinal and circular muscle layers of the rat's myometrium to oxytocin in vitro during pregnancy. Can J Physiol Pharmacol 1987;65:773-7.

8. Tuross N, Mahtani M, Marshall JM. Comparison of effects of oxytocin and prostaglandin $F_{2\alpha}$ on circular and longitudinal myometrium from the pregnant rat. Biol Reprod 1987;37:348-55.

9. Riemer RK, Goldfien AC, Goldfien A, Roberts JM. Rabbit uterine oxytocin receptors and in vitro contractile response: abrupt changes at term and the role of eicosanoids. Endocrinology 1986;119:699-709.

10. El Alj A, Breuiller M, Jolivet A, et al. β_2-adrenoceptor response in the rat uterus at the end of gestation and after induction of labor with Ru486. Can J Physiol Pharmacol 1989;67:1051-7.

11. Crankshaw DJ, Gaspar V. 1990; unpublished.

12. Bennett PR, Elder MG, Myatt L. The effects of lipoxygenase metabolites of arachidonic acid on human myometrial contractility. Prostaglandins 1987;33:837-44.

13. Dyal RY, Crankshaw DJ. The effects of prostanoids on the human lower uterine segment in vitro [Abstract]. Symposium on Uterine Contractility, Serono Symposia, USA, St. Louis, MO, 1990.

14. Fleckenstein A, Grun G, Tritthart H, Byon K. Uterus-relaxation durch hochaktive Ca^{++}-antagonistische Hemmstoffe der elektromechanischen Koppelung wie Isoptin (verapamil, Iproveratril), Substanz D600 und Segontin (Prenylamin). Klin Wochenschr 49:32-41.

15. Csapo AI, Puri CP, Tarro S, Henzl MR. Deactivation of the uterus during normal and premature labor by the calcium antagonist nicardipine. Am J Obstet Gynecol 1982;142:483-91.

16. Melin P, Trojnar J, Johansson B, et al. Synthetic antagonists of the myometrial response to oxytocin and vasopressin. J Endocrinol 1986;111:125-31.

17. Dyal R, Crankshaw DJ. The effects of some synthetic prostanoids on the contractility of the human lower uterine segment in vitro. Am J Obstet Gynecol 1988;58:281-5.

18. Holton P. A modification of the method of Dale and Laidlaw for standardization of posterior pituitary extract. Br J Pharmacol 1948;3:328-34.

19. Rudinger J, Pliska V, Krejci I. Oxytocin analogs in the analysis of some phases of hormone action. Recent Prog Horm Res 1972;28:131-66.

20. Crankshaw DJ. Muscarinic cholinoceptors in the rabbit's myometrium: a study of the relationship between binding and response. Eur J Pharmacol 1984;101:1-10.

21. Moore GJ. Photoaffinity labelling of angiotensin receptors: functional studies on responding tissues. Pharmacol Ther 1987;33:349-81.

22. Wiqvist N, Bryman I, Lindblom B, et al. The role of prostaglandins for the coordination of myometrial forces during labor. Acta Physiol Hung 1985;65:313-22.

23. Willman EA, Collins WP, Clayton SG. Studies in the involvement of prostaglandins in uterine symptomatology and pathology. Br J Obstet Gynaecol 1976;83:337-41.

24. Ke R, Vohra M, Casper R. Prolonged inhibition of human myometrial contractility by intermittent isoproterenol. Am J Obstet Gynecol 1984;149:841-4.

25. Casper RF, Lye SJ. Myometrial desensitization to continuous but not to intermittent β-adrenergic agonist infusion in the sheep. Am J Obstet Gynecol 1986;154:301-5.
26. Anderson G, Kawarabayashi T, Marshall JM. Effect of indomethacin and aspirin on uterine activity in pregnant rats: comparison of circular and longitudinal muscle. Biol Reprod 1981;24:359-72.
27. Furchgott RF, Zawadzki JV. The obligatory role of endothelial cells in the relaxation of arterial smooth muscle by acetylcholine. Nature 1980;288:373-6.
28. Goldie RG, Fernandes LB, Farmer SG, et al. Airway epithelium-derived inhibitory factor. TIPS 1990;11:67-70.
29. Sharma SC, Fitzpatrick RJ. Effect of oestradiol-17β and oxytocin treatment on prostaglandin F-alpha release in the anoestrous ewe. Prostaglandins 1974;6:97-105.
30. Roberts JS, McCracken JA, Gavagan JE, Soloff MS. Oxytocin-stimulated release of prostaglandin $F_{2\alpha}$ from ovine endometrium in vitro: correlation with estrous cycle and oxytocin-receptor binding. Endocrinology 1976;99:1107-976.
31. Chan WY. Relationship between the uterotonic action of oxytocin and prostaglandins: oxytocin action and release of PG-activity in isolated nonpregnant and pregnant rat uteri. Biol Reprod 1977;17:541-8.
32. Kenakin TP. The classification of drugs and drug receptors in isolated tissues. Pharmacol Rev 1984;36:165-222.
33. Moncada S, Flower RJ, Vane JR. Prostaglandins, prostacyclin, thromboxane A_2, and leukotrienes. In: Gilman AG, Goodman LS, Rall TW, Murad F, eds. Goodman and Gilman's The pharmacological basis of therapeutics. 7th ed. New York: MacMillan, 1985:660-73.
34. Maigaard S, Forman A, Andersson KE. Relaxant and contractile effects of some amines and prostanoids in myometrial and vascular smooth muscle within the human uteroplacental unit. Acta Physiol Scand 1986;128:33-40.
35. Aleem F, Shulman H, Saldana L, et al. the effect of prostaglandin $F_{2\alpha}$ on the placental progesterone level in midtrimester abortion. Am J Obstet Gynecol 1975;123:202-5.
36. Thorburn GD, Challis JRG. Control of parturition. Physiol Rev 1979;59:863-918.
37. Currie WB, Jeremy JY. In vitro action of progesterone on myometrium, 1. Reversible modulation of the resistance of rabbit uterus to excitation-contraction uncoupling. Biol Reprod 1979;21:945-52.
38. Garfield RE, Merrett D, Grover AK. Gap junction formation and regulation in myometrium. Am J Physiol 1980;239:C217-28.
39. Sherwood OD, Crnekovic VE, Gordon WL, et al. Radioimmunoassay of relaxin throughout pregnancy and during parturition in the rat. Endocrinology 1980;107:691-8.
40. Regoli D, Marceau F, Barabé J. De novo formation of vascular receptors for bradykinin. Can J Physiol Pharmacol 1978;56:674-7.
41. Bouthillier J, Deblois D, Marceau F. Studies on the induction of pharmacological responses to des-Arg^9-bradykinin in vitro and in vivo. Br J Pharmacol 1987;92:257-64.
42. Mitchell HW, Sparrow MP. The relevance of pharmacological dose-response curves to airway narrowing. TIPS 1989;10:488-91.
43. Samples DR, Sprague EA, Harper MJK, et al. In vitro adsorption losses of arachidonic acid and calcium ionophore A23187. Am Physiol Soc 1989;C1166-70.
44. Feyerabend PK. Problems of empiricism. Philosophical Papers, vol 2. Cambridge: Cambridge University Press, 1981.

45. Wainman BC, Burcea I, Crankshaw DJ. The effects of prostanoids on estrogen-dominated rat myometrial longitudinal muscle. Biol Reprod 1988;39:221-8.

46. Molnar M, Asem EK, Hertelendy F. Differential effects of prostaglandin $F_{2\alpha}$ and of prostaglandins E_1 and E_2 on cyclic 3', 5'-monophosphate production and intracellular calcium mobilization in avian uterine smooth muscle cells. Biol Reprod 1987;36: 384-91.

47. Krejci I, Polacek I. Effect of magnesium on the action of oxytocin and a group of analogues on the uterus in vitro. Eur J Pharmacol 1968;2:393-8.

48. Crankshaw DJ, Ruzycky AL. Characterization of putative beta-adrenoceptors in the myometrium of the pregnant ewe: correlation between the binding of [^{3}H]dihydroalprenolol and the inhibition of myometrial contractility in vitro. Biol Reprod 1984;30:609-18.

49. Greenburg S, Gaines K, Sweatt D. Evidence for circulating factors as a cause of venous hypertrophy in spontaneously hypertensive rats. Am J Physiol 1981;241:H421-30.

50. Garfield RE, Beier S. Increased myometrial responsiveness to oxytocin during term and preterm labor. Am J Obstet Gynecol 1989;161:454-61.

51. Alexandrova M, Soloff MS. Oxytocin receptors and parturition, I. Control of oxytocin receptor concentration in the rat myometrium at term. Endocrinology 1980;106: 730-5.

52. Soloff MS. Oxytocin receptors and mechanisms of oxytocin action. In: Amico JA, Robinson AG, eds. Oxytocin: clinical and laboratory studies. Amsterdam: Excerpta Medica, 1988:259-76.

53. Fuchs AR, Poblete VF Jr. Oxytocin and uterine function in pregnant and parturient rats. Biol Reprod 1970;2:387-400.

54. Soloff MS. The role of oxytocin in the induction of labor and oxytocin-prostaglandin interactions. In: McNellis D, Challis JRG, MacDonald PC, Nathanielsz PW, Roberts JM, eds. The onset of labor: cellular and integrative mechanisms. Ithaca, NY: Perinatology Press, 1988:87-110.

55. Goren HJ, Geonzon RM, Hollenberg MD, Lederis K, Morgan DO. Oxytocin action: lack of correlation between receptor number and tissue responsiveness. J Supramol Struct 1980;14:129-38.

56. Ruzycky AL, Crankshaw DJ. Role of inositol phospholipid hydrolysis in the initiation of agonist-induced contractions of rat uterus: effects of domination by 17β-estradiol and progesterone. Can J Physiol Pharmacol 1988;66:10-7.

57. Nissenson R, Flouret G, Hechter O. Opposing effects of estradiol and progesterone on oxytocin receptors in rabbit uterus. Proc Natl Acad Sci USA 1978;75:2044-8.

58. Pliska V, Heiniger J, Muller-Lhotsky A, Pliska P, Ekberg B. Binding of oxytocin to uterine cells in vitro. J Biol Chem 1986;261:16984-9.

59. Crankshaw DJ, Gaspar V, Pliska V. Multiple [^{3}H]oxytocin binding sites in rat myometrial plasma membranes [Abstract]. Symposium on Uterine Contractility, Serono Symposia, USA, St Louis, MO, 1990.

60. Aronstam RS, Triggle DJ, Eldefrawi ME. Structural and stereochemical requirements for muscarinic receptor binding. Mol Pharmacol 1978;15:227-34.

61. Lederis K, Goren MJ, Hollenberg MD. Oxytocin: an insulin-like hormone. In: Amico JA, Robinson AG, eds. Oxytocin: clinical and laboratory studies. Amsterdam: Excerpta Medica, 1985:284-302.

62. Soloff MS, Sweet P. Oxytocin inhibition of $(Ca^{2+} + Mg^{2+})$-ATPase activity in rat myometrial plasma membranes. J Biol Chem 1982;257:10687-93.
63. De Lean A, Stadel JM, Lefkowitz RJ. A ternary complex model explains the agonist-specific binding properties of the adenylate cyclase coupled β-adrenergic receptor. J Biol Chem 1978;255:7108-17.
64. Black JW, Leff P. Operational models of pharmacological agonism. Proc R Soc Lond 1983;220:141-62.
65. Rodbell M. Signal transduction in biological membranes. In: Poste G, Crooke ST, eds. Mechanisms of receptor regulation. New York: Plenum Press, 1985:65-73.
66. Roberts JM, Riemer RK, Bottari SP, et al. Myometrial post receptor responses: targets for steroidal regulation. In: McNellis D, Challis JRG, MacDonald PC, Nathanielsz PW, Roberts JM, eds. The onset of labor: cellular and integrative mechanisms. Ithaca, NY: Perinatology Press, 1988:37-50.
67. MacKay D. Agonist potency and apparent affinity: interpretation using classical and steady state ternary-complex models. TIPS 1990;11:17-22.

8

Receptor-Linked Phospholipase C Activity in Myometrium

R. Kirk Riemer

Department of Obstetrics, Gynecology, and Reproductive Sciences, and Reproductive Endocrinology Center, University of California, San Francisco

PHOSPHOLIPASE C AND CALCIUM MOBILIZATION

Myometrial contraction depends upon an increase in the intracellular ionized calcium concentration. Many stimulatory agents initiate this intracellular process via their specific receptors through the activation of a specific receptor-operated phospholipase C (1) (PLC), which selectively hydrolyzes phosphatidylinositol 4,5-bisphosphate (PIP_2) to generate two second messengers, inositol 1,4,5-trisphosphate (IP_3); and 1,2-diacylglycerols (DAG) containing predominantly arachidonate at the second carbon position. Inositol trisphosphate triggers an increase in intracellular calcium concentration through release of limited stores from the sarcoplasmic reticulum. This Ca^{++} transient is followed by an increase in Ca^{++} influx, and subsequent activation of the contractile apparatus. Thus, PLC activation is the initial post receptor event leading to myometrial contraction.

Forms of PLC

There are known to be at least five different molecular forms of PLC in mammalian cells (2) occurring in soluble as well as membrane-localized forms. It is not known which of the cloned PLCs are the receptor-operated PLC(s), but the membrane-attached forms are likely candidates because receptors and G-proteins also reside in the membrane. However, the primary structures of many receptors are known, and commonly have rather extensive structures capable of interacting with "soluble" cytoplasmic entities. Of the three PLC isozymes known to associated with the plasma membrane (α, β, and γ), one (β form) is also found in cytosol fractions. Thus PLCs might be translocated from the cytoplasm to the membrane in the

Acknowledgments: This work was supported by NIH Grant HD-26152.

process of receptor activation (analogous to protein kinase C, PKC activation). For the purposes of the present discussion, the term PLC will refer to the PIP_2 hydrolyzing activity that is stimulated by agonists and detected by metabolic labeling with radioactive inositol. The measured agonist-stimulated response could conceivably be the result of the activation of more than one enzyme isoform.

Metabolism of IP_3

The fate of IP_3 generated from PLC action on PIP_2 has been found to vary substantially from tissue to tissue, but some patterns are evident (Fig. 1). The shortest inactivation route is via a 5-phosphatase conversion to biologically inactive (so far as is currently known) 1,4-IP_2, followed by sequential dephosphorylation to myo-inositol, which can re-form Pi by reaction with CDP-DAG. The other route of IP_3 metabolism is much more complex and still poorly understood in terms of its biologic relevance. The key enzyme in the branch point is an IP_3 3-kinase that generates inositol 1,3,4,5-tetrakisphosphate (IP_4). The activity of the 3-kinase is increased by Ca^{++}; thus there appears to be a shunting of IP_3 to IP_4 as intracellular Ca^{++} concentration rises. IP_4 is subsequently dephosphorylated by the same 5-phosphatase that acts on IP_3, and generates a second IP_3, inositol 1,3,4-trisphosphate. The 1,3,4-isomer of IP_3 is found in abundance following agonist stimulation of PLC in many tissues and cells, although with a characteristic lag, consistent with conversion from 1,4,5-IP_3 via IP_4. Thus, while the intracellular level of 1,4,5-IP_3 declines after about 60 sec in most systems, the level of 1,3,4-IP_3 continues to increase after the initial lag, so that beyond 60 sec, the bulk of the IP_3

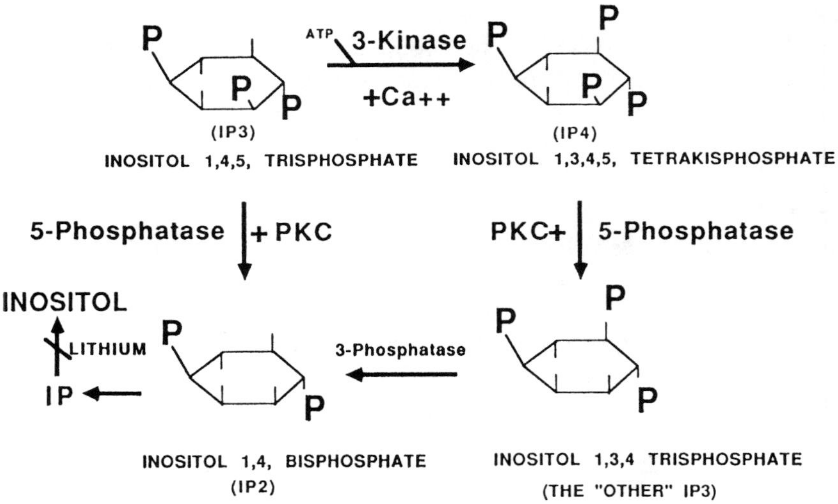

Fig. 1. Metabolism of inositol trisphosphate. See text for details of the steps. Note that the 5-phosphatase enzyme is a substrate for PKC, and its activity is increased by phosphorylation.

present is the 1,3,4-isomer. Two other inositol phosphate isomers, IP_5 and IP_6, are present in high concentrations in many tissues, including rabbit myometrium, although their levels change little upon agonist stimulation

Effects of IP_3 and IP_4 on Intracellular Calcium

Inositol 1,4,5,-trisphosphate binds to specific receptor sites causing a transient release of a limited amount of calcium from sarcoplasmic reticulum-like Ca^{++} storage sites. The cellular location of these storage sites and the mechanism for their release and replenishment is still unclear, although some interesting models have been suggested. As shown in Figure 2, GTP and IP_4 may be involved in the regulation of the Ca^{++} storage sites, which may actually be replenished via transfer from the extracellular space rather than uptake from the cytoplasmic space.

In many cell types, prolonged agonist stimulation causes not sustained elevation of intracellular Ca^{++}, but rather regular oscillatory elevations peaking in the range of 500 nM Ca^{++} with a period of 5–60 sec. Since prolonged depolarization (e.g., with KCl) can elicit these oscillations, it is thought that this may be a general homeostatic response to Ca^{++} overload in the cytoplasm which is caused by activation of voltage-operated Ca^{++} gating along with receptor-operated and IP_3-operated Ca^{++} gating mechanisms.

The brief intracellular calcium transient elicited by IP_3 is considered to be the initial or triggering event in the contractile activation process of smooth

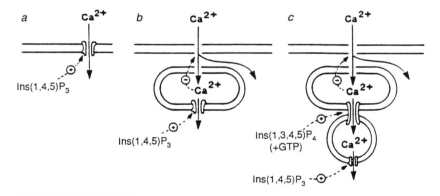

Fig. 2. Ca^{++} mobilization. The exact mechanism by which IP_3 regulates the gating of extracellular Ca^{++} is not known. Three possible models are depicted here. In model a, IP_3 simply controls a Ca^{++} channel in the plasma membrane. Model b depicts a capacitance model in which the concentration of Ca^{++} in a submembranous compartment is feedback-regulated by Ca^{++} and IP_3 controls the release from this compartment (this model originally proposed by J. Putney). Model c represents an extension of the Putney model, with two Ca^{++} pools, and IP_4 controlling the flux from the IP_3-insensitive pool to the IP_3-sensitive pool. (From Berridge MJ, Irvine R, Inositol phosphates and cell signalling, Nature (Lond) 1989;341:197–205, with permission.)

muscles, while the influx of calcium from the extracellular space is required for full activation of the contractile apparatus. This gating is probably regulated by the IP_3-induced transient via a Ca^{++}-induced Ca^{++} conductance mechanism that would modulate voltage-operated Ca^{++} gating mechanisms. While this mechanism is far from proven, it does allow for modulation of the Ca^{++} signal by the degree of PLC activation and hence provides the graded response to agonists characteristic of smooth muscles.

Second-Messenger Action of Diacylglycerol

The other second messenger generated by PLC activity against PIP_2 is 1,2-diacylglycerol, (DAG). DAG acts together with Ca^{++} to promote the interaction of a cytoplasmic protein serine kinase, protein kinase C (PKC), with membranous phosphatidylserines, "translocation" to the sarcolemma. The translocation of PKC to the sarcolemma increases its sensitivity to Ca^{++}, which translates to increased kinase activity even without elevation of intracellular Ca^{++} concentration (reviewed in reference 4). The role of PKC activation in uterine or other smooth-muscle contractility remains unclear, primarily because many of the endogenous substrates for PKC are still uncharacterized. However, PKC activation (implied by phorbol ester or exogenous DAG treatment) can influence the Ca^{++} signal. It is known that PKC phosphorylates and increases the activity of the 5-phosphatase that inactivates IP_3 and IP_4. This would suggest a homeostatic feedback inhibitory role for PKC to promote IP_3 and IP_4 degradation, thereby terminating the receptor signal. Another way in which PKC may regulate intracellular Ca^{++} concentration is by promoting Ca^{++} removal by the Ca^{++} pumping ATPase and Na/Ca^{++} exchange mechanisms (reviewed in reference 5). It is also known that PKC phosphorylates the regulatory light-chains of myosin, although at a site(s) distinct from that of myosin light-chain kinase (6). Recent evidence suggests, however, that PKC-mediated phosphorylation of myosin may not be a component of the process initiated through agonist stimulation of PLC (7; also see Chapter 4).

The sources and the metabolic fates of DAGs also have implications for their PLC signaling pathway. It has recently become clear that agonist-coupled PLCs can break down phosphatidylcholine as well as PIP and Pi lipids, thereby producing DAGs without accompanying IP_3 production (3). This would have the effect to maintain PKC activation without concomitant IP_3 production. Diacylglycerols are somewhat heterogenous compounds in terms of the lipids on carbon atoms 1 and 2. However, most DAG molecules contain arachidonate at the second carbon atom. This is significant because most cells have enzymes (mono- and diacylglycerol lipases) that can release this arachidonate, enabling its metabolism to eicosanoids, which can then act as third-order messengers to alter the initial signal. Thus, agonist activation of PLC can produce DAG from other lipids besides PIP_2, and this DAG may be metabolized to eicosanoids.

Summary: PLC in Smooth-Muscle Contraction

Agonist-stimulated IP_3 production is the initial intracellular event in myometrial contraction, leading to transiently elevated intracellular Ca^{++} levels through release from subcellular stores. This is followed by a greater elevation in intracellular Ca^{++} via gated influx, and the activation of contraction by stimulation of the key control enzyme, Ca^{++}- and calmodulin-dependent myosin light-chain kinase (MLCK). The spread of the activation process among cells in the tissue would be expected by virtue of the distribution of agonist among the cells as well as through the movement of Ca^{++} or perhaps IP_3 among cells via gap junctions. The DAG generated in parallel with IP_3 activates PKC, which may serve to terminate the IP_3 signal by activation of IP_3 5-phosphatase as well as by promoting Ca^{++} extrusion by the Ca^{++} pump and exchange mechanisms.

RECEPTOR ACTIVATION OF PLC

Several types of hormones stimulate PLC activity in myometrium, including oxytocin (OT), arginine vasopressin (AVP), norepinephrine (NE), acetylcholine, prostaglandin E_2 and other eicosanoids, angiotensin II, PAF, and numerous other agents that also have in common the ability to activate uterine contractions.

Molecular Organization of Receptors with PLC

PLC activation is a graded response that is dependent on receptor density and agonist concentration. While the molecular configuration of the receptor-PLC effector units is not known, it is known that a guanyl nucleotide sensitive protein(s) probably couples receptors to PLC. The evidence for G-protein control is illustrated in Figure 3. The implication of this receptor-coupler-effector configuration (by

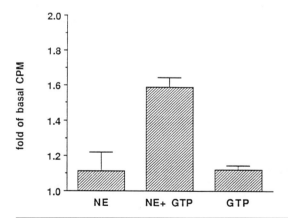

Fig. 3. G-proteins and PLC activation. The effect of GTP to augment agonist activation of PLC is shown in a typical experiment from rabbit uterine primary myocytes. The cells were labeled with [$_3$H]inositol (16 µCi/ml for 24 h), permeabilized by a 1-h exposure to ATP (0.1 mM), then exposed to the effector or combination of effectors indicated. (NE = norepinephrine, 0.1 mM; GTP = GTP gamma thiophosphate, 0.1 mM.) The response measured was a 15-min accumulation of IPs in the presence of 20 mM LiCl. The data are mean ± SEM of triplicates. (From R. K. Riemer, unpublished data.)

analogy with other G-protein-coupled systems) is that an agonist-occupied receptor could activate more than one PLC effector unit and also that there is a finite lifetime to the activation process that is governed by the rate of GTP hydrolysis. This configuration, therefore, provides another level of control over the efficacy of an agonist-occupied receptor: Changing the stoichiometry of receptor to G-protein and or G-protein to PLC can give an enormous change in the degree of signal amplification (i.e., in the rate of IP_3 production).

The nature of the G-protein(s) coupling PLC to receptors is not clear. A Gi-like protein has been implicated for some agonists responses in some tissues, including the uterus (see Chapter 6) through the ability of pertussis toxin to inhibit agonist response. However, other investigators have been unable to demonstrate an effect of pertussis toxin (e.g., see Chapter 10). Also, some investigators have reported that cholera toxin can inhibit some agonist responses [8]. However, some caution is warranted because these toxins may have other effects that complicate the interpretation of the results (e.g., a reduction in receptor concentration secondary to cholera-toxin treatment [9]).

Interactions Among Receptors Coupled to PLC

We find that the magnitude of the myometrial PLC responses to different agents (measured in terms of maximal response compared to vehicle control) varies from a common range of 2- to 3-fold for many agonists (e.g., NE, acetylcholine, and PAF) to 6-fold or greater for angiotensin II (R. K. Riemer, unpublished observations). Thus the PLC response differs quantitatively for different agonists, suggesting that receptors (or coupling proteins) probably determine the number of enzymatic units activated from a generally larger cellular pool of PLC units. This configuration is also suggested from examinations of the interaction of combinations of two different agonists. If receptors or coupling proteins are limiting, then the maximal response to two agonists should be additive. This is the case for catecholamine and cholinergic receptors in myometrium (Fig. 4). Thus each receptor appears to control a fraction of the total cellular PLC activity, rather than any one receptor type activating all PLCs. This configuration suggests that the magnitude of response mediated by a specific receptor can be regulated independent of other receptor-PLC configurations.

HETEROLOGOUS REGULATION OF PLC IN MYOMETRIUM

If ovarian steroid hormones increase the ability of agents to activate PLC, then this should be manifest as an increased rate or magnitude of IP_3 production. This hormonal effect would likely be observed as an increased sensitivity for contraction and/or an increased maximal response, depending on whether the rate of IP_3 production or the cumulative amount of IP_3 governs subsequent steps (Ca^{++} influx, phosphorylation of myosin). The ability to modify the effectiveness of receptor activation by changing the postreceptor responses constitutes a mechanism for fine tuning myometrial responses to discrete stimuli.

The myometrium presents a special opportunity to examine the question of

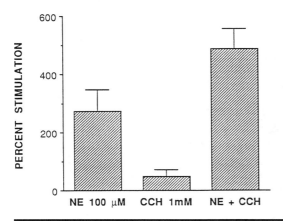

Fig. 4. Agonist interactions with uterine PLC. Shown are the responses of uterine minces to the effector or combination of effectors indicated. (NE = norepinephrine, 0.1 mM; CCH = carbachol, 1 mM.) The tissue was labeled for 2 h at 37°C with 16 µCi/ml of [^{3}H]inositol in Krebs solution. The response measured was a 30 min accumulation of IPs in the presence of 20 mM LiCl. The data are mean ± SEM of triplicates from a typical experiment. (From R. K. Riemer, unpublished data.)

whether hormones regulate PLC activity as a way to modulate agonist potency (i.e., contractile sensitivity). Increasing receptor concentration is a demonstrated means for heterologously augmenting responses. However, responses can be increased without apparent receptor changes (Table 1).

Table 1. The effect of estrogen on rabbit uterine contractile sensitivity to norepinephrine and α1 adrenoceptor concentration.

	Treatment			
	Ovex	Mature	Ovex-E$_2$	E$_2$-Ovex
EC$_{50}$ (nM)[a]	746 ± 139[c] (7)	176 ± 18 (5)	164 ± 16 (9)	131 ± 12 (7)
α1 receptors (fmol/mg)[b]	46 ± 14 (5)	46 ± 7 (14)	99 ± 16[d] (8)	46 ± 10 (8)

Note: Values are mean ± SE for (n) animals.

[a]EC$_{50}$ values from cumulative dose-response curves for norepinephrine (see reference 10).

[b]α1 adrenoceptor concentration determined by saturation analysis (see reference 10).

[c]Significantly different from all other treatments; P < 0.001 by one-way ANOVA.

[d]Significantly different from all other treatments; P < 0.01 by one-way ANOVA.

Ovex = ovariectomized (hormone withdrawn) and sacrificed 10 days postsurgery following 4 days of treatment with oil vehicle; mature = untreated rabbits (ca. 7 lb in weight); Ovex-E$_2$-treated with estradiol benzoate (50 µg/kg IM) in oil vehicle for 4 days; and E$_2$-Ovex = treated as above with estradiol prior to ovariectomy.

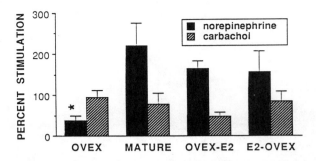

Fig. 5.   Comparison of estrogen effects on PLC stimulation in uterine minces. The tissue was labeled for 2 h at 37°C with 16 µCi/ml of [^{3}H]inositol in Krebs solution. The response measured was a 30-min accumulation of IPs in the presence of 20 mM LiCl. Agonist concentrations were norepinephrine, 0.1 mM, and carbachol, 1 mM. (* = P < 0.05 versus all other treatment groups.) Treatments are described in Table 1. (Data from Riemer RK, Roberts J, Estrogen increases adrenergic but not cholinergic mediated production of inositol phosphates in rabbit uterus, Mol Pharmacol 1987;32:663–8.)

Estrogen increases the sensitivity of myometrium to both OT and NE. This is accompanied by an increase in receptor concentration in the former case, but not the latter. We have examined NE-stimulated PLC activity in uterine minces from rabbits treated in vivo with estrogen or oil vehicle following ovariectomy (11). Estrogen increases maximal PLC response to NE but not carbamylcholine (CCH), a stable analog of acetylcholine (Fig. 5). Increased contractile response without changes in receptor concentration or affinity suggests changes in the molecular events occurring distal to receptor occupancy, such as IP$_3$ production, Ca^{++} gating, and phosphorylation events. Thus, increased contractile sensitivity to norepinephrine is associated with increased IP$_3$ production. This effect of estrogen is also agonist selective: Estrogen increases adrenergic but not cholinergic contractile sensitivity and also adrenergic, but not cholinergic, stimulation of PLC. These results demonstrate that second-messenger production is a process that can be discretely regulated by heterologously acting agents such as estrogen.

The response to OT increases near term of pregnancy in rabbits (12). Studies conducted with uterine minces from pregnant rabbits reveal that there is increased IP$_3$ production at day 31 (term) compared with day 27 (Fig. 6). We have previously shown that myometrial OT receptor concentrations increase approximately 10-fold within 24 h of term (13). This is an example of a increase in PLC activation that is probably receptor-dependent.

We are presently conducting studies of agonist-stimulated PLC activity in primary cultures of uterine myocytes from rabbits treated in vivo with estrogen or oil vehicle to establish the response as a property of the uterine smooth-muscle cell. We find that estrogen increases oxytocin response of the myocytes (Fig. 7). These data demonstrate that the effects of E$_2$ on PLC activation are mediated directly upon uterine smooth-muscle cells.

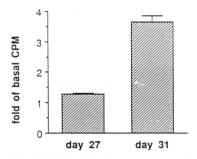

Fig. 6. PLC activation by oxytocin in pregnant rabbit uterus. Shown are the responses of uterine minces to 1 μM oxytocin before term (day 27) and at term (day 31). The tissue was labeled for 2 h at 37°C with 16 μCi/ml of [³H] inositol in Krebs solution. The response measured was a 30-min accumulation of IPs in the presence of 20 mM LiCl. The data are mean ± SEM of triplicates from a typical experiment. (From R. K. Riemer, unpublished data.)

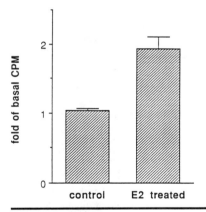

Fig. 7. PLC activation in myocytes: Effects of estrogen on the response to 0.1 μM oxytocin. Rabbits were ovariectomized and treated as described in Table 1. Primary myocytes were obtained by enzymatic dispersion. The responses were measured exactly as described for Figure 3. The data are mean ± SEM of triplicates from a typical experiment. (From R. K. Riemer, unpublished data.)

OVERVIEW

These studies demonstrate that agonist-stimulated PLC activity can be modified by the hormonal environment. Comparing the effect of estrogen on oxytocin and norepinephrine responses reveals that it is not necessary to increase receptor concentration to increase PLC activation by an agonist. Increased PLC activity is associated with increased contractile sensitivity to the agonists. Much is still to be learned about the mechanisms through which these changes occur, and their role in the maintenance of uterine quiescence and the initiation of labor.

REFERENCES

1. Berridge MJ, Irvine R. Inositol phosphates and cell signalling. Nature (Lond) 1989;341:197-205.
2. Rhee SG, Suh P, Ryu S, Lee S. Studies of inositol phospholipid-specific phospholipase C. Science 1989;244:546-50.
3. Exton JH. Signalling through phosphatidylcholine breakdown. J Biol Chem 1990;265:1-5
4. Nishizuka Y. The molecular heterogeneity of protein kinase C and its implications for cellular regulation. Nature (Lond) 1988;334:661-5.
5. Nishizuka Y. Studies and perspectives of protein kinase C. Science 1986;233:305-12.
6. Stull JT, Taylor D, MacKenzie L, Casey L. Biochemistry and physiology of smooth muscle contractility. In: McNellis D, Challis J, MacDonald P, Nathanielsz P, Roberts J, eds. The onset of labor: cellular and integrative methods. Ithaca, NY: Perinatology Press, 1988:17-32.
7. Kamm KE, Hsu L, Kubota Y, Stull J. Phosphorylation of smooth muscle myosin heavy and light chains. J Biol Chem 1989;264:21223-9.
8. Ruzycky AL, Crankshaw D. Role of inositol phospholipid hydrolysis in the initiation of agonist-induced contractions of rat uterus: effects of domination by 17 beta-estradiol and progesterone. Can J Physiol Pharmacol 1988;66:10-7.
9. Guillon G, Balestre M, Lombard C, Rassendren F, Kirk, C. Influence of bacterial toxins and forskolin upon vasopressin-induced inositol phosphate accumulation in WRK 1 cells. Biochem J 1989;260:665-72.
10. Riemer RK, Goldfien A, Roberts J. Rabbit myometrial adrenergic sensitivity is increased by estrogen but is dissociated from changes in alpha adrenoceptor concentration. J Pharmacol Exp Ther 1987;117:44-50.
11. Riemer RK, Roberts J. Estrogen increases adrenergic but not cholinergic mediated production of inositol phosphates in rabbit uterus. Mol Pharmacol 1987;32:663-8.
12. Riemer RK, Goldfien A, Roberts J. Rabbit myometrial oxytocin receptors and in vitro contractile response: abrupt changes at term and the role of eicosanoids. Endocrinology 1986;119:699-709.
13. Jacobsen L, Riemer R, Goldfien A, Lykins D, Siiteri P, Roberts J. Rabbit myometrial oxytocin and alpha-2 adrenergic receptors are increased by estrogen but are differentially regulated by progesterone. Endocrinology 1987;120:1184-9.

9

Receptor-Linked Adenylyl Cyclase: Role in Myometrial Contraction

James M. Roberts, Andre Ruzycky, and R. Kirk Riemer

Department of Obstetrics, Gynecology, and Reproductive Sciences, and Cardiovascular Research Institute, University of California, San Francisco

T he cAMP-mediated inhibition of myometrial contractions is the best established and most extensively studied pathway involved in the inhibition of uterine contractility. The linkage of receptors to stimulation of adenylyl cyclase is also extremely well characterized (1) and presents several potential sites for regulation. This receptor G-protein interaction is a model for several other G-protein-linked responses, including the activation of myometrial contraction through phosphatidyl inositol bis-phosphate specific phospholipase C (2). In this presentation, we review the role of cAMP as an inhibitor of myometrial contractility, but concentrate most attention on the transduction of stimulatory receptor occupancy to the activation of adenylyl cyclase. The points of potential regulation and examples of this modulation are considered. We review evidence of this regulation primarily for the uterus. Work from our laboratory that is presented examines the modulation of adrenergic-mediated adenylyl cyclase activation in rabbit myometrium.

KINASE A AND INHIBITION OF MYOMETRIAL CONTRACTIONS

Most, if not all, of the actions of cAMP in eukaryotic cells are mediated by phosphorylation events catalyzed by the cAMP-dependent protein kinase, kinase A (3). Alterations in protein structure and function by kinase A-mediated phosphorylation are proposed to reduce myometrial contractility at several levels. In in vitro systems, cAMP acting through kinase A increases the binding of calcium to plasma membrane and microsomal vesicles, apparently by increasing the affinity of these proteins for calcium (4). The increased binding of calcium reduces the concentration of intracytoplasmic free calcium (Fig. 1). Cyclic AMP is also purported to reduce

Acknowledgments: Special thanks to David Lykins for technical assistance and Louvina Forkin for manuscript preparation. This work was supported by NIH grant HD-21785.

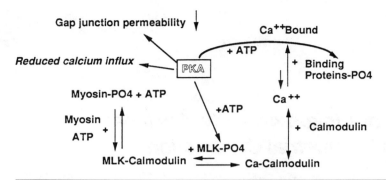

Fig. 1. Putative mechanisms by which cAMP reduces myometrial contractions. The actions of cAMP are mediated by kinase A activation of several intracellular processes. Two mechanisms are postulated to reduce intracellular free-calcium concentration: reduced calcium influx and increased binding of calcium to intracellular sites. In addition, cAMP can phosphorylate myosin light-chain kinase, decreasing its affinity for calcium calmodulin and reducing activation of this enzyme. Closure of gap junctions interferes with intercellular communication and propagation of action potentials.

intracytoplasmic calcium by reducing entry of calcium into cells (5). Acting at another site, cAMP or the kinase A catalytic subunit can activate the phosphorylation of myosin light-chain kinase (MLK), the enzyme responsible for phosphorylating and activating myosin (6). When myosin light-chain kinase is phosphorylated by kinase A, its affinity for calmodulin, the second-message molecule responsible for activating this enzyme, is decreased. The reduced interaction of MLK with calmodulin decreases myosin light-chain phosphorylation inhibiting smooth-muscle contraction. In addition the propagation of contraction between cells may also be affected by cAMP, which has the capability to close gap junctions (7).

Thus, cAMP has the potential to inhibit myometrial contraction by several mechanisms acting on at least three targets. It must be pointed out, however, that the physiological relevance of these mechanisms is currently a subject of debate as some of these mechanisms have not been demonstrated in vivo. For example, although the phosphorylation of MLK by kinase A is an attractive hypothesis, Stull and coworkers point out that concentrations of cAMP sufficient to accomplish the activation are unlikely to occur in intact tissues (8).

THE TRANSDUCTION OF RECEPTOR OCCUPANCY TO SECOND-MESSAGE GENERATION

The steps between β-receptor occupancy and adenylyl cyclase activation have been elegantly demonstrated (1). Initially felt to be generalizable to other receptors activating cyclase, it is now clear that the receptor/G-protein interactions of this system are present with minor modifications in several other response cascades.

The schema is illustrated in Figure 2. The components of the system are the receptor, the G-protein heterotrimer, and the catalytic component of adenylyl cyclase. When the receptor is unoccupied, it interacts minimally with the G-protein complex. In this setting the G-protein is present as a heterotrimer, $G_{s\,\alpha,\beta,\gamma}$ The guanylnucleotide binding site on the α-subunit is occupied by GDP and there is

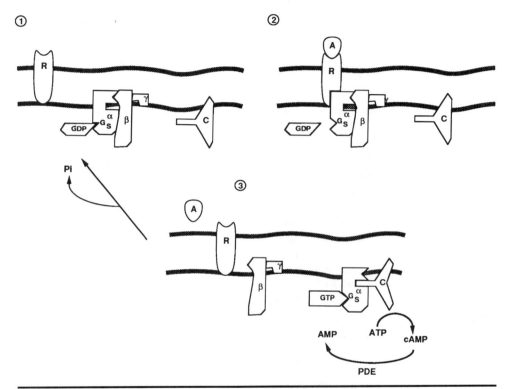

Fig. 2. Receptor-mediated activation of adenylyl cyclase. In the unstimulated state in panel 1, there is minimal interaction between the receptor (R) and the guanyl nucleotide sensitive regulatory heterotrimer ($G_{s\,\alpha,\beta,\gamma}$). In the heterotrimeric state, GDP is bound to $G_{s\alpha}$, and there is minimal interaction with the catalytic component of adenylyl cyclase (C). With the binding of an agonist to the receptor in panel 2, the interaction between R and the heterotrimer is facilitated. As a result of the interaction of R and ($G_{s\,\alpha,\beta,\gamma}$) the affinity of GDP is reduced and GDP dissociates. This form of G_s is very transient, as GDP is rapidly replaced by GTP, present at high concentrations intracellularly in panel 3. GTP reduces the affinity of $G_{s\alpha}$ for $G_{s\beta\gamma}$ and the heterotrimer dissociates, allowing the interaction of $G_{s\alpha}$ with C. This activates C, which catalyzes the conversion of ATP to cAMP, which is then subject to degradation by phosphodiesterases (PDE). Also note that GTP reduces the affinity of R for G_s and the agonist for the receptor. The system is recycled by the hydrolysis of GTP to GDP and inorganic phosphorus (Pi).

minimal interaction of the G-protein with the catalytic component. Receptor occupancy increases its interaction with G-protein, decreasing the affinity of the α-subunit for GDP, which dissociates from its binding site. In isolated membrane preparations that are depleted of GTP, it is possible to demonstrate high affinity-binding of β-adrenergic agonists to the G-protein devoid of guanyl nucleotide, which has been exploited as an index of this interaction. However, in the intact system, GTP, which is present in excess intracellularly, replaces GDP with important consequences. With GTP in the binding site, the G-protein/receptor complex dissociates, as does the $G_{s\,\alpha,\beta,\gamma}$ complex. (The G-protein subunits, β and γ, are virtually always found together and will be referred to as βγ.) Unliganded α-subunits now activate the catalytic subunit. The reaction is recycled by the hydrolysis of GTP by a specific GTPase present on $G_{s\alpha}$.

The model as presented provides several potential sites for regulation: Receptor concentration could be increased or decreased as could the affinity of agents activating the receptor, by covalent modification of the receptor or by changes in other factors acting on the receptor. The ability of the receptor to interact with the G-protein complex could be altered by changes in concentration or affinity of the receptor or G-protein or by modification of the membrane or cytoskeleton. The dissociation of the G-protein complex could be altered by changes in the affinity of GDP and/or GTP for the α-subunit. The ability of the α-subunit to interact with C would change with changing concentration or affinity of either component. As the model is presented (Fig. 2), the βγ-subunit is a regulatory component serving to reduce α-subunit/cyclase interactions. Thus, another level of regulation for this response system is alteration in the concentration of unliganded βγ. This could be accomplished by either discordant (stoichiometrically) synthesis or degradation of $G_{s\alpha}$ and $G_{s\beta\gamma}$ or by the release of βγ from other G-proteins. It can be demonstrated in several systems that βγ-subunits isolated with all of the α-subunits thus far identified are structurally quite similar and functionally identical (1).

MODIFICATION OF RABBIT MYOMETRIAL ADRENERGIC RESPONSES BY STEROIDS

The rabbit uterus provides a useful model in which to examine the modulation of adenylyl cyclase activation. Miller and Marshall demonstrated that the adrenergic contractile response of this organ is strikingly altered by sex steroids (9). The uterus of the estrogen-treated animal responds to hypogastric nerve stimulation in the intact animal or to norepinephrine as muscle strips in isolated muscle bath, with myometrial contraction through activation of α1-adrenergic receptors. However, if estrogen treatment is followed by progesterone, the response to the same stimulators is inhibition of spontaneous contractions mediated by β-adrenergic interactions.

We demonstrated that the β-adrenergic predominance of contractile response in the progesterone-treated animal is accompanied by increased cAMP generation by β-adrenergic agonists in myometrial minces (10) (see Fig. 3). How-

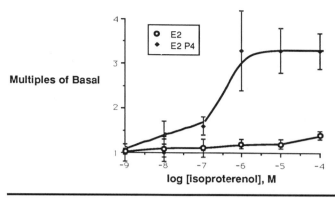

Fig. 3. Reduced β-receptor-stimulated myometrial cAMP generation after estrogen treatment. Virgin rabbits were treated for 4 days with estradiol benzoate, (E_2) 50 μg/kg, or by this treatment followed by progesterone (E_2P_4), 50 mg/kg, for 4 days. Minces prepared from these uteri were incubated with the β-agonist isoproterenol and cAMP measured by radioimmunoassay. Results are the mean of triplicate determinations in four rabbits in each group.

ever, in minces prepared from estrogen-treated animals there is no increase in cAMP generation with β-adrenergic stimulation. This difference in β-adrenergic response was much more striking than the reduced response to activation by PGE_2 or by forskolin, which acts distal to the receptor (Fig. 4).

Since all experiments were performed in the presence of a phosphodiesterase inhibitor, it did not seem likely that these differences were secondary to

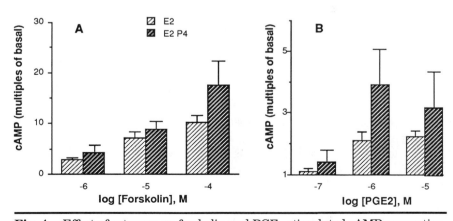

Fig. 4. Effect of estrogen on forskolin and PGE_2-stimulated cAMP generation. Cyclic AMP generation in response to PGE_2 and forskolin, an agent that activates adenylyl cyclase at sites beyond the receptor, were compared in the uterine minces described in Figure 3. Although mean values of generation were lower in E_2 rabbits, these did not achieve statistical significance.

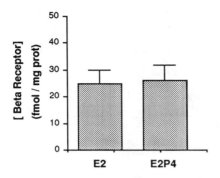

Fig. 5. Similar β-receptor concentration with different hormonal treatments. Membrane particulates from myometrium of rabbits treated as described in Figure 3 were incubated with increasing concentrations of the radioligand [^{125}I]hydroxypindolol and receptor concentration determined by an iterative nonlinear curve-fitting program. Data are the mean and standard error of the mean of 5 experiments with each treatment.

differences in cAMP degradation with the different treatments. We also measured ATP in the myometrium of the differently treated animals and found no differences (10).

This combination of findings suggested that the change with estrogen was at the level of the β-adrenergic receptor. However, the β-receptor concentration was not different in membranes prepared from myometrium of the different animals (11) (see Fig. 5). Similarly, the affinity of isoproterenol was not different nor was the ability of isoproterenol to form high affinity HRG complexes an indirect measure of receptor G_s interactions (12) (see Fig. 6). Therefore, we looked for differences beyond the receptor.

We found that the concentration of $G_{s\alpha}$ as indicated by cholera-toxin-stimulated ADP-ribosylation was reduced in membranes prepared from the myometrium of estrogen treated animals (10) (see Fig. 7). This finding was confirmed by immunoblots using an antibody specific for $G_{s\alpha}$ in membrane preparations of myometrial minces. Since this change was modest compared to the striking decrease in isoproterenol-activated adenylyl cyclase, we attempted to determine changes in functional properties of $G_{s\alpha}$. Two approaches were used. We extracted $G_{s\alpha}$ from the membranes of myometrium from estrogen- and estrogen-progesterone-treated animals and inserted them in the membranes of the S49 lymphoma variant cyc- that lacks functional $G_{s\alpha}$ (10). In these studies, $G_{s\alpha}$ from both treatment groups resulted in coupling of β-receptor occupancy to adenylyl cyclase (Fig. 8). There did, however, appear to be differences in the reconstituted membranes.

In other studies we attempted to use cholera-toxin labeling of $G_{s\alpha}$ as an indicator of G-protein function. We examined the kinetics of cholera-toxin labeling in

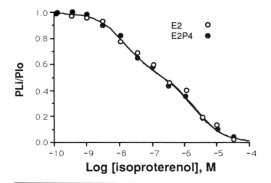

Fig. 6. Lack of effect of estrogen on high-affinity binding of agonists to the β-receptors. Myometrial membrane particulates were prepared from rabbits treated as described in Figure 3. Increasing concentrations of isoproterenol were incubated with particulate and 50 pM [^{125}I]cyanopindolol. Data was analyzed by an iterative nonlinear curve-fitting program and revealed no difference in best fit with the two treatments. In both cases, data described a two-site interaction with the high-affinity binding similar after either treatment (Kh = 6.8 nM for E_2 and 7.5 nM for E_2P_4) as was the percentage of high-affinity binding (% Rh = 48% for E_2 and 42% for E_2P_4).

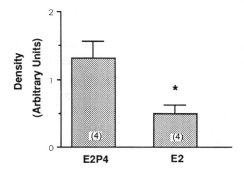

Fig. 7. Cholera-toxin-catalyzed ADP-ribosylation of rabbit myometrial membranes. Data are presented as arbitrary units of integrated area determined by laser scanning densitometry. Data was compared by paired testing of densities of autoradiograms from the same gel after loading similar amounts of protein in each lane. Data is the mean and standard error of the mean of results from 3 separate gels.

membranes from the estrogen- and progesterone-treated rabbits. There was a striking difference in the rate of ADP-ribosylation in these two settings. The half-time of labeling for the estrogen-treated animals was significantly slower ($t_{1/2}$ = 20 min) compared to that of estrogen-progesterone-treated animals ($t_{1/2}$ = 0.5 min). These differences could reflect reduced accessibility of $G_{s\alpha}$ for GTP with estrogen

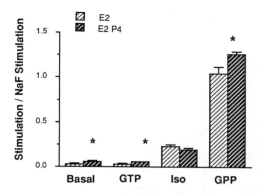

Fig. 8.   Expression of uterine G_s in S49 cyc- membranes. G_s was extracted from uterine membranes from the differently treated rabbits and recombined into cyc-membranes. Adenylyl cyclase activity in response to different effectors was then determined. Data is normalized to NaF-stimulated cyclase activity. ($P < 0.05$.)

treatment consistent with the reduced receptor mediated activation of adenylyl cyclase. However, cholera-toxin ADP-ribosylation is a complex reaction. In addition to $G_{s\alpha}$ and cholera toxin another potentially regulatable protein, ADP-ribosylation factor (ARF), is also required. Thus these findings support altered $G_{s\alpha}$ function with estrogen treatment but may also have other explanations.

In recent experiments we extended these studies to membranes prepared from acutely dispersed myocytes to further probe the mechanisms involved in the regulation of adenylyl cyclase by sex steroids. After enzymatic dispersion and separation on a Percoll gradient, we were able to isolate a preparation of myocytes with less than 15% contamination with other cell types. The use of myocytes allowed the determination that alterations of adenylyl cyclase were in the cell of interest. Additionally, with these isolated cells we were able to prepare a membrane-rich particulate fraction that maintained β-adrenergic responsiveness, which we had not been able to accomplish successfully using membrane preparations of homogenates of intact myometrium. Studies with these membranes confirmed that the difference in cAMP generation was at the level of activation of adenylyl cyclase which was significantly blunted in membranes from estrogen-treated animals.

The β-receptor concentration in these isolated myocytes was not different with the different treatments. However, in preliminary experiments, immuno-blotting of myocyte membrane preparations indicate a much greater reduction of $G_{s\alpha}$ than had previously been appreciated in membranes containing all uterine cell types.

SUMMARY

Receptor-linked adenylyl cyclase acting through kinase A inhibits uterine contractions by several putative mechanisms. The activation of adenylyl cyclase through these receptors present several sites of potential regulation. Our findings have demonstrated that such regulation does occur. Although the exact mechanisms are not yet fully determined, it is apparent that in the rabbit uterus this regulation does not occur by alteration of β-receptor concentration. One likely site of regulation supported by our data is at the level of the transducing G-protein G_s. It is quite likely, however, that the regulation is more complex than simple regulation of the concentration of $G_{s\alpha}$ Regulation of postreceptor responses mediated by G-protein transducers is undoubtedly not limited to the β-adrenergic response system or $G_{s\alpha}$.

REFERENCES

1. Gilman AG. G proteins: transducers of receptor-generated signals. Annu Rev Biochem 1987:615-50.
2. Magnusson MK, Halldorsson H, Kjeld M, Thorgeirsson G. Endothelial inositol phosphate generation and prostacyclin production in response to G-protein activation by AIF. Biochem J 1989;264:703-11.
3. Blackshear PJ, Nairn AC, Kuo JF. Protein kinases 1988: a current perspective. FASEB J 1988;2:2957-69.
4. Korenman SG, Krall JF. The role of cyclic AMP in the regulation of smooth muscle cell contraction in the uterus. Biol Reprod 1977;16:1-17.
5. Meisheri KD, Van Breemen C. Effects of β-adrenergic stimulation on calcium movements in rabbit aortic smooth muscle: relationship with cAMP. J Physiol 1982;331:429-41.
6. Conti MA, Adelstein RS. The relationship between calmodulin binding and phosphorylation of smooth muscle myosin kinase by the catalytic subunit of 3:5 cAMP-dependent protein kinase. J Biol Chem 1981;256:3178-81.
7. Garfield RE. Structural and functional studies of the control of myometrial contractility and labor. In: McNellis D., Challis JRG, MacDonald PC, Nathanielsz PW, Roberts JM, eds. The onset of labor: cellular and integrative mechanisms. Ithaca, NY: Perinatology Press, 1988:55-85.
8. Kamm KE, Stull JT. Regulation of smooth muscle contractile elements by second messengers. Annu Rev Physiol 1989;51:299-313.
9. Miller MD, Marshall JM. Uterine response to nerve stimulation: relation to hormonal status and catecholamines. Am J Physiol 1965;209:859-65.
10. Riemer RK, Wu YY, Bottari SP, Jacobs MM, Goldfien A, Roberts J. Estrogen reduces the function and labelling of the guanyl nucleotide regulatory protein, G_s, in rabbit myometrium. Mol Pharmacol 1988;33:389-95.
11. Roberts JM, Insel PA, Goldfien A. Regulation of myometrial adrenoreceptors and adrenergic response by sex steroids. Mol Pharmacol 1981;20:52-8.
12. Roberts JM, Lewis V, Riemer RK. Hormonal control of uterine adrenergic response. In: Bottari S, Thomas JP, Vokaer A, Vokaer R, eds. Proceedings of the international symposium on uterine contractility. Paris: Masson Publishers, 1982:161-173.

10

Multiple Regulation of the Generation of Inositol Phosphates and cAMP in Myometrium

S. Harbon, S. Marc, O. Goureau, Z. Tanfin, D. Leiber, A. Mokhtari, and L. Do Khac

Endocrinologie et Régulations Cellulaires, Université Paris Sud, Orsay Cédex, France

I n the myometrium as in many other smooth-muscle preparations, Ca^{++} and cAMP, the two major intracellular second messengers, exert opposite effects at the level of contractility. A rise in intracellular Ca^{++} is required to initiate contraction (1, 2), while increase in cAMP content has been demonstrated to contribute to uterine relaxation (3, 4). The increase in intracellular Ca^{++} evoked by stimulatory agonists is considered to originate at least in part from intracellular stores (2, 5, 6). In this regard the phosphoinositide-phospholipase C transducing mechanism that is consistently associated with Ca^{++}-mobilizing receptors (7, 8) has recently been demonstrated to be activated by contracting agonists in different myometrial preparations (9–11). Additionally, a number of recent reported findings provide satisfactory correlations between the increased generation of inositol phosphates, the ability of inositol 1,4,5-trisphosphate to release Ca^{++} from intracellular stores (12, 13) and the accompanying Ca^{++}-induced uterine contractions (10, 13, 14). The objective of this chapter is to summarize some results of our own recent studies that emphasize different mechanisms that may contribute to the modulation of the levels of both inositol phosphates and cAMP in rat and guinea pig myometrial preparations.

Acknowledgments: This work was supported by grants from the Centre National de la Recherche Scientifique (URA 1131) and by a contribution from the Institut National de la Santé et de la Recherche Médicale (CREN 874008). We would like to thank M. H. Sarda and G. Delarbre for carefully preparing the manuscript.

METHODS

Uteri were obtained from immature female Wistar rats (4 weeks old) and Hartley guinea pigs (5 weeks old), pretreated with 30 µg and 160 µg of estradiol, respectively, for 2 days and used the following day. Myometrium was prepared by stripping away the endometrium. For the pregnant rats (at days 12 and 20–21 of gestation), the uterine horns were excised longitudinally, and after removal of fetuses, their sites of attachment, and placenta tissues, myometrium was prepared free of endometrium essentially as reported (15). We have previously described the various methods utilized in this work, including incubation of myometrial strips for the estimation of cAMP (15–17), as well as [^{3}H]inositol phosphate accumulation (9, 10) and the immunological characterization of the α-subunits of G-proteins (18). Specific details are reported in the legends to figures and tables.

MODULATION OF THE GENERATION OF INOSITOL PHOSPHATES IN ESTROGEN-TREATED GUINEA PIG MYOMETRIUM

Receptor and G-Protein Regulation of Phospholipase C

In the intact estrogen-treated guinea pig myometrium prelabeled with [^{3}H]inositol, carbachol and oxytocin were found to cause an enhancement of inositol phosphate accumulation that was potentiated in the presence of 10-mM LiCl (EC$_{50}$ = 15 µM and 20 nM, respectively). Stimulations by carbachol were abolished by atropine, an antagonist of muscarinic receptors. The stimulatory response of oxytocin was markedly attenuated in the presence of the synthetic analog d(CH$_2$)$_5$-D-Phe^2,Ile^4 arginine vasopressine (500 nM), which is an antagonist for both oxytocin and vasopressin receptors (19). However, arginine vasopressin and lysine vasopressin, although causing an accumulation of inositol phosphates, were much less effective than oxytocin. On the other hand, [Thr^4,Gly^7]OT, a specific oxytocin receptor agonist, which is inactive at vasopressin receptors (20), exhibited a potency similar to (if not higher than) oxytocin. These observations strongly suggested that activation of phospholipase C by oxytocin is predominantly an oxytocin receptor-mediated event. It was also found that with both carbachol and oxytocin, there was a rapid increase in IP$_3$ which preceded that of IP$_2$ and IP, with a sequential precursor-product relationship, supporting the interpretation that the primary substrate for receptor-mediated activation of phospholipase C is most probably PtdIns(4,5)P$_2$ (9, 10).

In order to assess the possible role played by a guanine nucleotide binding protein (21–23) in mediating activation of phospholipase C, the ability of NaF plus AlCl$_3$ to affect inositol phosphate generation was examined. We took advantage of the fact that muscarinic receptor activation in the guinea pig myometrium is also coupled to inhibition of adenylate cyclase (14, 17) and demonstrated that treatment of the myometrium with 10 mM NaF plus AlCl$_3$ was able to reproduce the muscarinic receptor-mediated activation of G$_i$ resulting in an attenuation of cAMP accumulation caused by prostacyclin.

Under similar conditions of fluoride treatment and in the presence of Li$^+$, there was an accumulation of each of the 3 inositol phosphates (Fig. 1). Compared with the muscarinic and oxytocin receptor-mediated effects, which were very rapid in onset, a significant delay was observed in response to NaF plus AlCl$_3$. Then the extent of the labeling of total inositol phosphates, reflecting mainly [^{3}H]IP$_2$ + [^{3}H]IP, was roughly linear over 30 min. Nonetheless the accumulation of [^{3}H]IP$_3$ (inset) reached a plateau more rapidly (at 15 min), similar to the situation with carbachol and oxytocin, although in the latter cases the plateau was reached earlier. It was further demonstrated that the increases in inositol phosphates caused by NaF plus AlCl$_3$, which were obtained during tissue incubation in the Li$^+$-containing buffer, could hardly be ascribed to a "Li$^+$-like" effect of F$^-$ on inositol phosphate phosphatases, but were rather consistent with NaF-mediated stimulation at the level of phosphoinositide degradation (i.e., phospholipase C activation) (10). AlCl$_3$ enhanced the fluoride effect, supporting the concept that AlF$_4^-$ was the active species (23). It was thus proposed that a G-protein showing structural

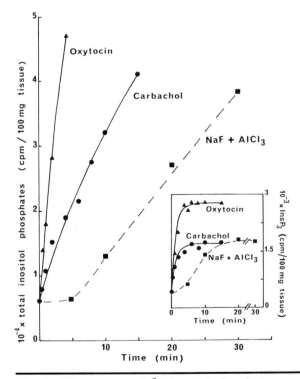

Fig. 1. Time-course of [^{3}H]inositol phosphate accumulation in response to 50 μM carbachol, 0.2 μM oxytocin or 10 mM NaF + 10 μM AlCl$_3$. Values correspond to the combined inositol phosphate peaks. The inset shows the time-dependent accumulation of IP$_3$. (From Marc S, Leiber D, Harbon S, Fluoroaluminates mimic muscarinic- and oxytocin-receptor mediated generation of inositol phosphates and contraction in the intact guinea-pig myometrium, Biochem J 1988;255: 705–13, with permission.)

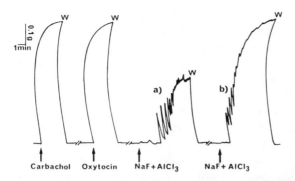

Fig. 2. Tracing of isometric contractions of isolated guinea pig myometrium in response to 5 µM carbachol, 10 mM oxytocin, and 2 mM *(a)* and 10 mM *(b)* NaF in the presence of 10 µM AlCl$_3$. (W = washing.) (From Marc S, Leiber D, Harbon S, Fluoroaluminates mimic muscarinic- and oxytocin-receptor mediated generation of inositol phosphates and contraction in the intact guinea-pig myometrium, Biochem J 1988;255:705–13, with permission.)

resemblance to the well-characterized G-proteins (G$_s$, G$_i$, and transducin) contributes to the activation of phospholipase C in the guinea pig myometrium and that this relevant protein may be involved in the coupling of oxytocin and muscarinic receptors to phospholipase C (10). NaF applied at millimolar concentrations plus 10 µM AlCl$_3$ was able to cause contractions of the guinea pig myometrium (Fig. 2). As was the case with the production of IP$_3$, contraction induced by AlF$_4$- was delayed compared with carbachol- and oxytocin-mediated responses.

Another interesting observation was that maximal contraction could be obtained with NaF (at 10 mM), under conditions where only submaximal increases in inositol phosphates could be observed. This correlates with our previous observations (9) that a small generation of IP$_3$ triggered by carbachol and oxytocin would be sufficient to activate contraction maximally. The data further suggested that contraction elicited by AlF$_4$- may be causally related to its ability to increase IP$_3$ via the activation of the putative G-protein linked to phospholipase C.

Additional experiments illustrated in Figure 3 demonstrated that treatment of myometrial strips with pertussis toxin (21, 22) prevented the activation of G$_i$, which couples muscarinic receptors to inhibition of adenylate cyclase (i.e., the inhibitory effect of carbachol on the rise in cAMP due to prostacyclin could no longer be expressed). In contrast, treatment with pertussis toxin under similar conditions did not affect the receptor-mediated stimulations of inositol phosphates (IP$_3$, IP$_2$, as well as IP), whether elicited by carbachol or oxytocin. Contractions caused by carbachol and oxytocin were similarly unaffected in the pertussis-toxin-treated tissues. The findings clearly suggest that the muscarinic and oxytocin receptors in the guinea pig myometrium are coupled to the activation of phospholipase C and contraction through a pertussis-toxin-insensitive G-protein, which can thus be considered to differ from G$_i$ and probably from G$_o$ (21, 22). Thus, the estrogen-

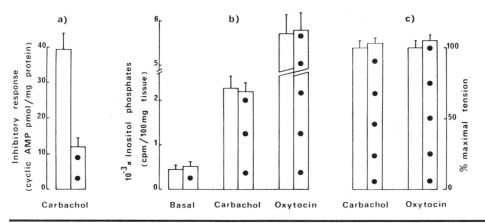

Fig. 3. Differential effects of pertussis toxin on carbachol-induced inhibition of cAMP accumulation and receptor-mediated generation of inositol phosphates and tension. Guinea pig myometrial strips were incubated for 6 h in the absence (open bars) or the presence (dotted bars) of 200-ng of pertussis toxin/ml. When used [^{3}H]inositol was present during the last $3^1/_2$ h of the pertussis-toxin treatment. For the determination of cAMP *(a)*, incubations were carried out for 10 min in the presence of 150-µM IBMX with 1-µM prostacyclin added individually or simultaneously with 1-µM carbachol. For the determination of total [^{3}H]inositol phosphates *(b)*, [^{3}H]inositol prelabeled strips were incubated for 5 min with 100-µM carbachol or 1-µM oxytocin in the presence of 10-mM LiCl. The contractile activity *(c)* was integrated during a 2-min exposure to 5-µM carbachol or 20-nM oxytocin. (From Marc S, Leiber D., Harbon S, Fluoroaluminates mimic muscarinic- and oxytocin-receptor mediated generation of inositol phosphates and contraction in the intact guinea-pig myometrium, Biochem J 1988;255:703–13, with permission.)

treated guinea pig myometrium (10) offers an additional model similar to that reported in the majority (but not all) of cells (24), where Ca^{++}-mobilizing receptors are found to be coupled to phospholipase C through a pertussis-toxin-insensitive G-protein. In this regard, it is worth mentioning a recent report demonstrating that in the estrogen-treated rat myometrium, oxytocin-induced increases in inositol phosphates were affected, although partially, by pertussis toxin (25). The nature of the G-protein involved in receptor-mediated activation of phospholipase C is yet to be established (24).

Role of Ca^{++}

We next examined the role of extracellular Ca^{++} and its influx into cells in controlling the generation of inositol phosphates in the guinea pig myometrium, although in our previous preliminary experiments, a Ca^{++} effect could hardly be detected (9). Omission of Ca^{++} from the incubating medium resulted in a slight (30%) but consistent attenuation of the increased generation of inositol phosphates provoked by carbachol, oxytocin (Fig. 4) and also AlF_4^- (not shown). Basal levels of inositol phosphates were also reduced when Ca^{++} was omitted. Although total inositol phosphate accumulation was attenuated, the degree of stimulability by the specific agonist remained virtually unchanged. It was thus evident that the cascade of the signaling system involving receptor G-protein–phopholipase C interactions was not regulated by an influx of extracellular Ca^{++}. Nevertheless, substantial depletion of intracellular Ca^{++} by treatment of the myometrium in the absence of Ca^{++} with 1 mM EGTA did not only lower basal levels of inositol phosphates but altered severely the stimulation of inositol phosphate accumulation due to carbachol and oxytocin. A minimum content of Ca^{++} was required for an optimal expression of phospholipase C activity (7–9).

High K^+ stimulation, which provokes membrane depolarization and uterine contractions, is the most common method to introduce Ca^{++} into the cells without receptor stimulation. As shown in Figure 4, incubation of myometrial strips in a high (60 mM) K^+ buffer resulted in an increased generation of total inositol phosphates. Stimulations could be demonstrated at the level of each individual inositol phosphate with an early production of IP_3 prior to IP_2 and IP (not shown), indicating that the primary effect of K^+ is on the hydrolysis of $PtdIns(4,5)P_2$, as is the case

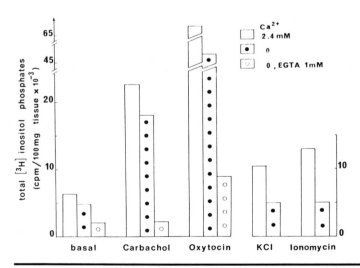

Fig. 4. Effects of ionomycin and high K^+ on inositol phosphate levels in the guinea pig myometrium. Role of Ca^{++} in the receptor-mediated stimulations. [^3H]inositol-labeled myometrial strips were incubated in normal medium (2.4-mM Ca^{++}), a medium without Ca^{++}, or a medium without Ca^{++} and with 1-mM EGTA for 5 min before the addition of 10-mM LiCl. After 10-min further incubation, tissues were treated with 15-µM carbachol, 20-nM oxytocin, 1-µM ionomycin, or 60-mM KCl for 15 min. Values correspond to the combined inositol phosphate peaks (see reference 10).

for agonist- and fluoroaluminate-mediated increases in inositol phosphates. An enhancement in the production of inositol phosphates was similarly provoked by the calcium ionophore ionomycin. Maximal stimulations caused by both ionomycin and high K^+ were lower (3- to 6-fold) than that normally evoked by carbachol or oxytocin. A more important difference was the observation that omission of Ca^{++} from the medium virtually abolished the elevation of inositol phosphates in response to ionomycin and high K^+, a result consistent in both cases with a requirement for influx of extracellular Ca^{++}. It was also found that K^+ and ionomycin-induced increases in inositol phosphates persisted in the presence of inhibitors of the cyclo-oxygenase and lipoxygenases, ruling out the possibility that the Ca^{++}-induced stimulations resulted from the generation of an endogenous arachidonic acid metabolite that might have activated the phospholipase C through the receptor G-protein cascade.

Our findings rather support the contention that two distinct mechanisms contribute to the activation of phospholipase C degrading $PtdIns(4,5)P_2$ in the myometrium, one triggered by a direct receptor coupling via a G-protein and a second induced by rises in intracellular Ca^{++} probably due to an increased influx of the cation. It remained still possible to consider that the Ca^{++} entry-dependent process might also contribute to the 30% attenuation of the overall agonist-induced increases in inositol phosphates detected in myometrial strips when Ca^{++} was withdrawn from the incubation medium. The interpretation was further supported by data in Table 1, illustrating the ability of inhibitors of the voltage-gated Ca^{++} channels—namely, nifedipine and verapamil—to cause an attenuation of the accumulation of inositol phosphates promoted by carbachol and oxytocin. Nifedipine also decreased the inositol phosphate stimulations evoked by fluoroaluminate which bypass receptor interaction. In all cases the degree of inhibition (30%) was quite similar to that elicited by Ca^{++} withdrawal from the medium. Both inhibitors were without effect on basal inositol phosphates accumulated in the presence of Li^+.

Table 1. Inhibitory effects of nifedipine and verapamil on receptor- and AlF_4^--mediated increases in inositol phosphates in the guinea pig myometrium.

Additions	Total Inositol Phosphates (cpm/100 mg of Tissue)		
	0	Nifedipine (250 nM)	Verapamil (50 µM)
Control	$8,791 \pm 975$	$8,212 \pm 811$	$7,612 \pm 800$
Carbachol	$39,802 \pm 2,502$	$21,220 \pm 1,560$	$21,634 \pm 2,000$
Oxytocin	$121,034 \pm 11,800$	$78,218 \pm 4,919$	$81,041 \pm 7,100$
AlF_4^-	$212,713 \pm 22,493$	$164,969 \pm 14,969$	

Note: $[^3H]$inositol-labeled myometrial strips were incubated in the absence and presence of nifedipine or verapamil for 1 min and treated for 20 min with carbachol (15 µM), oxytoxine (20 nM) and AlF_4^- (20-mM NaF + 10-µM $AlCl_3$) in the presence of 10-mM LiCl. Values correspond to total inositol phosphates (see references 9 and 10).

The cumulative data agree with the recent proposal made by Eberhard and Holz (25) for the presence in excitable tissues of two distinct mechanisms involved in the activation of phospholipase C degrading PtdIns(4,5)P$_2$. Our present findings would then tend to imply that in the guinea pig myometrium, beside the direct coupling of receptors (oxytocin, muscarinic) via a G-protein to phospholipase C activation (a process that contributes predominantly to the receptor-mediated increases in inositol phosphates), there is an additional functional coupling of cell surface receptors most probably through a G-protein (mimicked by fluoroaluminates) to the activation of voltage-operated Ca^{++} channels, the resulting rises in intracellular Ca^{++} being then responsible for the additional, although modest (30%), Ca^{++}-mediated phospholipase C activation. The mechanisms that link muscarinic and oxytocin receptors to the activation of voltage-operated Ca^{++} channels whether direct or indirect (e.g., as a consequence of the generation of a second messenger [2, 26, 27]) has yet to be clarified.

PHARMACOLOGICAL EVIDENCE FOR DISTINCT MUSCARINIC RECEPTOR SUBTYPES COUPLED TO INHIBITION OF ADENYLATE CYCLASE AND TO INCREASED GENERATION OF INOSITOL PHOSPHATES IN THE GUINEA PIG MYOMETRIUM

In recent years, pharmacological evidence has indicated the existence of multiple subtypes of muscarinic receptors. At least three subtypes, termed M$_1$, M$_2$, M$_3$, have been proposed. They can be differentiated on the basis of affinity for the antagonists pirenzepine, AF-DX116, and 4-DAMP (28). The classification of muscarinic receptor subtypes has further been extended by the cloning of a family of at least five distinct but highly homologous subtypes coded by five different genes (29). Our demonstration that in the estrogen-dominated guinea pig myometrium, stimulation of muscarinic receptors is associated, via G$_i$, with the inhibitory pathway of the adenylate cyclase and via G$_p$, a pertussis-toxin-insensitive G-protein, with an increased generation of inositol phosphates, provided an interesting model to address the question of whether a single receptor subtype is coupled to a single effector, or whether each muscarinic receptor subtype can interact with multiple effectors. Our findings (Fig. 5) demonstrate that the muscarinic receptors coupled to the adenylate cyclase and phospholipase C can be differentiated by virtue of their sensitivity to the full agonist, carbachol, and the efficiency by which two partial agonists— oxotremorine and pilocarpine—elicit the receptor-mediated second-messenger response. This was clearly illustrated, first, by the greater potency of carbachol in inhibiting cAMP formation (EC$_{50}$ = 8 nM) than in stimulating the accumulation of inositol phosphates and tension (EC$_{50}$ = 15 μM and 2 μM, respectively) and, second, by the weak ability of oxotremorine and pilocarpine to activate phospholipase C versus their apparently full efficacy in inhibiting cAMP accumulation. In addition, both oxotremorine and pilocarpine were able to attenuate the stimulations normally evoked by carbachol at the level of inositol phosphate generation.

Data shown in Table 2 summarize the effects of discriminating antagonists—pirenzepine, AF-DX116, and 4-DAMP—at the level of functional and

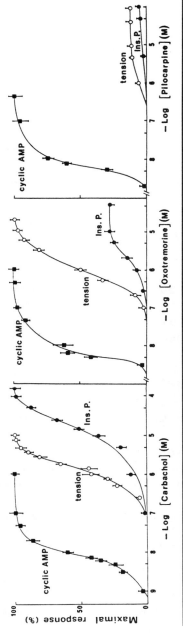

Fig. 5. Differential effects of carbachol, oxotremorine, and pilocarpine on the inhibition of cAMP accumulation and on the generation of inositol phosphates and tension in the guinea pig myometrium. Results are expressed as the percentage of each specific response to a maximal effective concentration of carbachol. The maximal response elicited by carbachol was for cAMP inhibition (53-pmol cAMP) and for total inositol phosphates (280% percent stimulation above basal). (From Leiber D, Marc S, Harbon S, Pharmacological evidence for distinct muscarinic receptor subtypes coupled to the inhibition of adenylate cyclase and to the increased generation of inositol phosphates in the guinea pig myometrium, J Pharmacol Exp Ther 1990;252:800–809, with permission.)

Table 2.   Differential Ki values for atropine, pirenzepine, AF-DX116, and
4-DAMP to antagonize carbachol-mediated responses in estrogen-dominated
guinea pig myometrium.

	Ki (nM)		
	cAMP	Inositol Phosphates	Tension
Atropine	0.37 ± 0.02	1.15 ± 0.1	0.8 ± 0.04
Pirenzepine	286 ± 31	92 ± 6	110 ± 9
AF-DX116	1.14 ± 0.15	346 ± 35	$K_H = 1 ± 0.07$ (24%)
			$K_L = 100 ± 5$ (76%)
4-DAMP	314 ± 12	0.3 ± 0.03	0.24 ± 0.04

Source: Data from from Leiber D, Marc S, Harbon S, Pharmacological evidence for distinct muscarinic receptor subtypes coupled to the inhibition of adenylate cyclase and to the increased generation of inositol phosphates in the guinea pig myometrium, J Pharmacol Exp Ther 1990;252:800–809, with permission.

biochemical (i.e., second-messenger generation) responses. As expected, atropine, the conventional antagonist, was equipotent in antagonizing the different muscarinic responses displaying Ki values in nanomolar ranges. Pirenzepine was unable to discriminate between the diverse muscarinic responses. Ki values of pirenzepine for inhibiting the generation of inositol phosphates and tension (92 and 110 nM, respectively) were almost identical to that (286 nM) for reversing cAMP attenuation. This relative moderate antagonistic activity displayed by pirenzepine allowed the interpretation that an M_1 receptor subtype does not contribute to any of the two signaling systems and likewise to the contractile response associated with muscarinic stimulations in the guinea pig myometrium. On the other hand, our findings obtained with AF-DX116 and 4-DAMP allowed us to discriminate between the muscarinic-mediated inositol phosphate and cAMP responses. Judging by its high sensitivity to AF-DX116 (Ki = 1.14 nM) and its relatively low sensitivity to both pirenzepine and 4-DAMP, carbachol-mediated attenuation of the cAMP response could be considered to reflect an interaction with the M_2 receptor subtype. Based on the low antagonistic properties of both AF-DX116 (Ki = 346 nM) and pirenzepine, as opposed to the high affinity displayed by 4-DAMP (Ki = 0.3 nM), it is possible to postulate that the M_3 receptor subtype is involved in carbachol-mediated activation of phospholipase C. In light of the involvement of both a low- and a high-affinity component in the inhibitory effect of AF-DX116 on uterine contractions, it is reasonable to propose that the M_2 receptor subtype, most probably through the accompanying decrease in cAMP, may contribute to the modulation of contraction which remained essentially (76%) triggered by the M_3 receptor subtype. Taken together, the data additionally support the contention for an exclusive second-messenger response associated with a defined muscarinic receptor subtype interacting with a specific regulatory G-protein (14).

MODULATORY MECHANISMS REGULATING LEVELS OF INTRACELLULAR cAMP IN PREGNANT RAT MYOMETRIUM

Cross-Talk Between Stimulatory and Inhibitory Pathways of Adenylate Cyclase Signals

In the estrogen-dominated rat myometrium (15, 16, 30), the adenylate cyclase cAMP forming system can be enhanced by way of receptor activation (β-adrenergic, prostaglandin E_2, prostacyclin) via the stimulatory regulatory protein G_s by cholera toxin, which activates G_s, as well as by forskolin, which interacts with the catalytic unit of the adenylate cyclase (16, 30, 31). The responsiveness to these agonists of myometrial strips obtained at different stages of gestation is illustrated in Figure 6. In all cases, the onset of gestation was accompanied by a progressive decline in the cAMP responses, compared to the corresponding maximal responses observed in the estrogen-dominated myometrium (considered as day 0), with no more than 10% stimulations being expressed in the day-12 tissue. The phase of attenuated responsiveness to the diverse stimulations in terms of cAMP accumulation was followed by a gradual and total restoration phase just before parturition, except for PGs, whose cAMP stimulatory responses remained impaired during the whole gestation period. The decline in isoproterenol-mediated cAMP accumulation could not be

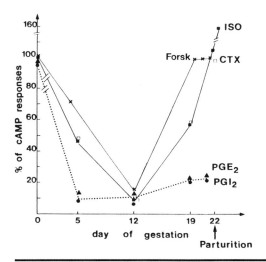

Fig. 6. Evolution of cAMP accumulation in the rat myometrium throughout gestation. Myometrial strips obtained from rats at the indicated day of gestation were incubated for 7 min with 240-μM IBMX in the presence of 0.1-μM isoproterenol (Iso, solid square), 10-μM PGE_2 (solid triangle), 5-μM PGI_2 (solid circle), 10 μM forskolin (Forsk, X). Treatment with cholera toxin (CTX, open square) was for 120 min. Results are expressed as the percentage of control responses (day 0: estrogen-treated). (From Tanfin Z, Harbon S, Heterologous regulations of cAMP responses in pregnant rat myometrium: evolution from a stimulatory to an inhibitory prostaglandin E_2 and prostacyclin effect, Mol Pharmacol 1987;32:249–57, with permission.)

ascribed to alterations in either β-adrenergic receptor density or coupling properties (15). Of much interest was the finding that treatment of day 12-myometrium
(midgestation) with pertussis toxin, which is known to alter the function of G_i,
improved markedly the β-adrenergic-elicited cAMP accumulation as well as the
stimulations caused by cholera toxin (Fig. 7).

Using the ability of cholera toxin to specifically label, via an ADP-
riboysylation reaction, the α_s-subunits, it was possible to demonstrate the existence
in different myometrial membranes of a major 52 kD and two minor 45 kD/53 kD
corresponding to the α_s-subunits. Data pertaining to the extent of incorporation of
ADP-ribose due to cholera toxin suggested that the level of α_s was consistently
lower in day-12 membranes compared to the day-0 preparations (15). Riemer et al.
(32) recently reported a modulatory effect of estrogen on the extent of labeling of
α_s-subunits by cholera toxin in rabbit myometrium. Using varied α_i-subunit specific antisera (33, 34), we further identified G_{i2} as a major G_i form in rat
myometrium (Fig. 8). Immunoblotting of rat myometrial membranes with an
antiserum (SG1), which recognizes the α-subunits of both G_{i1} and G_{i2} (see the brain
membranes), indicated the presence of detectable levels of an apparently single
polypeptide form with an electrophoretic mobility identical to brain α_{i2}. A second
antiserum (LE$_2$) specific for G_{i2} also recognized this protein, confirming its identity

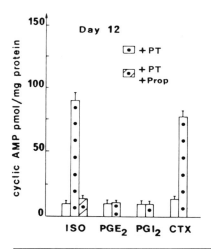

Fig. 7.   Effect of pertussis-toxin (PT) pretreatment of isoproterenol-, cholera
toxin-, and PG-mediated cAMP accumulation in day-12 rat myometrium. Treatment with PT (200 ng/ml) was for 6 h. This was followed by a 7-min incubation
with 0.1-μM isoproterenol (Iso) or 0.1-μM Iso + 1-μM propranolol (Prop), 10-μM
PGE$_2$ or 5-μM PGI$_2$. Cholera toxin (CTX) at 30 nM was present during the last 2
h of PT treatment. (From Tanfin Z, Harbon S, Heterologous regulations of cAMP
responses in pregnant rat myometrium: evolution from a stimulatory to an
inhibitory prostaglandin E$_2$ and prostacyclin effect, Mol Pharmacol 1987;32:
249–57, with permission.)

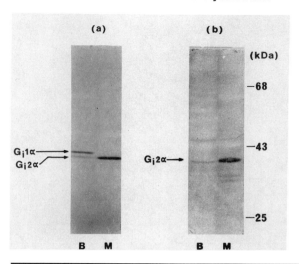

Fig. 8. Identification of $G_i2\alpha$ and absence of $G_i1\alpha$ in rat myometrium. Membrane from either rat brain (B) or estrogen-treated rat myometrium (M) were resolved on SDS-polyacrylamide gel (12.5% [w/v] acrylamide) and immunoblotted as described (18). The blot was developed using antiserum SGl (1:200 dilution), which recognizes the α-subunit of both G_{i1} and G_{i2} as the primary reagent *(a)*. A similar experiment was performed except that the primary antiserum was a 1:200 dilution of LE_2, which displays specificity for $G_i2\alpha$ *(b)*. (From Milligan G, Tanfin Z, Goureau O, Unson C, Harbon S, Identification of both G_{i2} and a novel immunologically distinct form of G_o in rat myometrial membranes, FEBS Lett 1989;244:411–6, with permission.)

(18). Recent findings (unpublished) now demonstrate that G_{i3} is additionally present in the rat myometrial preparations. Of relevance was the increase (75%) noted for G_{i2} at the midgestation phase, which together with the apparent decrease in G_s may provide an explanation for the amplified expression of G_i (i.e., altered G_s-mediated activation of cAMP and its reversal by pertussis toxin).

The latest phase of gestation (day 21) was characterized by a full restoration of adenylate cyclase responsiveness toward isoproterenol and cholera toxin. In marked contrast, the inability of PGE_2 (and similarly of PGI_2), which emerged at the onset of gestation, was still retained and coincided with the development of a G_i-mediated inhibitory PG effect. This is illustrated (Fig. 9) by the findings that in day-21 myometrium, PGE_2 and $PGF_{2\alpha}$ attenuated markedly the rises in cAMP caused by isoproterenol with a half-maximal effect at 2 nM. Pretreatment of the myometrium with pertussis-toxin-suppressed PGE_2-mediated inhibition of cAMP accumulation, indicative of a functional interaction of PG receptors with the inhibitory pathway of the cyclase. Thus the PG-mediated effect at the level of cAMP which was exclusively stimulatory in the day-0 myometrium appeared exclusively inhibitory at the end of gestation. The differential characteristics of both effects (dose dependency, agonist specificity) would suggest the presence in the myo-

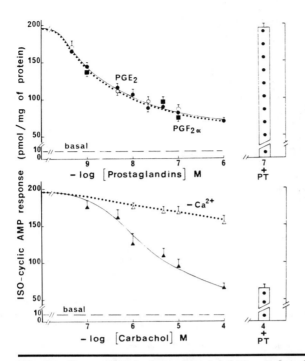

Fig. 9. Concentration-dependent inhibition induced by prostaglandins (PGE$_2$, PGF$_{2\alpha}$) and carbachol on cAMP accumulation due to isoproterenol in the pregnant, day-21 rat myometrium. Differential effects of Ca^{++} and pertussis toxin. Myometrial strips were incubated for 15 min in a normal (2.4 nM) Krebs buffer (closed symbols) or in a Ca^{++}-deprived medium containing 1-mM EGTA. Incubations were for 7 min in the presence of 240-µM IBMX with 0.3 µM isoproterenol alone or combined with carbachol (solid triangle, open triangle), PGE$_2$ (open circle, closed circle), or PGF$_{2\alpha}$ (solid square). Treatment with pertussis toxin (PT, 200 ng/ml) was for 6 h.

metrium of distinct types of PG receptors, namely, stimulatory and inhibitory, coupled to the adenylate cyclase as well as control mechanisms operating during gestation at the level of their functional expression.

Interactions Between cAMP and Ca^{++} Signals

In the day-21 myometrium, carbachol was similarly able to attenuate the rise in cAMP caused by isoproterenol in the presence of 240-µM IBMX, with an EC$_{50}$ at 2 µM (Fig. 9). In marked contrast to PGE$_2$-induced inhibition, the attenuation of cAMP due to carbachol was insensitive to pertussis toxin, suggesting that the inhibitory pathway of the cyclase was not involved. Moreover, the muscarinic receptor-mediated decreases in cAMP were abolished in Ca^{++}-depleted preparations under conditions where both the stimulatory (isoproterenol-activated) and inhibitory (PGE$_2$-activated) pathways of the cyclase were not affected. These findings substantiated the interpretation that the muscarinic receptor-mediated attenuation of cAMP in the day-21 myometrium did not involve the inhibitory pathway of the cyclase but could rather be due, at least in part, to a Ca^{++}-mediated activation of cAMP degradation. In additional experiments (not reported), it was possible to demonstrate that a Ca^{++}-dependent phosphodiesterase activity could be expressed in the intact myometrial strips stimulated by carbachol.

Data in Figure 10 further illustrate that the ability of carbachol to attenuate cAMP accumulation coincided with the capacity of the muscarinic agonist to increase the generation of inositol phosphates. Both effects displayed a superposable dose dependency and were similarly unaffected by pertussis toxin. Oxotremorine, which produced a partial increased generation of inositol phosphates, was similarly able to cause only a partial attenuation of the cAMP response

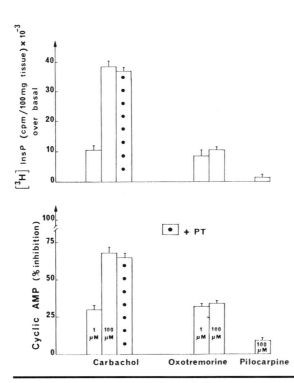

Fig. 10. A comparative effect of different muscarinic agonists on the attenuation of cAMP accumulation and on the increased generation of inositol phosphates in the pregnant, day-21 rat myometrium. For the estimation of cAMP, tissue strips were incubated, as in Figure 9, with 0.3-μM isoproterenol alone or combined with the indicated concentration of carbachol, oxotremorine, or pilocarpine. For the accumulation of total inositol phosphates, [^{3}H]inositol-labeled strips were incubated in the presence of 10-mM LiCl and stimulated for 10 min with the muscarinic agonist.

compared to the full muscarinic agonist carbachol. Finally, pilocarpine at concentrations as high as 100 μM was unable to elicit any increase in the generation of inositol phosphates and concurrently failed to cause any attenuation in the accumulation of cAMP. These data support our proposal for a carbachol-mediated enhancement of a Ca^{++}-dependent phosphodiesterase activity, compatible with the rises in Ca^{++} associated with muscarinic-induced increased generation of inositol phosphates (35). They further illustrate that a cross-talk between the two second-messenger generating systems contributed to an ultimate decrease in cAMP. The combined rises in Ca^{++} and decline in cAMP would tend to enhance the contractile activity of the uterus at the onset of parturition.

REFERENCES

1. Izumi H. Changes in the mechanical properties of the longitudinal and circular muscle tissues of the rat myometrium during gestation. Br J Pharmacol 1985;86: 247-57.
2. van Breemen C, Saida K. Cellular mechanisms regulating $[Ca^{2+}]$ in smooth muscle. Annu Rev Physiol 1989;51:315-29.
3. Hardman JG. Cyclic nucleotides and smooth muscle contraction: some conceptual and experimental considerations. In: Bulbring E, Braching AF, Jones AW, Tomita T, eds. Smooth muscle: an assessment of current knowledge. London: Edward Arnold, 1981:249-62.
4. Do Khac L, Mokhtari A, Harbon S. A re-evaluated role for cAMP in uterine relaxation. Differential effect of isoproterenol and forskolin. J Pharmacol Exp Ther 1986;239: 236-42.
5. Somlyo AP, Himpens B. Cell calcium and its regulation in smooth muscle. FASEB J 1989;3:2266-76.
6. Mironneau C, Mironneau J, Savineau JP. Maintained contractions of rat uterine smooth muscle incubated in a Ca^{2+}-free solution. Br J Pharmacol 1984;82:735-43.
7. Berridge MJ, Irvine RF. Inositol trisphosphate, a novel second messenger in cellular signal transduction. Nature (Lond) 1984;312:315-21.
8. Berridge MJ. Inositol trisphosphate and diacylglycerol: two interacting second messengers. Annu Rev Biochem 1987;56:159-93.
9. Marc S, Leiber D, Harbon S. Carbachol and oxytocin stimulate the generation of inositol phosphates in the guinea pig myometrium. FEBS Lett 1986;201:9-14.
10. Marc S, Leiber D, Harbon S. Fluoroaluminates mimic muscarinic- and oxytocin-receptor mediated generation of inositol phosphates and contraction in the intact guinea-pig myometrium. Biochem J 1988;255:705-13.
11. Anwer K, Hovington JA, Sanborn BM. Antagonism of contractants and relaxants at the level of intracellular calcium and phosphoinositide turnover in the rat uterus. Endocrinology 1989;124:2995-3002.
12. Carsten ME, Miller JD. Ca^{2+} release by inositol trisphosphate from Ca^{2+}-transporting microsomes derived from uterine sarcoplasmic reticulum. Biochem Biophys Res Comm 1985;130:1027-31.
13. Kanmura Y, Missiaen L, Casteels R. Properties of intracellular calcium stores in pregnant rat myometrium. Br J Pharmacol 1988;95:284-90.
14. Leiber D, Marc S, Harbon S. Pharmacological evidence for distinct muscarinic recep-

tor subtypes coupled to the inhibition of adenylate cyclase and to the increased generation of inositol phosphates in the guinea pig myometrium. J Pharmacol Exp Ther 1990;252:800-9.

15. Tanfin Z, Harbon S. Heterologous regulations of cAMP responses in pregnant rat myometrium: evolution from a stimulatory to an inhibitory prostaglandin E_2 and prostacyclin effect. Mol Pharmacol 1987;32:249-57.

16. Vesin MF, Do Khac L, Harbon S. Prostacyclin as an endogenous modulator of adenosine cyclic 3'5'-monophosphate levels in rat myometrium and endometrium. Mol Pharmacol 1979;16:823-40.

17. Mokhtari A, Do Khac L, Harbon S. Forskolin alters sensitivity of the cAMP-generating system to stimulatory as well as to inhibitory agonists. Eur J Biochem 1988;176:131-7.

18. Milligan G, Tanfin Z, Goureau O, Unson C, Harbon S. Identification of both G_{i2} and a novel immunologically distinct form of G_0 in rat myometrial membranes. FEBS Lett 1989;244:411-6.

19. Manning M, Olma A, Klis WA, Seto J, Sawyer WH. Potent antagonists of the antidiuretic responses to arginine-vasopressin based on modifications of [1-(β-mercapto-β,β-cyclopentamethylene propionic acid),2-D-phenylalanine, 4-valine] arginine-vasopressin at position 4. J Med Chem 1983;26:1607-13.

20. Lowbridge J, Manning M, Haldar J, Sawyer WH. Synthesis and some pharmacological properties of [4-threonine,7-glycine] oxytocin, [1-(L-2-hydroxy-3-mercaptopropanoic acid), 4-threonine, 7 glycine] oxytocin, (hydroxy[Thr^4,Gly^7] oxytocin, and [7-glycine] oxytocin, peptides with high oxytocic-antidiuretic selectivity. J Med Chem 1977;20:120-23.

21. Gilman AG. G proteins: transducers of receptor-generated signals. Annu Rev Biochem 1987;56:615-49.

22. Casey PJ, Gilman AG. G protein involvement in receptor-effector coupling. J Biol Chem 1988;263:2577-80

23. Bigay J, Deterre P, Pfister C, Chabre M. Fluoride complexes of aluminium of beryllium act on G proteins as reversibly bound analogues of the γ phosphate of GTP. EMBO J 1987;6: 2907-13.

24. Boyer JL, Hepler JR, Harden TK. Hormone and growth factor receptor-mediated regulation of phospholipase C activity. Trends Pharmacol Sci 1989;10:360-4

25. Eberhard DA, Holz RW. Intracellular Ca^{2+} activates phospholipase C. Trends Neurosci 1988;11:517-20.

26. Yatani A, Codina J, Imoto Y, Reeves JP, Birnbaumer L, Brown AM. A G protein directly regulates mammalian calcium channels. Science 1987;238:1288-92.

27. Rosenthal W, Hescheler J, Trautwein W, Schultz G. Control of voltage-dependent Ca^{2+} channels by G protein-coupled receptors. FASEB J. 1988;2:2784-90.

28. Doods HN, Mathy MJ, Davidesko D, van Charldorp KJ, De Jonge A, van Zwieten PA. Selectivity of muscarinic antagonists in radioligand and in vivo experiments for the putative M_1, M_2 and M_3 receptors. J Pharmacol Exp Ther 1987;242:257-62.

29. Bonner TI. The molecular basis of muscarinic receptor diversity. Trends Neurosci 1989;12:148-51.

30. Mokhtari A, Do Khac L, Tanfin Z, Harbon S. Forskolin modulates cAMP generation in the rat myometrium. Interaction with isoproterenol and prostaglandins E_2 and I_2. J Cyclic Nucleotide Protein Phosphor Res 1985;10:213-28.

31. Seamon KB, Daly JW. Forskolin: its biological and chemical properties. Adv Cyclic Nucleotide Protein Phosphor 1986;20:1 -150.

32. Riemer RK, Wu YY, Bottari SP, Jacobs MM, Goldfien A, Roberts JM. Estrogen reduces β-adrenoreceptor-mediated cAMP production and the concentration of the guanyl nucleotide-regulatory protein, G_s, in rabbit myometrium. Mol Pharmacol 1988;33:389-95.

33. Milligan G. Techniques used in the identification and analysis of function of pertussis toxin-sensitive guanine nucleotide binding proteins. Biochem J 1988;255:1-13.

34. Goldsmith P, Gierschik P, Milligan G, et al. Antibodies directed against synthetic peptides distinguish between GTP-binding proteins in neutrophil and brain. J Biol Chem 1987;262:14683-8.

35. Nakakata N, Martin MW, Hughes AR, Hepler JR, harden TK. H1-histamine receptors on human astrocytoma cells. Mol Pharmacol 1986;29:188-95.

THE CHANGING HORMONAL ENVIRONMENT

11

Distribution of Prostaglandin Synthesizing and Metabolizing Enzymes in Intrauterine Tissues

J. R. G. Challis,[1] R. A. Jacobs,[1] S. C. Riley,[1] D. P. Boshier,[2] V. K. Han,[1] W. Smith,[3] P. Y. C. Cheung,[1] D. Langlois,[1] and L. J. Fraher[1]

[1]*Lawson Research Institute, St. Joseph's Health Centre, MRC Group in Fetal and Neonatal Health and Development, London, Ontario, Canada;* [2]*Department of Anatomy, University of Auckland, New Zealand; and* [3]*Department of Anatomy, Michigan State University, East Lansing*

A central role for prostaglandins (PG) in the stimulus to myometrial contractility at term has been suggested by many investigators (1, 2). However, at the present time there remains conjecture about which PGs are involved in this process, whether bioactive agents other than PGs may have an obligatory role, and which intrauterine tissues are major sites of stimulatory PG biosynthesis. The use of in vitro systems to examine controls of PG output is conducted with loss of in vivo cellular architecture, and in homogenate or subcellular fractions without knowledge of the activities of particular cell types. Further, the cell types present in in vitro culture systems are often not characterized. Different results are obtained for different periods in culture; for example, as placental trophoblast cells form a syncytium and as amnion cells may reach confluency (3). For these reasons, we initiated a series of studies to examine the localization of prostaglandin H_2 synthase (PGHS) and 15-hydroxy prostaglandin dehydrogenase (PGDH) by immunocytochemistry in intrauterine tissues from sheep and women during pregnancy. In sheep, control of PG synthesis prepartum is generally considered to reflect the systemic influence of circulating steroids (4). In women, a vast body of evidence suggests that the fetal membranes and decidua are

Acknowledgments: This work was supported by the Canadian Medical Research Council (Group Grant in Fetal and Neonatal Health and Development, JRGC; and by grants from the Lawson Research Institute). We gratefully acknowledge the provision of purified human placental PGDH from D. Tai, University of Kentucky.

major sources of PG output, and regulation is effected through paracrine and/or autocrine influences.

DISTRIBUTION OF PG BIOSYNTHETIC AND METABOLIC ENZYMES IN SHEEP

In sheep, the PG content of the fetal membranes, endometrium, and cotyledons increases with progressive gestation (5), correlating with increased capacity for PG output by dispersed cell preparations from these tissues in vitro (6) and an increase in PG concentrations in amniotic fluid (7) and fetal plasma (8). Amnion seems unlikely to be the major source of PGs prepartum in this species. The amnion does not extend into a nonpregnant horn in singleton pregnancies yet uterine activity evolves similarly in both horns (9). In addition, amnion is separated from chorion over much of its surface by the allantois (10). The cotyledons have been identified biochemically as sources of PG production. Their distribution throughout the uterus situates them ideally to produce PGs that might act in a paracrine fashion on underlying endometrium and myometrium. Alternatively, PG produced in the cotyledons may reach the myometrium through the systemic circulation (11).

At euthanasia we obtained amnion and cotyledons from sheep at different stages of pregnancy. Tissues were fixed in Bouin's fluid, and embedded in paraffin. The paraffin blocks were sectioned at 5 μ, deparaffinized, rehydrated, and stained for prostaglandin H_2 synthase (PGHS) or 15-hydroxy prostaglandin dehydrogenase (PGDH), using the avidin-biotin procedure (Vector ABC Dimension Laboratories, Mississauga, Ontario). The PGHS antibody was raised in rabbits against PGHS purified from ram seminal vesicles and, at specificity, determined by Western blot analysis (12). It was used at a final dilution of 1:1000 to 1:2000. The PGDH antibody (Cayman Company, Ann Arbor, Michigan), raised in rabbits against purified human placental PGDH, was used at a final dilution of 1:2000 to 1:3000. Purified PGHS was obtained from Cayman Company. Purified human placental PGDH was a generous gift from D. Tai (University of Kentucky). Sections were counterstained with Carrazzi's hematoxylin. As negative controls, sections were incubated in the absence of primary antibody, with nonimmune rabbit serum instead of the primary antibody, or after pre-absorption with 1–5μM purified antigen.

By day 45 of gestation (term = day 145), positive staining for PGHS was present in sheep cotyledons, but it was confined to single cells or small clusters of cells in the maternal villous epithelial syncytium (13). There was no immuno-reactive PGHS in the villous trophoblast epithelium or stromal tissue, nor in binucleate cells. This pattern of staining persisted until day 80. Between day 80 and day 100, positive PGHS immunostaining had virtually disappeared. By day 100 there was little or no PGHS immunoactivity in either maternal or fetal tissue components of the placenta, although immunoactive PGHS was localized to endo-thelial cells of blood vessels in the endometrium underlying the placenta. By day 125 immunoreactive PGHS was again expressed in the cotyledon but was now present exclusively in the epithelium of the villous trophoblast. Positive staining was absent from maternal tissue and absent from the binucleate cells. This pattern of immunostaining, confined to the villous trophoblast epithelium within the zona intima and zona intermedia of the cotyledon, persisted until term. Within approximately 7 days of term, two additional subsets of cells appeared which stained positively for PGHS. These subsets were localized at tips of fronds of maternal villous tissue projecting into the hemophagus zone of the placenta and in a subset of cells localized at the base of the cotyldeon in regions where maternal villi originate from the underlying endometrium. PGHS immunoactivity was abolished by preabsorbing the primary antibody with 1-μM purified PGHS, and positive staining was absent when the sections were incubated with nonimmune rabbit serum or in the absence of the primary antibody.

We also sought PGHS immunoactivity in sheep amnion (13). There was no positive staining in tissue collected at day 45 of gestation. PGHS immunoactivity was expressed by day 65, but was confined to a subepithelial population of fibroblasts. There was no PGHS staining in the amniotic epithelium. This pattern persisted at day 100 and at term: PGHS staining in amnion remaining in the subepithelial layer and never appearing in the epithelium.

Thus, the pattern of PGHS immunostaining in sheep cotyledons and amnion shows discrete tissue-specific patterns. In the placenta, immunoactive PGHS is present only in maternal villi during the first half of pregnancy. PGHS expression decreases, only to be promoted in the trophoblast epithelium after days 110–115. In contrast, PGHS is expressed in amnion by day 65, but in a subepithelial population of cells, and remains throughout gestation. This different pattern might indicate that amnion and placental PGHS expression are controlled by different factors. In particular, the inhibition and later expression of PGHS in the placenta may reflect paracrine control mechanisms. At this time, one can only speculate on what these may be. Interferon α (IFN α) inhibits PGE_2 and $PGF_{2\alpha}$ output from cultured ovine endometrial cells by direct and indirect actions on PGHS activity/expression (14). IFN α reproduces the effects of ovine trophoblast protein 1 (oTP 1) in inhibiting endometrial PG synthesis. There is a high sequence homology between these polypeptides, and the current view is that IFN α is responsible for the suppression of endometrial PG production necessary to protect the corpus luteum of early pregnancy (14). It is possible that the effects of IFN α persist until day 60 to day 80. Alternatively, TGF β inhibits PG production from human amnion cells and A431 cells (15) and could exert a similar effect in the sheep uterus. The factors responsible for turning on PGHS expression during the last 40 days of pregnancy are unclear. The prepartum increase in systemic PGE_2 and $PGF_{2\alpha}$ concentrations have been attributed to the influences of an altered relative output of estradiol and progesterone from the placenta, consequent upon fetal hypothalamic-pituitary-adrenal (HPA) activation (16). But, expression of PGHS by days 110–115 in the placenta precedes HPA activation, and an alternate induction mechanism must be invoked. It should be noted that all previous measurements of PG synthetic activity using dispersed cells, cultured cells, homogenates, and microsomal preparations of tissue have failed to identify the subtle, yet presumably important, switch in PGHS expression from maternal to villous trophoblast.

The output of bioactive PG from the placenta depends on PG synthetic and PG metabolic activities. Therefore, we sought localization of PGDH in sections of sheep placental tissue throughout pregnancy (17). By days 45–54 PGDH immunostaining was present in the placenta, localized to both trophoblast epithelium and diffused throughout the stromal core tissue of the maternal villi. PGDH activity was not present in binucleate cells. Through pregnancy there was a gradual diminution in relative staining in the maternal villi, and at term immunoactive PGDH was localized almost exclusively to the trophoblast epithelium. This pattern is consistent with measurements suggesting that PGDH activity in the fetal cotyledon increases during pregnancy, whereas maternal PGDH activity decreases with labor (18). Unfortunately, the technical difficulties associated with separating the fetal and maternal components of the cotyledon compromised interpretation of this information.

Most attention has favored on cyclo-oxygenase products of arachidonate metabolism in relation to parturition. However, in subhuman primates it is now clear that birth can occur without changes in amniotic fluid concentrations of either PGE_2 or $PGF_{2\alpha}$, but with increases in the products of lipoxygenase pathways of arachidonate metabolism (19). Arachidonate lipoxygenase products are generated by human intrauterine tissues (20), stimulate myometrial activity (21), and are elevated in the amniotic fluid of patients with intra-amniotic infection and preterm labor (22). The possibility has been raised that the onset of parturition may be characterized by a switch in intrauterine arachidonate metabolism from lipoxygenase to cyclooxygenase products although it also seems likely that imposition of other uterotonins on a lipoxygenase-driven uterus could be an effective stimulus to myometrial contractility (21, 23).

In sheep, 5-, 12-, and 15-lipoxygenase activities are present in the cotyledon, myometrium, and endometrium (24). LTB_4 was the major product formed in the fetal membranes, whereas the maternal caruncle and myometrium produced mainly 12-HETE. Unfortunately, these experiments were performed only using tissues obtained at days 125–135 of gestation, and comparison with term tissues has not been made.

Therefore, we incubated homogenates of whole cotyledons, endometrium, and fetal membranes obtained from sheep in early active labor for 15 min at 37°C with 0.45-μCi [^{3}H]arachidonic acid (AA) (25). Following incubation, tissue homogenates were denatured with an equal volume of methanol:acetonitrile (1:1, v/v) and centrifuged at $1000 \times g$ to remove precipitated material. The supernatants were acidified to pH 3.0 with H_3PO_4 and injected directly onto a Rad-Pak C18 column (100×8 mm, 5-μm particles, Waters Chromatography). The various metabolites of arachidonic acid were then eluted with water/organic (methanol and acetonitrile) mixtures including pH gradients (from 3.0 to 5.5) at a flow rate of 2.0 ml/min. This HPLC system is capable of separating cyclo-oxygenase products from hydroxy acids (HETEs, LTB_4, and isomers) at pH 3.0, followed by separate elution of the peptidoleukotrienes at pH 5.5.

In term amnion, 15-HETE was the major product formed from [^{3}H]AA, but represented <1% of the starting radioactivity. There was little metabolism of AA by endometrium. However, placenta converted [^{3}H]AA extensively to 12-HETE, 15-HETE, LTB$_4$ and to primary PGs. These results support the contention that placenta is the major intrauterine site of arachidonate metabolism in the late pregnant sheep. Further studies are required to determine the extent to which the profile of metabolites at labor reflects an altered pathway of AA metabolism peculiar to late pregnancy.

PG SYNTHESIZING METABOLIZING ENZYMES IN HUMAN PREGNANCY

In women, the fetal membranes and placenta are major sites of PG production during late pregnancy, and the different activities of these structures have been described in detail (26, 27). Briefly, amnion produces mainly PGE$_2$, and this output increases with labor. There is little PGDH activity in amnion. In contrast, chorion metabolizes PGs extensively, has high PGDH activity, and produces mainly PGFM and PGEM in vitro from endogenous precursors or exogenous PGE$_2$ (28). Decidua produces PGE$_2$ and PGF$_{2\alpha}$ de novo from arachidonic acid and has some limited PGDH and 9-ketoreductase activity. The basal output of PGs from short-term cultures of decidual cells is higher in tissues taken from patients at spontaneous labor than at term-elective cesarean section. It is likely that amnion and/or decidua are the major sources of stimulatory PG to the myometrium at the time of parturition. It has been suggested that PGE$_2$, produced in amnion, may not be metabolized in chorion but may reach the decidua and/or myometrium, where further PG production is stimulated. In vitro studies have shown the passage of small amounts of [^{3}H]PGE$_2$ across full-thickness human fetal membranes from fetal to maternal side (29, 30). The similarity with transfer rates for inulin suggests that the major route of transfer is through the extracellular space. An alternate explanation is that PGDH is not uniformly expressed throughout chorion. To examine this issue, we used immunocytochemistry to examine the localization of PGDH in human fetal membranes and placenta obtained at term cesarean section and at spontaneous labor. We examined whether this activity changed with labor, and we compared the distribution of PGDH with that of PGHS. Staining procedures were conducted as described above.

Epithelial derived cells were localized by the presence of immunoactive cytokeratin. Positive cells included the amniotic epithelium, trophoblast cells in the chorion and invading trophoblast in the decidua, cytotrophoblasts and syncytiotrophoblasts in the placenta, and intermediate trophoblasts located within the fetal villi, and in maternal septal tissue and decidua.

PGHS staining in the human fetal membranes and placenta has been reported recently by Price et al. (31), and our own observations (32) essentially confirm their results. Positive PGHS staining was localized heterogeneously to the amniotic epithelium and extensively to the trophoblast layer of the chorion (31). Invading trophoblasts in the decidua and decidual stromal cells also stained positive for PGHS. In the placenta, PGHS immunoactivity was present in cytotrophoblasts, in syncytiotrophoblasts, and in intermediate trophoblast cells in the anchoring villi and basal decidua. Price et al. (31) did not establish any difference in the pattern of PGHS staining between tissue from patients in labor or not in labor.

In contrast to PGHS and in agreement with the biochemical information, there was no PGDH staining in the amniotic epithelium or in the subepithelial layer. However, we found extensive immunoactive PGDH in the trophoblast layer of chorion. Staining was localized to 50%–60% of the nonvacuolated trophoblast cells, but only to 5%–10% of vacuolated trophoblasts. The cellular distribution of PGDH in chorion suggested that despite the high PGDH activity observed in homogenate and dispersed cell preparations, this was not spread uniformly throughout the tissue (32). Thus, the potential clearly exists for PGE_2 to escape metabolism during any transmembrane transfer. PGDH was also localized to invading trophoblast cells of the decidua, but not to decidual stromal cells. This observation suggests the possibility that previous reports of decidual PGDH activity may reflect some contamination by trophoblast cells of chorionic origin. In the placenta, PGDH was localized to intermediate trophoblasts and with weak staining to syncytiotrophoblasts. We did not observe immunoactive PGDH in the sparse number of cytotrophoblasts that were present in the sections. The distribution of PGDH did not change with labor in either the fetal membranes or in the placenta.

Placental PGDH type I activity in man is significantly greater than in the sheep (18), and may, in part, be under fetal rather than maternal endocrine control (33). Placental PGDH activity develops early in pregnancy, and by midgestation the activity is similar to that at term. Early reports had failed to demonstrate any change in PGDH activity with labor, although this result may reflect the wide variation found between individual patients (34). Localization of PGDH to both intermediate trophoblasts and syncytiotrophoblasts points to the need to characterize cell populations carefully in tissue culture experiments, since during short-term cultures mostly mononucleated trophoblasts are collected for culture, although these form a syncytium with time.

CHANGES IN PGHS ACTIVITY WITH TIME AND CULTURE

A variety of peptide and steroid influences on PG output by human intrauterine tissues have been studied, and results, primarily with amnion, are summarized in Table 1. We have recently examined effects of two of these factors, namely cortisol and CRH, on PG output in more detail.

In monolayer cultures of amnion grown to confluence, several groups have demonstrated that glucocorticoids stimulate PGE_2 output. This effect is believed to be mediated through increased gene expression for PGHS and was blocked by the glucocorticoid receptor antagonist RU38486 (35). Recently, however, Gibb and Lavoie (36) reported that this effect of glucocorticoids was dependent on the length of time that the cells had been maintained in culture. Amnion cells, cultured for up to 48 h produced less PGE_2 after exposure to glucocorticoids, whereas glucocorticoids were stimulatory to PGE_2 output in confluent cultures. We (37) found that

Table 1. Factors affecting prostaglandin production in intrauterine tissues.

Stimulatory	Inhibitory
Ca^{++}	Lipocortin
Platelet activating factor	Endogenous inhibitor of
β-agonists	prostaglandin synthesis
Estrogen	(EIPS)
Cortisol	Chorion phospholipase A_2
Epidermal growth factor	inhibitor (lipocortin VI)
Transforming growth factor α	Cortisol
Interleukin-1α and β	Progesterone
Lipopolysaccharide	Estrogen
Tumor necrosis factor	Interferon α
Adrenocorticotrophin	
Corticotrophin-releasing factor	
Placental PGDH inhibitor	

dexamethasone inhibited PGE_2 output in a dose-dependent fashion by amnion and mixed placental cell cultures for up to 96 h. This effect was not influenced by concurrent treatment with progesterone. At the end of a 48-h culture period in the presence of dexamethasone, the medium was replaced with one containing 2-µM arachidonic acid. Arachidonate stimulated PGE_2 output, but this conversion was inhibited in a dose-dependent manner according to the concentration of dexamethasone to which the cells had been exposed during the previous 48 h. These results would be consistent with dexamethasone having a direct inhibitory effect on PGHS gene expression and/or activity. Several previous reports (38, 39) have suggested that glucocorticoids may inhibit PGHS activity in macrophages, endothelial cells, and vascular smooth-muscle cells, where PGHS mRNA levels were also suppressed by glucocorticoids (40).

It is possible that glucocorticoids may also influence PG production in human fetal membranes and placenta indirectly through corticotrophin-releasing hormone (CRH). CRH is produced in these tissues, and in short-term (48 h) culture, its output and pre-pro CRH mRNA levels are increased by glucocorticoid treatment (41, 42). CRH also stimulates PG output by fetal membranes and placental tissue, and this effect may be antagonized by co-administration of an antibody to $ACTH_{1-39}$, suggesting that in part it may be mediated through ACTH. We have proposed elsewhere (43, 44) that human parturition may result from a positive cascade interaction of glucocorticoids, CRH and PG, that is broken by down regulation of placental CRH receptors or by the process of birth. However, this scheme revolves around enhanced CRH gene expression with exposure to glucocorticoids. While this is true for short-term placental cultures, at 12–14 days in culture glucocorticoids inhibit CRH output from the placenta (42), similar to the inhibition of CRH mRNA levels in the hypothalamus.

Thus, there is a need to characterize precisely the cell types in these cultures, since these results imply that glucocorticoids may influence CRH output from intermediate trophoblasts and perhaps cytotrophoblasts in a different fashion to their action on syncytiotrophoblasts.

CONCLUDING COMMENTS

We have used immunocytochemistry to determine the localization of PGHS and PGDH in intrauterine tissues of sheep and women during pregnancy. This approach has revealed major alterations in the cell populations expressing these enzymes during pregnancy and has delineated unexpected patterns in the distribution of cells expressing the enzymes in different tissues. These studies have shown the necessity to remain cognizant of cell-cell interaction while performing studies with whole-tissue homogenates or subcellular fractions and has emphasized the necessity of characterizing carefully the cell types that are being studied under different culture conditions.

REFERENCES

1. Challis JRG, Olson DM. Parturition. In: Knobil E, Neill J, eds. New York: Raven Press, 1988:2177-215.
2. Casey ML, Cox SM, Word RA, MacDonald PC. Prostaglandins and pregnancy—a 1989 review. Reprod Fertil Develop 1990 (in press).
3. Kliman HJ, Feinman MA, Strauss JF II. Cellular biology and pharmacology of the placenta. In: Miller RK, Thiede HA, eds. Trophoblast research. New York: Plenum, 1985:407-21.
4. Liggins GC, Fairclough RJ, Grieves SA, Kendall JZ, Knox BS. The mechanism of initiation of parturition in the ewes. Rec Prog Horm Res 1973;29:111-50.
5. Evans CA, Kennedy TG, Challis JRG. Gestational changes in prostanoid concentrations in intrauterine tissues and fetal fluids from pregnant sheep, and the relation to prostanoid output in vitro. Biol Reprod 1982;127:1-11.
6. Olson DM, Lye SJ, Skinner K, Challis JRG. Early changes in prostaglandin concentrations in ovine maternal and fetal plasma, amniotic fluid and from dispersed cells of intrauterine tissues before the onset of ACTH-induced pre-term labour. J Reprod Fert 1984;71:45-55.
7. Evans CA, Kennedy TG, Patrick JE, Challis JRG. The effects of indomethacin on uterine activity and prostaglandin (PG) concentrations during labor induced by administering ACTH to fetal sheep. Can J Physiol Pharmacol 1982;60:1200-9.
8. Challis JRG, Dilley SR, Robinson JS, Thorburn GD. Prostaglandins in the circulation of the fetal lamb. Prostaglandins 1976;11:1041-52.
9. Lye SJ, Sprague CL, Mitchell BF, Challis JRG. Activation of ovine fetal adrenal function by pulsatile or continuous administration of adrenocorticotrophin-(1-24), I. Effects on fetal plasma corticosteroids. Endocrinology 1983;113:770-82.
10. Wintour EM, Laurence BM, Lingwood BE. Anatomy, physiology and pathology of the amniotic and allantoic compartments in the sheep and cow. Aust Vet J 1986;63:216-21.

11. Thorburn GD, Challis JRG. Endocrine control of parturition. Physiol Rev 1979; 59:863-918.

12. Smith, W. 1989. Personal communication.

13. Boshier DP, Jacobs RA, Han VK, Smith W, Challis JRG. Immunocytochemical localization of PGHS (cyclo-oxygenase) activity in the sheep placenta. Soc Study Fertil Annu Conf 1990 (in press).

14. Salamonsen LA, Manikhot J, Healy DL, Findlay JK. Ovine trophoblast protein-1 and human interferon alpha reduce prostaglandin synthesis by ovine endometrial cells. Prostaglandins 1989;38:289-306.

15. Berchuk A, MacDonald PC, Milewich L, Casey ML. Transforming growth factor-β inhibits prostaglandin production in amnion and A431 cells. Prostaglandins 1989;38:453-64.

16. Challis JRG, Brooks AN. Maturation and activation of hypothalamic-pituitary-adrenal function in fetal sheep. Endocr Rev 1989;10:182-204.

17. Riley SC, Herlich J, Boshier DP, Jacobs RA, Challis JRG. Localization of 15-hydroxy prostaglandin dehydrogenase in the sheep placenta throughout gestation. Soc Study Fertil Annu Conf 1990 (in press).

18. Erwich JJHM, Keirse MJNC. Species differences in placental 15-hydroxy-prostaglandin dehydrogenase. 1st European Congress on Prostaglandins in Reproduction. Vienna, 1988.

19. Walsh SW. 5-hydroxyeicosatetraenoic acid, leukotriene C_4, and prostaglandin $F_{2\alpha}$ in amniotic fluid before and during term and preterm labor. Am J Obstet Gynecol 1989.

20. Mitchell MD, Grzyboski CF. Arachidonic acid metabolism by lipoxygenase pathways in intrauterine tissues of women at term of pregnancy. Prostaglandins, Leukotrienes Med 1987;28:303-12.

21. Bennett PR, Elder MG, Myatt L. The effects of lipoxygenase metabolites of arachidonic acid on human myometrial contractility. Prostaglandins 1987;33:837-44.

22. Romero R, Wu YK, Mazor M, Oyarzun E, Hobbins JC, Mitchell MD. Amniotic fluid arachidonate lipoxygenase metabolites in preterm labor. Prostaglandins, Leukotrienes Essential Fatty Acids 1989;36:69-75.

23. Carraher R, Hahn DW, Ritchie DM, McGuire JL. Involvement of lipoxygenase products in myometrial contractions. Prostaglandins 1983;26:23-32.

24. Mitchell MD, Grzyboski CF, Dedhar CM, Hunter JA. Arachidonic acid metabolism by lipoxygenase pathways in uterine and intrauterine tissues of pregnant sheep. Prostaglandins, Leukotrienes Med 1987;27:197-207.

25. Langlois D, Fraher LF, Challis JRG. Patterns of arachidonic acid metabolism by sheep fetal membranes and placenta with late pregnancy. (in preparation).

26. McNellis D, Challis JRG, MacDonald PC, Nathanielsz PW, Roberts JM, eds. The onset of labor: cellular and integrative mechanisms. Ithaca, NY: Perinatology Press.

27. Bleasdale JE, Johnston JM. Prostaglandins and human parturition: regulation of arachidonic acid mobilization. Rev Perinatal Med 1985;5:151-91.

28. Cheung PYC, Challis JRG. Prostaglandin E_2 metabolism in the human fetal membranes. Am J Obstet Gynecol 1990;161:1580-5.

29. Nakla S, Skinner K, Mitchell BF, Challis JRG. Changes in prostaglandin transfer across human fetal membranes obtained after spontaneous labour. Am J Obstet Gynecol 1986;155:1337-41.

30. Bennett PR, Chamberlain GVP, Myatt L, Patel L, Elder MG. Mechanisms of parturition: the transfer of prostaglandins across fetal membranes. In: Jones CT, ed.

Research in perinatal medicine: fetal and neonatal development. Ithaca, NY: Perinatology Press, 1988:407-9.

31. Price TM, Kauma SW, Curry Jr TE, Clark MR. Immunohistochemical localization of prostaglandin endoperoxide synthase in human fetal membranes and decidua. Biol Reprod 1989;41:701-5.

32. Cheung PYC, Walton JC, Tai D, Riley SC, Challis JRG. Immunocytochemical distribution and localization of 15-hydroxy prostaglandin dehydrogenase in human fetal membrane, decidua, and placenta. Am J Obstet Gynecol 1990 (submitted).

33. Erwish JJHM, Keirse MJNC. Human placental 15-hydroxy-prostaglandin dehydrogenase activity is under fetal genetic control. Prostaglandins 1988;35:123-31.

34. Hansen HS. 15-hydroxyprostaglandin dehydrogenase. A review. Prostaglandins 1976;12:647-79.

35. Potestio FA, Zakar T, Olson DM. Glucocorticoids stimulate prostaglandin synthesis in human amnion cells by a receptor-mediated mechanism. J Clin Endocrinol Metab 1988;67:1205-10.

36. Gibb W, Lavoie J-C. Effects of glucocorticoids on prostaglandin formation by human amnion. Can J Physiol Pharmacol 1990 (in press).

37. Riley SC, Schembri LA, Challis JRG. Dexamethasone inhibits prostaglandin E_2 output from human placental cells in culture by inhibition of prostaglandin H_2 synthase. Soc Study Fertil Annu Conf (in press).

38. Hullin F, Raynal P, Ragab-Thomas JMF, Fauvel J, Chap H. Effect of dexamethasone on prostaglandin synthesis and on lipocortin status in human endothelial cells. J Biol Chem 1989;264:3506-13.

39. Goppelt-Struebe M, Wolter D, Resch K. Glucocorticoids inhibit prostaglandin synthesis not only at the level of phospholipase A_2 but also at the level of cyclo-oxygenase/ PGE isomerase. Br J Pharmacol 1989;98:1287-95.

40. Bailey JM, Makheja AN, Pash J, Verma M. Corticosteroids suppress cyclooxygenase messenger RNA levels and prostanoid synthesis in cultured vascular cells. Biochem Biophys Res Commun 1988;157:1159-63.

41. Robinson BG, Emanual RL, Frim DM, Majzoub JA. Glucocorticoid stimulates expression of corticotropin-releasing hormone gene in human placenta. Proc Natl Acad Sci USA 1988;85:5244-8.

42. Jones SA, Brooks AN, Challis JRG. Steroids modulate corticotrophin-releasing factor production in human fetal membranes and placenta. J Clin Endocrinol Metab 1989;68:825-30.

43. Jones SA, Challis JRG. Local stimulation of prostaglandin production by corticotrophin-releasing hormone in human fetal membranes and placenta. Biochem Biophys Res Commun 1989;159:192-99.

44. Challis JRG, Hooper S. Endocrine mechanisms in the control of birth. In: Jones CT, ed. Perinatal endocrinology, Bailliere's clinical endocrinology and metabolism. New York: WB Saunders, 1989.

12

Studies on Labor-Conditioning and Labor-Inducing Effects of Antiprogesterones in Animal Models

Walter Elger,[1] Krzysztof Chwalisz,[1] Marianne Fähnrich,[1] Syed Hamiddudin Hasan,[1] Dirk Laurent,[1] Sybille Beier,[1] Eckhard Ottow,[1] Günter Neef,[1] and Robert Edward Garfield[2]

[1]Schering Research Laboratories, Berlin, and [2]Department of Biomedical Science, MacMaster University, Hamilton, Ontario, Canada

P rogesterone is considered an essential hormone of pregnancy and is necessary for maintaining an ideal uterine environment during gestation. Its actions in maternal tissues include the transformation of the endometrium from a proliferating into a secretory tissue capable of sustaining an implanted embryo, inhibition of uterine contractions, and induction of mammary gland growth and development. Csapo (1) concluded that there is a spontaneous tendency of the uterus to evacuate its contents unless its motor function is paralyzed by progesterone. According to Csapo, progesterone elevates the threshold to oxytocins present as intrinsic uterine stimulants. Consequently, one should expect that a blockade of the progesterone receptor due to a treatment with antiprogesterones should prompt an expulsion of the uterine contents.

ANTIPROGESTERONE COMPOUNDS

In this section, we briefly review studies with antiprogesterone compounds (antiprogestins, antigestagens, and progesterone antagonists).

Chemistry of Antigestagens. Figure 1 demonstrates the chemical structure of RU 486 and that of three analogs. RU 486 is a derivative of 19-nor-testosterone, with an alkylation in position C17, and an additional double bond between C-atoms 9 and 10 of the steroid skeleton. The most prominent chemical feature of RU 486 and the related compounds is a dimethyl/aminophenyl-moiety in position 11. The other compounds are related. They differ from RU 486 by alterations of the side chain or by steric changes of the steroid skeleton, respectively, in addition to side-chain modifications. ZK 112.993 is characterized by an acetyl-phenyl group in position 11.

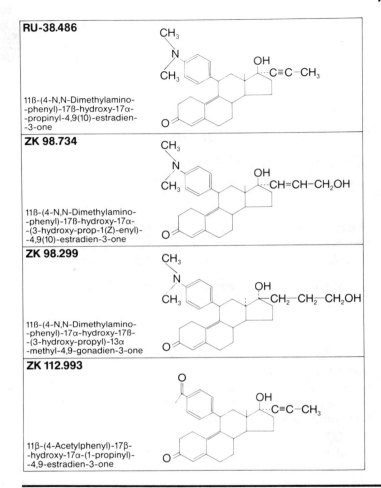

RU-38.486

11β-(4-N,N-Dimethylamino-
-phenyl)-17β-hydroxy-17α-
-propinyl-4,9(10)-estradien-
-3-one

ZK 98.734

11β-(4-N,N-Dimethylamino-
-phenyl)-17β-hydroxy-17α-
-(3-hydroxy-prop-1(Z)-enyl)-
-4,9(10)-estradien-3-one

ZK 98.299

11β-(4-N,N-Dimethylamino-
-phenyl)-17α-hydroxy-17β-
-(3-hydroxy-propyl)-13α
-methyl-4,9-gonadien-3-one

ZK 112.993

11β-(4-Acetylphenyl)-17β-
-hydroxy-17α-(1-propinyl)-
-4,9-estradien-3-one

Fig. 1. Chemical structure of investigated antiprogesterones.

Gestagenic/Antigestagenic Activity. In spite of the progesterone receptor affinity of the antigestagen compounds there was no progesterone-like effect after local intrauterine application of the test compounds in rabbits (see Figs. 2A and 2B). If the same experiment is done in progesterone-treated animals, there is a substantial reduction of endometrial transformation in a strictly local manner. These studies indicate that antigestagen agents have little progesterone (gestagenic) action, but are capable of blocking its effects (antagonistic activity).

Glucocorticoid/Antiglucocorticoid Activity. RU 486 and the other analogs have antiglucocorticoid activity; however, there are important quantitative differences in this respect (see Fig. 3). In order to evaluate this pharmacological property, adrenalectomized male rats were used. Thymus regression was induced by dexamethasone treatment. The capability of antigestagen compounds to abolish the

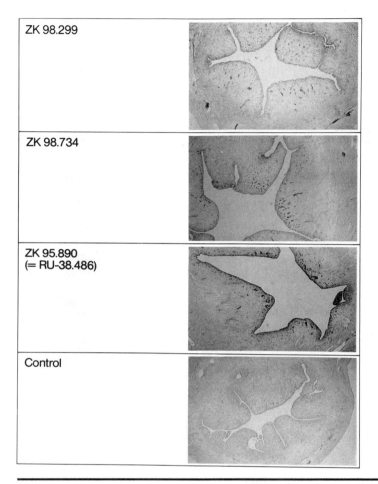

Fig. 2A. Evaluation of progesterone-agonistic and antagonistic activity by intrauterine application of antigestagens in sealed silastic tubes in rabbits: The test for agonistic activity showed no evidence of gestagenic activity. (IUD = days 1–9; autopsy = day 9.)

effects of dexamethasone on the thymus was used as a parameter of antiglucocorticoid activity. RU 486 was found to have higher antiglucocorticoid activity as indicated by a lower threshold and higher maximal effects. There was a general tendency for more pronounced antiglucocorticoid activity on oral application. This was particularly true for RU 486; there is no corresponding increase of antigestagenic activity on oral application. Active metabolites may play a role in this context. ZK 98.734 had the lowest level of antiglucocorticoid activity. It has only minor glucocorticoid activity at very high dose levels.

Miscellaneous Hormonal and Antihormonal Properties of Antigestagens. Comparing the effective threshold doses of different hormonal activities in rats, it

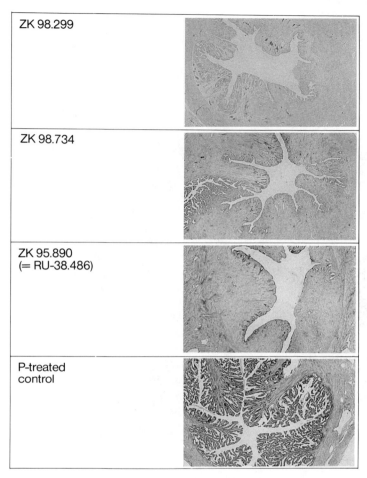

Fig. 2B. Evaluation of progesterone-agonistic and antagonistic activity by intrauterine application of antigestagens in sealed silastic tubes in rabbits: The test for antagonistic activity in progesterone (P)-treated animals showed a distinct inhibitory effect of antigestagens. (IUD = 1–9 days; P-treatment = 30 mg/day sc days 2–8; autopsy = day 9.)

becomes clear that these become manifest at rather different dose levels: Progesterone antagonistic activity becomes manifest at 5 mg/kg body weight, independent of oral or subcutaneous application. Antiglucocorticoid activity is generally seen at 6–20 times higher doses. This applies to antiandrogenic activity as well. There are some exceptions to this rule. In the case of RU 486, on oral application the antigestagenic and antiglucocorticoid threshold are very close to each other. ZK 98.734 has antimineralocorticoid activity at dose levels close to those that block nidation. There are few examples of agonistic properties: ZK 98.734 has some glucocorticoid and androgenic activity at high doses. Table 1 summarizes the reported and other experimental data. It shows the difference between compounds.

Mean % inhibition of DEX-induced thymus weight suppression

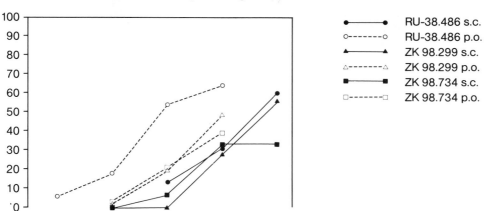

Fig. 3. Antithymolytic activity of antigestagens in adrenalectomized dexamethasone (DEX)-substituted male rats. (b.w. = 110–130 g; treatment = 4 days; autopsy = day 5.)

Table 1. Feature of the pharmacological properties of antiprogestins in rats: Comparison of effective threshold doses.

	mg/kg b.w.					
	RU 38.486		ZK 98.299		ZK 98.734	
	sc	po	sc	po	sc	po
Antagonistic activities						
antigestagenic[a]	~ 5.0	~ 5.0	~ 5.0	~ 5.0	~ 5.0	~ 5.0
antiglucocorticoid	~ 30.0	~ 10.0	~ 100.0	~ 30.0	~ 100.0	~ 30.0
antiandrogenic	≥ 30.0	≥ 100.0	≥ 300.0	≥ 100.0	> 300.0	> 300.0
antimineralocorticoid	> 50.0	> 50.0	nt	> 50.0	nt	≥ 7.0
antiestrogenic	nt	nt	nt	nt	nt	nt
Agonistic activities						
gestagenic[b]	Inactive		Inactive		Inactive	
glucocorticoid	> 100.0	> 100.0	nt	nt	≥ 300.0	nt
androgenic	nt	nt	> 200.0	nt	≥ 20.0	≥ 70.0
mineralocorticoid	> 50.0	> 50.0	nt	> 50.0	nt	> 50.0
estrogenic	> 50.0	> 50.0	> 50.0	> 50.0	> 50.0	> 50.0

[a]Antinidatory.   [b]Rabbit endometrium, local application.   nt = not tested.

Interaction of Antigestagens with Estrogen Actions. None of the antigestagens listed in Figure 1 has affinity to the estrogen receptor. This excludes estrogenicity or interactions with estrogen at this level. There were also no negative effects on estrogen secretion in various experiments. Nevertheless there is evidence of interactions with specific estrogen actions in the endometrium. In long-term ovariectomized estradiol-treated rabbits, antigestagens abolish the estradiol-induced gland proliferation. The increase in uterine weights was not affected. The uterine concentration of cytosolic and nuclear estrogen receptor and its mRNA was paradoxically significantly elevated (2).

Effects of Antigestagens in Pregnancy. The guinea pig was selected for these studies primarily because of some physiological similarities between its pregnancy and human pregnancy (see Fig. 4). In both species, there is a luteoplacental shift of progesterone secretion and a high level of circulating progesterone until parturition. Therefore, uterine motor activation leading to expulsion is obtained in the presence of high levels of circulating progesterone. Another aspect that seems to be a further analogy to human pregnancy is the development of practically absolute estrogen-resistance of pregnancy. The latter develops in the guinea pig around day 20 of pregnancy.

Inhibition of Nidation. Nidation is prevented by treatment with antigestagens on days 4–6 of pregnancy (i.e., before implantation). A collapse of nidation sites is also

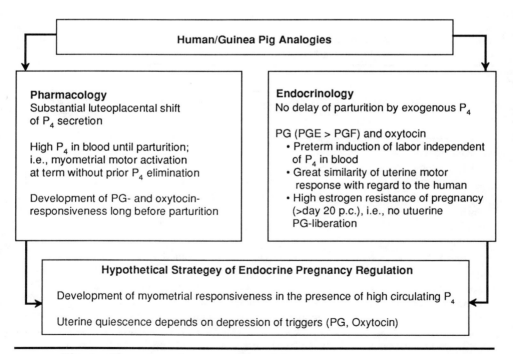

Fig. 4. The guinea pig pregnancy model.

induced by antigestagen treatment on days 8–11 of pregnancy (see Fig. 5). At both investigated perinidation stages, we found maximum effects at a dose of 10.0 mg/animal/day sc for all tested steroids. At a dose of 1.0 mg, there were no inhibitory effects. Incomplete and variable effects at a dose of 3.0 mg suggest that this is the threshold dose for all three compounds. This more or less comparable antigestagenic activity is in distinct contrast to different labor-inducing effects that were recorded in later stages of pregnancy. Histology revealed that embryonic tissue was still present at degenerating nidation sites. This finding of incomplete abortion indicates that myometrial activation and mechanical evacuation did not take place in perinidation stages. The unaffected serum progesterone furthermore suggests that uterine prostaglandin liberation, which would have exerted a luteolytic effect, was not induced. These results indicate that the antigestagens affect mainly the endometrium and deciduous tissues to end early pregnancy.

Induction of Expulsion in Advanced Pregnancy

RU 486 was the first effective progesterone antagonist in our hands that was able to induce abortion in the guinea pig by expulsion in advanced pregnancy. Several days elapse before expulsions occur after treatment. In this experimental situation, important differences between the tested compounds were found. In the case of RU 486, we noted that even very high doses, such as 30.0 mg/animal/day sc failed to induce expulsions in more than 50% of the animals. In contrast, ZK 98.734 showed dose-dependent effects and was faster acting than RU 486. All the animals aborted at the highest dose of 30.0 mg/animal/day sc (3). In this experimental situation, the low level of labor induction with some compounds compared to the rapid onset of labor and expulsion of conceptuses after sulprostone (an analog of PGE_2) prompted us to evaluate antigestagen/prostaglandin-combinations. There were strong synergistic effects of some antigestagen/sulprostone combinations. In the case of RU 486, a much higher number of animals aborted after simultaneous treatment with marginal sulprostone doses as compared to the effects of the progesterone antagonists alone. In addition, the expulsions occurred much earlier.

In order to establish the optimum duration of priming and optimum PG doses, we compared the effects of priming for 1 day versus 2 day's priming using a standard dose of 10.0-mg ZK 98.299/day sc and graded doses of sulprostone, injected 24 h after the last antigestagen application. There were no differences between the 1-day and the 2-day priming. These results show that complete sensitization of the uterus was obtained within 24 h after treatment with antigestagens. Above a well-defined threshold dose of sulprostone (0.01 mg sc), rapid expulsions and complete abortions were obtained. This elevation of sulprostone sensitivity may be estimated from Figure 6.

The uterine responsiveness to sulprostone following antigestagen treatment on day 43 is approximately 3 times higher than that established in control untreated guinea pigs in the immediate prepartum period and approximately 30 times higher than that in control animals on day 43. In spite of this extremely high myometrial responsiveness in antigestagen-treated animals, there was no tendency of spontaneous labor in the observed period. This indicates again that uterine

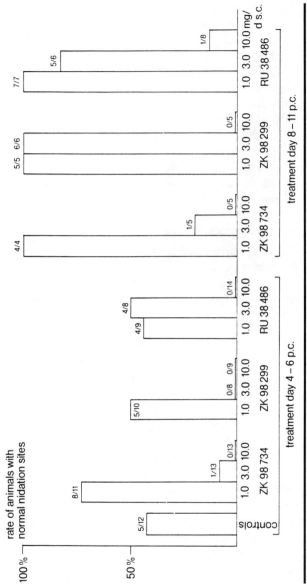

Fig. 5. Effects of antigestagens in perinidation stages of pregnancy in guinea pigs.

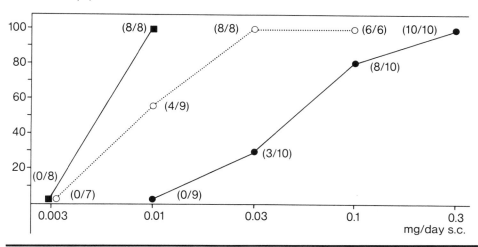

Fig. 6. Spontaneous changes of uterine responsiveness to sulprostone between days 43 and 63 of guinea pig pregnancy versus changes that occur following treatment with ZK 98.299 on day 43 of pregnancy. (Solid circles = dose-response curve S in midpregnancy; treatment days 43–44 postcoitum [pc]. Open circles = dose-response curve S in late pregnancy; treatment days 63–64 pc. Solid squares = dose-response curve after priming with 10.0-mg ZK 98.299/day in midpregnancy; treatment 1 or 2 days around day 43 pc.)

PG and other "intrinsic" uterine stimulants were not activated parallel to the development of uterine responsiveness (3).

Effects of Antigestagens on Myometrial Oxytocin Responsiveness

The effects of oxytocin in various species depends on the stage of pregnancy. Treatment with antigestagens alone on day 43 of pregnancy in guinea pigs stimulated cervical ripening and increased myometrial sensitivity for exogenous oxytocin, but did not effectively induce contractions. The prolonged labor and bleeding that were observed after treatment are evidence of the lack of sufficient expulsive activity. The sequential oxytocin injection after antigestagen treatment resulted in rapid delivery, which expresses the enhanced sensitivity of the myometrium and low cervical resistance (Fig. 7). These data agree with in vitro studies on rat uteri with oxytocin, showing substantially stronger mechanical responses with organs taken from ZK 98.299 primed rats compared to vehicle-treated controls (4).

A dramatic dilatation and softening of the cervix was recorded within 24 h after a single antigestagen treatment (ZK 98.299). Furthermore, mechanical studies indicate that extensibility of the cervix is much greater after antigestagen treatment (5). These changes certainly contribute to the observed synergism of antigestagens with prostaglandins and oxytocin.

cumulative rate of abortion (%)

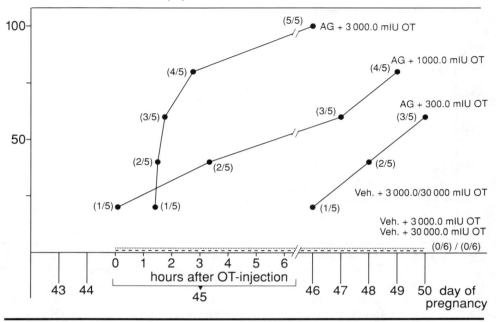

Fig. 7.   Effects of antigestagens on myometrial responsiveness to oxytocin.

MECHANISM OF ACTION

Studies on Uterine PG Generation

There is a lot of indirect evidence that the antigestagens fail to activate uterine prostaglandin production or liberation. Rather there is some direct evidence that the progesterone antagonists inhibit uterine PG.

After treatment with 10.0-mg ZK 98.299 there were no changes in PGF levels in uterine vein blood within 24 h. By contrast, a nonabortifacient dose of 1.0-mg PGE_2 administered subcutaneously significantly raised the prostaglandin levels (Fig. 8). Combining the same doses of antigestagens and PGE_2 in a sequential manner induced abortions within 6 h after PGE_2 injection in most of the guinea pigs. The described paradox—maximum elevation of myometrial sensitivity associated with an absence of "intrinsic uterine stimulants"—may have a surprising explanation. In the aforementioned inhibition of nidation studies, some nonpregnant females were treated with antigestagens on days 8–11 of the cycle. The measurement of serum progesterone by RIA revealed that in these ZK 98.299- and ZK 98.734-treated animals, the expected drop in progesterone levels at the end of the luteal phase did not occur. Instead, these animals showed a course of serum progesterone that is typical in pregnancy. In the meantime, we found that this antiluteolytic effect is due to an inhibition of uterine $PGF_{2\alpha}$ secretion. This is reflected by the PGFM (13,14-dihydro-15-keto-$PGF_{2\alpha}$) level in peripheral blood.

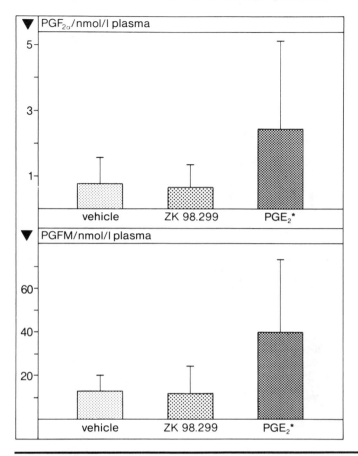

Fig. 8. Effects of ZK 98.299 on $PFG_{2\alpha}$ and PGFM concentrations in uterine vein plasma. Shown are $PGF_{2\alpha}$ and PGFM concentrations in uterine vein plasma in pregnant guinea pigs, day 44, 24 h after treatment with vehicle sc, 10.0-mg ZK 98.299 sc day 43 pc, and 1.0-mg PGE_2 sc day 44 pc. ($\bar{x} \pm SD$, n = 10/group; *P < 0.05 vs. vehicle.)

The typical PGFM elevation in peripheral blood during luteal regression after day 12 of the cycle in guinea pigs is completely abolished by progesterone antagonists (treatment started day 8 after ovulation). This antiluteolytic effect seems important under the aspect of uterine PG secretion because inhibiting progesterone action seems to inhibit the due uterine PG secretion.

In order to demonstrate that the uterus is the site of action for antiluteolytic effects, experiments with intrauterine silastic tubes, releasing minute amounts of ZK 98.299 (i.e., 10 μg/24 h), were performed. The findings of these experiments showed an inhibition of PGF release, which was seen in sham-treated control animals during luteolysis. There was no luteolysis in the antigestagen-treated animals (see Fig. 9). These findings suggest the importance of

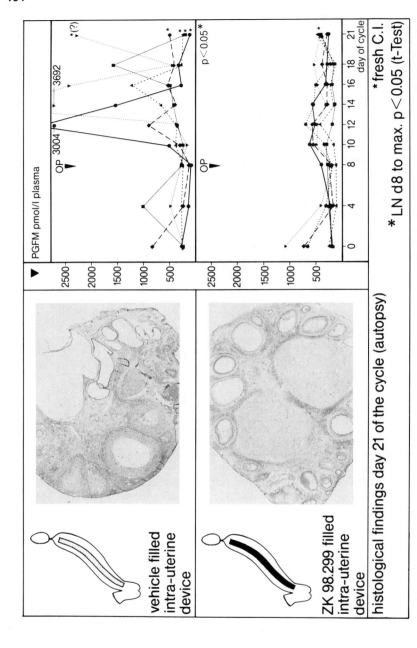

Fig. 9. Antiluteolytic effects of intrauterine microdoses of ZK 98.299 in unilaterally ovariectomized and/or hysterectomized guinea pigs. Insertion of ZK 98.299, resp. vehicle-filled silastic devices on day 8 of the cycle; medicated devices release ~10.0-μg ZK 98.299/24 h.

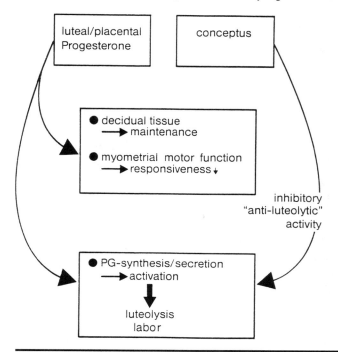

Fig. 10. Scheme of the hypothetical and paradoxical effects of progesterone with regard to myometrial motor function in guinea pig pregnancy.

direct uterine effects for the observed antiluteolytic effects of antigestagens rather than, for example, by an activation of luteotropic factor from the pituitary gland.

Important questions arise with regard to the role of progesterone in the control of uterine prostaglandins in this context. We can assume that progesterone is a stimulator of uterine prostaglandins in the guinea pig. The depression of uterine prostaglandins in pregnancy is a function of the embryo which first becomes manifest by its well-established antiluteolytic activity. Progesterone may represent a permanent stimulus of uterine prostaglandin generation in pregnancy which is under permanent embryonic suppression. Consequently, blockade of progesterone at this target in advanced pregnancy can be assumed to lead to paralyzed prostaglandin generation in analogy to that in the luteal phase.

The stimulatory role of progesterone on uterine PG secretion was also demonstrated by studies with Promegestone (R 5020), a potent and specific progesterone agonist (6). This compound was able to reverse the inhibitory effects of ZK 98.299 on uterine PG secretion, as reflected by elevated peripheral plasma PGFM levels. Treatment with R 5020 starting on day 8 of the cycle stimulated the uterine PGFM secretion above the level that was seen in cycling controls and for a much longer period of time, i.e., as long as the treatment was continued (day 22 of the cycle) (D. Laurent, unpublished observation).

Interaction of Antigestagens with Various Compounds

Interaction of Competitive Inhibitors of Progesterone and Compounds with Antisteroidogenic Activities (Epostane). Epostane is a highly potent enzyme inhibitor that blocks the activity of 3β-OH-Δ5-steroid-dehyrogenase with considerable selectivity for ovarian and placental steroidogenesis (7, 8). Clinical studies in early pregnancy show that Epostane leads to a substantial reduction of peripheral progesterone and estradiol levels (9, 10). The rate of complete abortion in animals treated with Epostane is comparable to that after RU 486 treatment at this stage of pregnancy (9, 11–15). As in humans, there is a substantial reduction of circulating progesterone in pregnant guinea pigs treated on days 43–44 of pregnancy (Figs. 11 and 13). There is also a reduction of circulating cortisol levels at the tested dose. In contrast to the findings in human pregnancy, however, we never recorded an abortion after treatment with Epostane alone. In combinations with sulprostone, abortions were only induced with relatively high doses of sulprostone (> = 0.1-mg sulprostone sc). In contrast with Epostane, 0.01-mg sulprostone was fully effective after 10.0-mg ZK 98.299 (16). Contrary to the progesterone-antagonist/sulprostone combinations, there was a low rate of complete abortions after corresponding sulprostone combinations with Epostane; in 3 of 4 animals one or more fetuses were retained in the uterus and were found intact at autopsy on day 50 (17). These data

Serum-Progesterone n mol/l

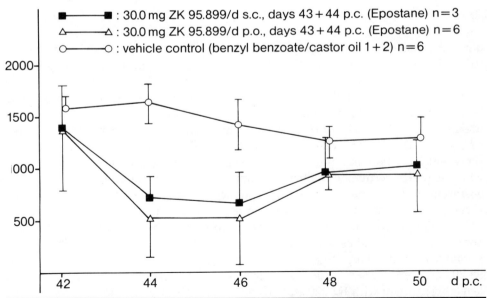

■━━━■ : 30.0 mg ZK 95.899/d s.c., days 43 + 44 p.c. (Epostane) n = 3
△━━━△ : 30.0 mg ZK 95.899/d p.o., days 43 + 44 p.c. (Epostane) n = 6
○━━━○ : vehicle control (benzyl benzoate/castor oil 1 + 2) n = 6

Fig. 11. Effect of Epostane on serum progesterone in pregnant guinea pigs (days 43–50 pc). Note: An intact pregnancy was recorded in all animals. (Autopsy = day 50 pc.)

show that the inhibition of progesterone secretion, and secondary to this the reduction in circulating progesterone, is a much less effective strategy to overcome the action of endogenous progesterone in guinea pigs than competitive inhibitors such as RU 486.

RU 486 was selected for our first studies with Epostane due to its low labor-inducing activity in the above standard experiment in guinea pigs. We combined a nonabortifacient dose of Epostane with an almost inactive dose of RU 486. Surprisingly, there was a remarkable effect on pregnancy. All treated animals expelled their uterine contents. There was a much shorter induction to abortion interval than ever observed after RU 486 or any of the antigestagens tested in the guinea pig (Fig. 12). There is no question that Epostane added a complementary labor-inducing component to the well-analyzed elevation of myometrial reactivity due to RU 486 (18). Studies with other antigestagens and Epostane revealed that the described synergistic action is a general phenomenon (17).

Mechanism of Antigestagen/Epostane Synergism

The rationale for the studies below is the assumption that the synergistic labor-inducing action of Epostane with RU 486 results from the antisteroidogenic action of Epostane. In view of other evidence that progesterone may have a stimulatory role on uterine prostaglandin F-secretion and in view of a broad spectrum of antisteroidogenic actions of Epostane, it was considered necessary to investigate

cumulative rate of abortion in %

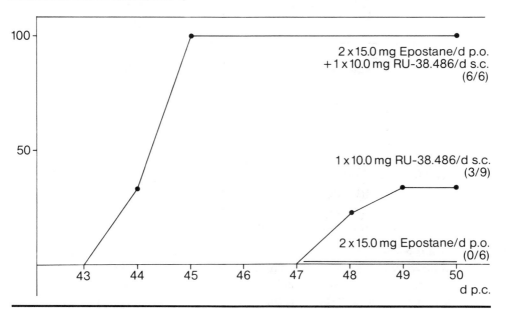

Fig. 12. Labor-inducing activity of RU 486/Epostane combinations in advanced pregnancy in guinea pigs. (Treatment = days 43–44 pc.)

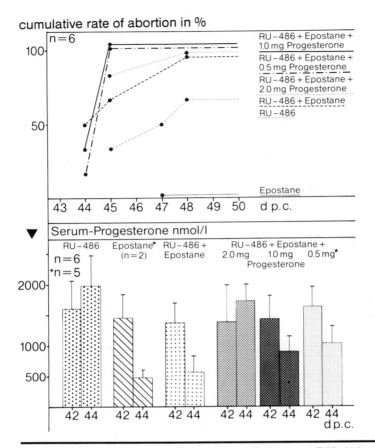

Fig. 13. Failure to abolish the effects of Epostane/RU 486 combination by substitution with progesterone in pregnant guinea pigs. (RU 486 = 10.0 mg/day sc, days 43–44 pc; Epostane = 2 × 15.0 mg/day po, days 43–44 pc; and progesterone = various doses sc, days 42–45 pc.)

the functional significance of different steroid hormone deficiencies. A loss of synergism was expected from the elimination of the hormone deficiency that promotes labor. The RU 486 and Epostane treatments were performed on days 43–44 as described above. Substitution treatments were uniformly given on days 42–45 in order to overlap the stimulatory antigestagen/Epostane treatments.

Progesterone Substitution Studies. It is reasonable to assume that the described superadditive synergism is due to simultaneous attacks on progesterone secretion and progesterone action We investigated this possibility by injections of various doses of progesterone (Fig. 13). The highest tested dose of progesterone (2.0 mg/day sc) abolished the lowering effect of Epostane on the serum progesterone levels. However, there was *no* inhibitory effect of exogenous progesterone on the antigestagen/Epostane synergism (Fig. 13). Rather the progesterone substitution promoted an even faster expulsion of uterine contents. The maintained synergism clearly demonstrates that the labor-inducing effect of Epostane in the above experiments is not due to its inhibitory effect on the progesterone secretion. The only reservation we have with regard to this interpretation is that it cannot be excluded that reductions of throphoblastic progesterone-secretion and progesterone concentrations in uterine tissues were not fully abolished by the above doses of progesterone.

Glucocorticoid Substitution Studies.   Cortisol and dexamethasone synergism was also evaluated. There were no inhibitory effects of 0.3 mg dexamethasone or 10-mg cortisol, respectively, on RU 486/Epostane-induced labor. If at all, one finds a gradual delay of the onset of labor due to the glucocorticoids. These data suggest that reduced cortisol levels play only a minor role or no role in the described antigestagen/Epostane synergism (17).

Substitution of Various C-19 Steroids.   Various steroids that are substrates or products of 3β-OH-Δ-5-steroid-dehydrogenase were also investigated for synergism. Dehydroepiandrosterone (DHEA, 10.0 mg/day sc), dehydroepiandrosterone-sulfate (DHEAS, 30.0 mg/day sc), and androstenedione (10.0 mg/day sc) are substrates of the 3β-OH-Δ-5-steroid-dehydrogenase and are suggested to compete with Epostane for this enzyme. Androstenedione is a product of 3β-OH-Δ-5-steroid-dehydrogenase and the most important substrate for the aromatase. In animals treated with C-19 steroids, serum estradiol levels were elevated, and contrary to the experiments with progesterone replacement, these treatments clearly blunted the antigestagen/Epostane synergism. There was a considerable delay of the onset of labor after DHEA and DHEAS treatment. Androstenedione led to a complete inhibition of the expected labor due to RU 486/Epostane treatment (17). These studies indicate that estrogens may inhibit the labor-inducing action of the treatments.

Estrogen Substitution Studies.   In order to be certain that estradiol mediates the inhibitory effects of androstenedione and DHEA it had to be shown that estradiol itself has similar inhibitory actions on the onset of labor in RU 486/Epostane-treated animals. In pilot experiments two doses of estradiol (0.01- or 0.1-mg estradiol/day sc on days 42–45 pc) were tested (Fig. 14). Indeed, not a single animal receiving the above doses of estradiol plus antigestagen/Epostane combination aborted. This result confirms the assumption that estrogens exert inhibitory effects on the onset of labor. Therefore, it is likely that Epostane acts synergistically with RU 486 not due to its effects on progesterone secretion but probably due to its inhibitory effects on estrogen biosynthesis. Rather than result from impaired aromatase activity, this estrogen deficiency could result from a reduction of substrates for aromatization. The increase in estradiol in serum following androstenedione supports this assumption. The behavior of estradiol in the RU 486/Epostane or ZK 112.993/Epostane-treated animals is consistent with this postulated effect. There is a decrease of estradiol in peripheral serum by day 44. A corresponding drop was not seen after RU 486 and other antigestagens, when given alone. Instead the antigestagens induce an elevation in serum estradiol by day 44 (data not shown).

Reconsideration of the Labor-Inducing Activity of Antigestagens: Do These Compounds Interact with Endogenous Estrogens? Antigestagens clearly differ in their labor-inducing activity (see above). Could these differences be explained by different "anti-estrogenic" activities? Is the onset of labor after antigestagens generally a reflection of an interaction with endogenous estrogens? The following experiments were done to study the possibility of such interactions using estrogens and anti-estrogens. Depending on the purpose of the interaction studies, different antigestagens were selected. ZK 98.734 and ZK 98.299 have a high labor-inducing activity and were therefore preferred for the evaluation of inhibitory effects of estrogens. RU 486 and ZK 112.993, on the other hand, have low labor-inducing activity. These antigestagens were considered as suitable to evaluate synergistic interactions. The abortifacient effect of ZK 98.734 (10.0 mg/day sc) was completely abolished by estradiol (0.1 mg/day sc, days 42–45 pc)(Fig. 14). In a second controlled study with ZK 98.299, it was found that as low as 0.001 mg/day estradiol clearly delays the onset of labor. Higher estradiol doses (i.e., 0.01 or 0.1 mg/day) further delay or abolish labor inducing activity of ZK 98.299 compared to antigestagen-treated controls (Fig. 15A).

　　According to these results it is tempting to conclude that ZK 98.734 and ZK 98.299 have more prominent anti-estrogenic activity than other antigestagens.

cumulative rate of abortion in %

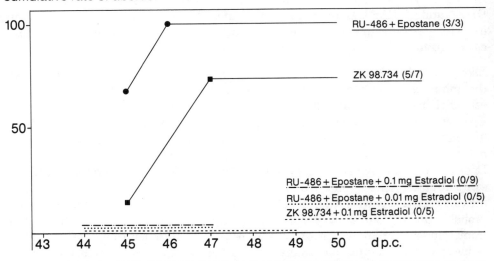

Fig. 14. Estradiol-17β abolishes the labor-inducing activity of RU 486/Epostane combination or that of ZK 98.734 completely. (AG [ZK 98.734, RU 486] = 10.0 mg/day sc, days 43–44 pc; Epostane = 30.0 mg/day sc, days 43–44 pc; and Estradiol = 0.1 mg resp. 0.01 mg/day sc, days 42–45 pc.)

cumulative rate of abortion in %

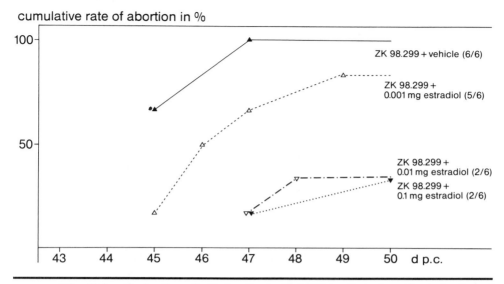

Fig. 15A. Evaluation of effects of estradiol-17β treatment on the induction of labor with the antigestagen ZK 98.299: Inhibition of spontaneous labor. (Antigestagen = 10.0-mg ZK 98.299/day sc, days 43–44 pc; estrogen doses = 0.001-mg, 0.01-mg, and 0.1-mg estradiol/day sc, days 42–45 pc.)

However, a mechanism of such actions is still obscure. There is no binding of RU 486 (19, 20), ZK 98.734, or ZK 98.299 (19) to the cytosolic estrogen receptor. Thus estradiol displacement from this site is very unlikely. There is also no evidence of decreased estrogen secretion following antigestagen treatment. There may be other mechanisms of estrogen interaction as discussed above.

RU 486/Tamoxifen, ZK 112.993/Tamoxifen Interaction Studies. The antiestrogen tamoxifen was used to study the significance of the "estrogen block." Tamoxifen (10 mg/day sc) itself had no adverse effect on pregnancy. However, when combined with marginally active doses (10 mg/day sc) of the above antigestagens it effectively promoted the expulsion of the uterine contents. Practically all animals aborted and in addition there was an earlier onset of labor compared to antigestagen-treated controls (17). These results confirm the conclusions drawn from the RU 486/Epostane studies. They seem to show that the estrogens in fact exert an inhibitory influence on the onset of labor in antigestagen-treated animals.

Evaluation of Myometrial Responses to Sulprostone in ZK 98.299-Treated "Estrogen-Blocked" Animals. It was the aim of these studies to localize the inhibitory effects of estrogen. In order to exclude other actions than those on the intrinsic trigger of labor, the myometrial prostaglandin reactivity in estrogen-blocked animals was tested. A single injection of ZK 98.299 around day 43 elevates the myometrial reactivity to such an extent that otherwise inactive doses of sulprostone

cumulative rate of abortion in %

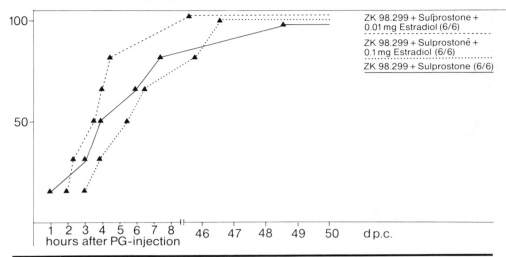

Fig. 15B. Evaluation of effects of estradiol-17β treatment on the induction of labor with the antigestagen ZK 98.299: There is no alteration of the myometrial reactivity to sulprostone. (Estradiol = 0.1 mg resp. 0.01 mg/day sc, days 43–44 pc; ZK 98.299 = 10.9 mg/day sc, day 44 pc; and sulprostone = 0.03 mg/day sc, day 45 pc.)

induces labor and abortion in high rates of animals (see above). In a controlled experiment 10.0-mg ZK 98.299 was injected on day 44 pc followed by 0.03-mg sulprostone sc on day 45 pc (controls). This regime induced an immediate expulsion of uterine contents in all animals (Fig. 15B). In two other groups, this treatment was combined with either 0.01- or 0.1-mg estradiol/day sc on days 43–44 pc. These doses of estradiol induce a long-lasting inhibition of labor when given in combination with ZK 98.299; however, they did not inhibit the effects of marginal sulprostone doses. These results show that exogenous estrogens block labor due to an interference with the intrinsic uterine trigger mechanism. The elevation in myometrial reactivity due to progesterone deprivation is not distinctly altered.

GENERAL DISCUSSION

Our studies in pregnant guinea pigs with antigestagens have shown that an effective inhibition of progesterone action in uterine tissues is not sufficient to induce effective labor. There is no question that the inhibition of progesterone induces an immediate and dramatic elevation of the capability of the myometrium to respond to prostaglandins. However, none of the tested antigestagens were able to induce a parallel increase in uterine prostaglandin F-secretion (21). Antigestagens have the capability to block the rising levels of uterine prostaglandin secretion at some stages of the reproductive cycle in guinea pigs. In rats there was a dose-dependent inhibition of the prepartal luteal regression indicating similar inhibitory effects in pregnancy as well (22). We tend to interpret some of the drawbacks that were encountered with the clinical use of RU 486 also as evidence of a uterine prostaglandin deficiency. The induction of labor by antigestagens is in general by a mechanism that converts the myometrium to a reactive tissue.

Some of our experiments identified other steroidal inhibitors of the "intrinsic uterine stimulant" rather than progesterone. Epostane, a potent inhibitor of the steroidogenic enzyme 3β-OH-Δ-5-steroid-dehydrogenase, was found to be a potent stimulator of labor in combination with RU 486 and various other antigestagens. The mode of synergism was interpreted as a complementary one. The antigestagen causes high myometrial reactivity and Epostane triggers the onset of labor. Surprisingly, progesterone substitution completely failed to antagonize this antigestagen/Epostane synergism. Our data suggest that inhibitory effects of Epostane on the estrogen biosynthesis plays a crucial role in the initiation of labor. Anti-estrogens (Tamoxifen) have the same facilitating effect in antigestagen-treated animals. Studies with exogenous estrogens and estradiol precursors led to similar conclusions. Their application abolished the labor-inducing activity of antigestagen/Epostane combinations. The labor-inducing component of antigestagens was reevaluated in light of the above findings. The question arose if antigestagens induce labor by interaction with endogenous estrogens. Indeed, the labor-inducing activity of antigestagens has been overcome by exogenous estrogens. The antigestagen effects on myometrial reactivity to prostaglandins, on the other hand, remain unaffected by estrogens. The problem that arises in this context is the lack of an established mechanism by which antigestagens could exert such anti-estrogenic actions. There are, however, other phenomena suggesting antigestagen interactions with estrogens. The endometrial effects of estrogens were effectively blocked by RU 486 treatment in cynomolgous monkeys (23). Differences in labor-inducing activity of antigestagens might reflect differences in anti-estrogenic activity by still unknown mechanisms of interaction with estrogens. An important question is the relevance of the employed guinea pig model.

REFERENCES

1. Csapo A I. Force of labor. In: Iffy L, Kaminestzky H A, eds. Principles and practice of obstetrics and perinatology, vol 2. New York: John Wiley & Sons, 1981:761-99.
2. Chwalisz K, Hegele-Hartung C, Fritzemeier KH, Putz B, Elger W. Selective inhibition of the estrogen-dependent endometrial gland formation by progesterone antagonists Onapristone (ZK 98.299) and Mifepristone (RU 486) in rabbits. Acta Endocrinol 1990;122(suppl 1):29.
3. Elger W, Faehnrich M, Beier S, Shi Shao Qing, Chwalisz K. Endometrial and myometrial effects of progesterone-antagonists in pregnant guinea pigs. International Symposium on Contraception (Singapore, 1986). Am J Obstet Gynecol 1987;157: 1065-74.
4. Garfield R, Beier S. Increased myometrial responsiveness to oxytocin during term and preterm birth. Am J Obstet Gynecol 1989;161:451-61.
5. Chwalisz K, Hegele-Hartung C, Louton T, Shi Shao Qing, Althof S, Elger W. Ripening

of the uterine cervix with the progesterone antagonist ZK 98.299. Acta Endocrinol 1989;120(suppl 1):186.

6. Raynaud JP. R 5020, a tag for the progestin receptor. In: McGuire WL, Raynaud JP. Progress in cancer research and therapy; vol 4. New York: Raven Press, 1977:9-22.

7. Christiansen RG, Neumann HC, Salvador UJ, Bell MR, Schane HP, Creange JE, Potts GO, Anzalone AJ. Steroidogenesis inhibitors, 1. Adrenal and interceptive activity of Trilostane and related compounds. J Med Chem 1984;27:928-31.

8. Creange JE, Anzalone AJ, Potts GO, Schane HP. WIN 32,729, a new, potent interceptive agent in rats and rhesus monkeys. Contraception 1981;24:289 pp.

9. Birgerson L, Odlind V, Johansson EDB. Contraception 1986;33:401 pp.

10. Pattison NS, Webster MA, Phipps SL, Anderson ABM, Gillmer MDG. Inhibition of 3β-hydroxysteroid dehydrogenase (3β-HSD) activity in first- and second-trimester human pregnancy and in luteal phase using Epostane. Fert Steril 1984;42:875 pp.

11. Odlind V, Birgerson L. Interruption of early pregnancy with antiprogestins. In: E Diszfalusy, M Bygdeman. Serono Symposia Publications from Raven Press 36: Fertility regulation today and tomorrow (Stockholm, 1986). New York: Raven Press, 1987:95-104.

12. Crooij MJ, de Nooyer CCA, Ramanath-Rao B, Berends GT, Gooren LJG, Janssens J. Termination of early pregnancy by the 3β-hydroxysteroid dehydrogenase inhibitor Epostane. N Engl J Med 1988;319:813-7.

13. Couzinet B, Schaison G. Mifegyne (Mifepristone), a new antiprogestin with potential therapeutic use in human fertility. DRUGS 1988;35:187-91.

14. Kovacs L, Sas M, Resch BA, et al. Termination of very early pregnancy by RU 486—an antiprogestational compound. Contraception 1984;29:399-410.

15. van Look PFA, Bygdeman M. Antiprogestational steroids: a new dimension in human fertility regulation. In: Milligal SR. Oxford Rev Reprod Biol 1989;11:1-60.

16. Elger W, Qing Shi Shao, Fähnrich M, Beier S, Chwalisz K, Henderson D, Neef G, Rohde R. The mechanism of action of new antiprogestins. In: Diszfalusy E, Bygdeman M. Serono Symposia Publications from Raven Press 36: Fertility regulation today and tomorrow (Stockholm 1986). New York: Raven Press, 1987:95-104.

17. Elger W, Neef G, Ottow E, Beier S, Chwalisz K, Fähnrich M, Kosub B, Hasan SH. Studies on interactions of antigestagens with prostaglandins and sex hormone-related agents at the myometrial level in pregnant guinea pigs. In: Puri CP, van Look PFA. Hormone antagonists for fertility regulation. Bombay: Good Print, 1989:105-21.

18. Elger W, Beier S, Chwalisz K, Fähnrich M, Hasan SH, Henderson D, Neef G, Rohde R. Studies on the mechanism of action of progesterone antagonists; XIIth Meeting of the International Study Group for Steroid Hormones (Rome, 1985). J Steroid Biochem 1986;25:835-46.

19. Pollow K, Juchem MJ, Grill HJ, Manz B, Beier S, Henderson D, Elger W. 3H-ZK 98.734, a new, 11β-aryl substituted antigestagen: binding characteristics to receptor and serum proteins. Acta Endocrinol 1989;120(suppl):161-2.

20. Baulieu E. Recent developments regarding steroid receptors and antihormones. Maturitas 1986;8:133-40.

21. Fähnrich M, Meyer B, Elger W. Evaluation of prostaglandins in uterine compartments after treatment with progesterone antagonists in advanced pregnancy in guinea pigs. Human reproduction, Abstracts from the 3rd meeting of the European Society of Human Reproduction and Embryology. Oxford: IRL Press, 1987:86.

22. Chwalisz K, Beier S, Hasan SH. Parturition induced with antigestagens in the rat is

associated with inhibition of prepartal luteolysis. Acta Endocrinol 1988;287(suppl 117):195-6.

23. van Uem JFHM, Hsiu JG, Chillik CF, Danforth DR, Uhlman A, Baulieu EE, Hodgen GD. Contraceptive potential of RU 486 by ovulation inhibition: pituitary versus ovarian action with blockade of estrogen induced endometrial proliferation. Contraception 1989;40:171 pp.

13

Oxytocin and Oxytocin Receptors: Maternal Signals for Parturition

Anna-Riitta Fuchs

Department of Obstetrics and Gynecology, Cornell University Medical College, New York

T he exact nature of the maternal and fetal signals that initiate parturition in primates and the way they are integrated and translated into uterine function are still incompletely understood. The fetal signals are best known in the sheep, where fetal pituitary and adrenal are the key factors (1). While there is no evidence that fetal ACTH and cortisol secretion play the same crucial role in primates as in sheep, the maturation of the fetal pituitary-adrenal axis as well as the pituitary-thyroid axis are important factors that contribute to the sequence of events culminating in birth.

In regard to the maternal signal(s) a substantial body of evidence points to oxytocin as the primary maternal factor that activates the uterus during labor in all mammals. (For review, see Fuchs [2, 3]). To be considered a primary stimulant of the myometrium during parturition, an agent must fulfill certain requirements listed in Table 1. It should be specific for the uterus, and the responsiveness of the myometrium to it should be controlled in a way that prevents preterm activation of the uterus. It should be released in a sufficiently precise manner to respond to clues from both the maternal and fetal organism in a timely fashion, and there should be an adequate supply ready for release at the appropriate time.

Oxytocin (OT) is the only endogenous uterus contracting agent that fulfills these requirements: (*a*) It is specific for the smooth muscles of the reproductive tract; (*b*) the myometrial responsiveness to OT is regulated in a purposeful way in that it is low during gestation and rises to maximal levels at term; (*c*) the release of OT is under neural control, which permits precise timing of the release; and (*d*) the pituitary content of OT in mother and fetus increases during pregnancy.

By contrast, the α-adrenergic compounds and prostaglandins stimulate all smooth muscles. The sensitivity of the uterus to α-adrenergic agonists decreases during gestation but does not rise until sometime after delivery, whereas the uterine sensitivity to prostaglandins is high throughout gestation. The release of α-adrenergic agents is of course neurally controlled and can be precisely regulated,

Table 1. Requirements for primary uterine stimulant during labor.

	Oxytocin	α-agonists	Prostaglandins
Specific for uterus	Yes	No	No
Release mechanism(s) permitting this precise control	Yes	Yes	No
End-organ sensitivity low in pregnancy, high in labor	Yes	No	No
Content(s) increase in mother and fetus during pregnancy	Yes	No	Yes
Systematic release, hence eliciting synchronous contractions	Yes	No	No

but during gestation the uterus is virtually depleted of its neurotransmitter content, which is not restored until some time postpartum. The capacity of uterine tissues to synthesize prostaglandins, on the other hand, increases during pregnancy, but the release mechanisms for prostaglandins are suffusive and nonspecific. While oxytocin is released systemically and therefore activates all parts of the myometrium simultaneously, prostaglandins are released locally and diffuse from the decidua to the inner layers only. Other mechanisms are therefore needed to transform these local contractions into propagated and synchronous contractions.

CIRCULATING OT LEVELS DURING PARTURITION

Animals

An increase in circulating oxytocin levels during parturition has been observed in all animal species studied (4, 5), and labor can be induced by OT in all species provided that the administration is properly timed. The doses required for labor induction result in maternal oxytocin levels that are quite similar to the levels observed during spontaneous labor (5, 6). Examples are shown in Figure 1 (rats) and Figure 2 (rabbits). The effectiveness of OT is in striking contrast to the failure of PGE_2, or $PGF_{2\alpha}$ to induce labor in many species (6).

The pattern of OT secretion and uterine activation during the course of labor varies dramatically in different species. In some, OT secretion is pulsatile and is associated with gradually increasing uterine activity over a period of several hours, as in rats; in others, OT is released as a surge that causes a sudden increase in uterine contractions and the expulsion of the fetuses within a short span of time, as in the rabbit. Parturition in the cow is also achieved by a sudden surge of OT, during which the calf is expelled. In rabbits, plasma OT levels fall to baseline values rapidly after delivery; in cows, OT levels remain high for 2–3 h throughout the first, second, and third stages of labor (5) (Fig. 3).

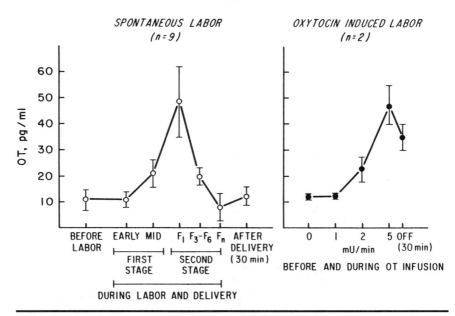

Fig. 1. Plasma OT levels in parturient rats measured in serial samples obtained by means of an in-dwelling atrial catheter before and during spontaneous (open circles) and OT-induced labor (closed circles). Note that the assay sensitivity was too low to detect a rise in plasma OT during infusion of 1-mU OT/min and during the first stage of labor. Uterine activity was measured in the same rats (values not shown; see Fuchs and Poblete, Biol Reprod 2:387, 1970). It increased in parallel with plasma OT in both situations. (From Fuchs A-R, Oxytocin in animal parturition, In: Amico J, Robinson AG, eds, Oxytocin: clinical and laboratory studies, Excerpta Medica, Intl Congr Ser 666, New York: Elsevier, 1985:207–35, courtesy of Elsevier Science Publishers.)

Women

In contrast to the clear-cut animal data, the data reported for plasma oxytocin levels in parturient women are conflicting. Some authors have found significant increases in plasma OT during both first and second stages of labor, whereas others have not found any increase, or an increase only in the second stage, or even a decrease (reviewed in references 3 and 5). This controversy has led some investigators to propose that OT is not functional in the sequence of events leading to parturition in women (7, 8). There are several reasons why such conflicting data are obtained. First, the measurement of circulating oxytocin in pregnant women is associated with unusual difficulties due to the extreme potency of OT and the presence of oxytocinase in pregnancy plasma of primates. The approximate plasma levels that are required to stimulate the human uterus at term have been calculated to be very low, in the range of 1–10 μU/ml (10^{-12}–10^{-11}M). The

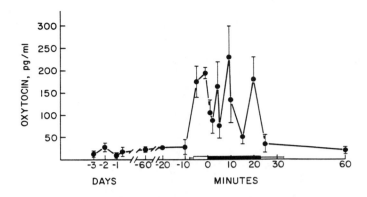

Fig. 2. Plasma OT levels during spontaneous labor measured in serial samples of jugular vein blood obtained from conscious, unrestrained animals. Uterine activity, measured in the same rabbits, increased abruptly in parallel with the rise in plasma OT. Both plasma levels and uterine activity could be mimicked with injections of 250–500 mU of OT IV. (From Fuchs A-R and Dawood MV, Endocrinology 1980;107:1117-26, by courtesy of the editors.)

endogenous oxytocin in a blood sample is subject to rapid degradation in vitro by the oxytocinase present in pregnancy plasma, making the measurement of these low concentrations extremely difficult. Second, the secretion of OT in women may occur in pulses, as in the ewe, rat, and cow, and the sampling frequency may not have been adequate in the previous studies.

We have therefore reexamined the secretory pattern of oxytocin in parturient women (9). Blood samples were collected at 1-min intervals during a 30-min period in 3 groups of women at term: (I) not in labor, (II) in the first stage of spontaneous labor (cervical dilatation on the average 4.5 cm), and (III) in the second and third stages of spontaneous labor. Oxytocin was extracted from 2-ml acidified EDTA plasma with heat-activated Florisil, and standards added to charcoal-treated pregnancy plasma were extracted with each assay to determine extraction recovery for which all results were corrected. A highly specific and sensitive antibody was used (donated by M. Morris from Bowman Gray School of Medicine, Winston-Salem, NC [10]). The results were calculated using logit-log transformed data and a computerized program provided by NIH (NIH RIA logit) (11). The detection limit during these studies was 0.15–0.2 µU/ml. Pulse limit was defined as $3 \times$ SD at the baseline that was calculated by the program.

The data indicated that OT is secreted in pulses in parturient women. The baseline values of all subjects were below the detection limit (mean 0.17 µU/ml) and were interspersed with pulses of short duration, 1–2 min. The pulse frequency in women not in labor was low, mean = 1.2/30 min. The pulse frequency was significantly increased in women sampled during the first stage of labor; mean = 4.5/30 min and a further increase to 6.7±/30 min occurred during the second and third

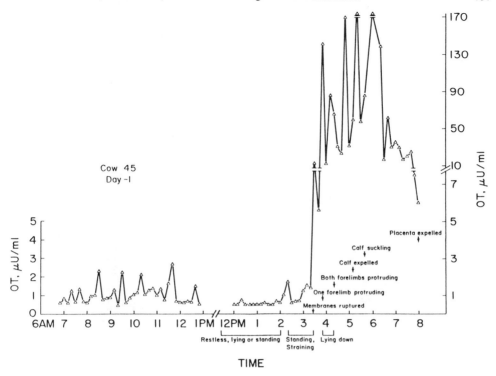

Fig. 3. Plasma OT before and during spontaneous parturition in a cow measured in serial samples of utero-ovarian vein blood. OT levels remained very high until the placenta was expelled, 2.5 h after delivery of the calf, which occurred 2 h after the surge of OT began. (From Fuchs A-R, Oxytocin in animal parturition, In: Amico J, Robinson AG, eds, Oxytocin: clinical and laboratory studies, Excerpta Medica, Intl Congr Ser 666, New York: Elsevier, 1985:207–35, courtesy of Elsevier Science Publishers.)

stages of labor (Fig. 4). The differences were highly significant, P < 0.001 (ANOV). The mean pulse height also increased from 0.9 µU/ml to 1.4 µU/ml as labor progressed, but the differences were not significant. Considerable variations were observed in pulse amplitude in some patients, whereas in others the pulses were of relatively constant magnitude. The proportion of samples below detection limit was dramatically decreased during labor, from 85% in women not in labor to 30% in women in the first stage and 10% in women in the second or third stages of labor.

These results show conclusively that the secretion of OT is significantly increased during labor in women, both in early and in advanced labor.

Response to Exogenous OT Pulses

The functional significance of the observed OT pulses was assessed by measuring plasma OT levels after bolus injections of 2-, 4-, 8-, and 16-mU of OT and by

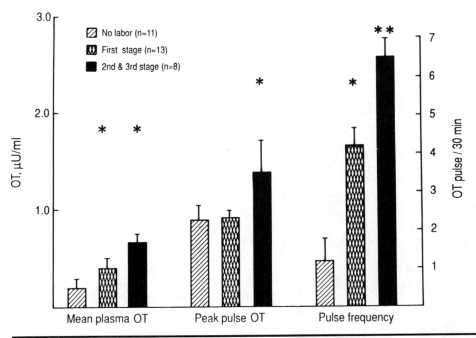

Fig. 4. Parameters of OT secretion measured in serial samples taken at 1-min intervals for 30 min from 3 groups of pregnant women: (I) term not in labor = hatched columns; (II) first stage of term spontaneous labor = crosshatched columns; (III) second and third stage of term labor = black columns. Mean concentration for all samples, mean level considered a pulse (>3 SD over baseline), and pulse frequency were calculated for each subject. (Values are mean ± SE for each group of women; * indicates significant difference from no labor values; ** indicate values between first stage and second stage.) (Modified from Fuchs A-R, Romero R, Parra M, et al., Am J Obstet Gynecol 1990 [in press].)

monitoring uterine activity by external tocography. In the 2-mU group, only 1 patient out of 5 had a significant rise in plasma OT, whereas in the 4-, 8-, and 16-mU groups, a rise was detectable in all women. The peak levels increased in a dose-related manner, and in the 16-mU group, the pulse duration was also increased. The majority of the spontaneous pulses observed during labor resembled those produced by 4- to 8- mU OT, and some, those produced by 16 mU; a few were greater (Fig. 5). The rise in plasma OT was associated with uterine contractions in most women. In the 2-mU group, only the patient who had an OT spike had a contraction. In the 4-mU and 8-mU groups, all but 1 in each group of 5 responded with uterine contractions and 1 woman went into labor after receiving 8-mU OT. One of the 2 receiving 16 mU responded with contractions. Thus, pulses of 0.5–1.5 µU/ml in magnitude are effective in stimulating uterine contractions in women at term.

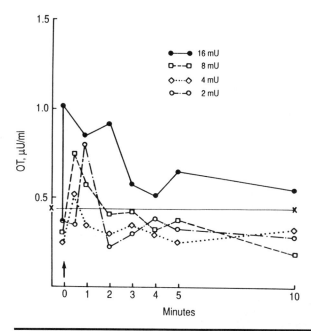

Fig. 5. Plasma OT levels in pregnant women at term before and after an injection (at arrow) of 2-, 4-, 8-, and 16-mU synthetic OT (Pitocin R). The level above which endogenous OT peaks were considered pulses is indicated by the horizontal line. (Modified from Fuchs A-R, Romero R, Parra M, et al., Am J Obstet Gynecol 1990 [in press].)

The variations observed among the experimental subjects in the uterine responsiveness to OT are in accordance with clinical observations (12, 13). The timing of the attainment of maximal uterine sensitivity varies in individual women, but common to all is that the onset of spontaneous labor is associated with increased uterine responsiveness to oxytocin. This was shown in a study we conducted on 28 normal pregnant women in whom daily OT sensitivity tests were performed beginning on the expected day of delivery and continued until the day labor began (14). The uterine sensitivity to oxytocin was increased in each subject on the day labor began. A concomitant increase occurred in the cervical scores (Fig. 6).

MYOMETRIAL OT RECEPTORS

The myometrial responsiveness to oxytocin plays a crucial role in the initiation of labor. The response to OT is in turn mediated by cell membrane receptors that have been demonstrated in myometria of all species (15). We have shown that OT-receptor concentrations in pregnant human uterus increase markedly during gestation; whereas the affinity of the OT receptors does not change significantly. In

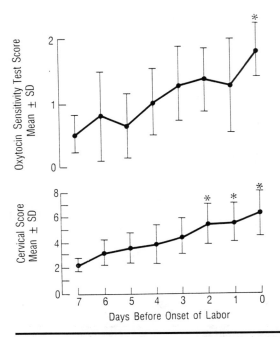

Fig. 6. Changes in uterine OT sensitivity during the last days of pregnancy measured daily in 28 normal pregnant women beginning on the expected delivery date and continued until the day labor began. 10-mU OT was injected IV and the uterine responses, measured by external CTG, were given a score of 0, 1, or 2 (0 = no response, 1 = one contraction of less than 30-sec duration, 2 = one or more contractions of over 30-sec duration). (Values are mean ± SE; * indicates significant difference from initial values.) (From Fuchs A-R and Fuchs F, Br J Obstet Gynaecol 1984;191:948–67, courtesy of the editors.)

early labor, a further increase in OT-receptor concentrations was observed (Fig. 7). The changes in myometrial OT-receptor concentrations during gestation and at term parallel the changes in uterine responsiveness to oxytocin (13, 14, 17), indicating that the concentration of OT receptors is the main factor regulating uterine responsiveness to oxytocin in women as in other species. Near maximal responses to OT are produced at plasma levels that are lower than the Kd for the receptors (approximately 1×10^{-9} M). This indicates the presence of "spare" receptors. This situation is not unique for oxytocin; other agents are known to have spare receptors, and they, too, show biological responses that are related to the total receptor density (18).

How OT-receptor concentrations are regulated in the human myometrium is not known at the present time. In the rat uterus, their formation is estrogen dependent (19). Progesterone exerts a strong suppressive effect on OT receptors in rat, rabbit, hamster, and sheep uteri, probably mediated by its action on estrogen

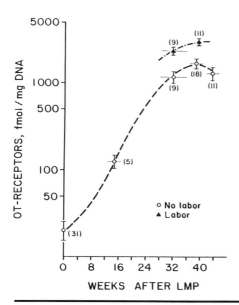

Fig. 7. Changes in human myometrial OT-receptor concentrations during pregnancy and labor measured in samples obtained at hysterectomy from premenopausal, nonpregnant women, and at cesarean section from pregnant and parturient women before (open circles) and after the onset of labor (closed circles). Note the logarithmic scale. (From Fuchs A-R, Fuchs F, Br J Obstet Gynaecol 1984;191:948–67, courtesy of the editors.)

receptors (19, 20). Clearly, progesterone does not suppress OT-receptor formation in women, since the rise in OT-receptor concentrations in pregnant women parallels the rise in plasma progesterone. Distention of the uterus is another factor that regulates OT-receptor concentrations in the rat and acts synergistically with estrogens, causing a significant increase in comparison to a nondistended uterus (21).

The human pregnant uterus is subject to considerable distention, which accelerates near term, when conceptus growth outpaces myometrial growth. Distention may therefore be an important factor in the regulation of OT-receptor concentrations in the human.

INTERACTION WITH PROSTAGLANDINS

Important as oxytocin receptors and oxytocin are, they are not the only factors concerned with uterine activation. Labor contractions can be inhibited by administering either ethanol (2, 3), an OT-release inhibitor, or an OT antagonist (22), or prostaglandin synthetase inhibitors (23), implicating both OT and prostaglandins in the activation of the uterus during labor. Many observations indicate that the production of PGE_2 and $PGF_{2\alpha}$ increases during parturition (24); however, the increase occurs in the active stage of labor and has not been observed at the onset of labor (8, 24). While oxytocin release is an early event, prostaglandin release is a later event in the process of parturition.

The prostaglandin $F_{2\alpha}$ produced during labor derives mostly from the decidua, since the myometrium produces mainly prostacyclin (PGI_2) and amnion produces mainly PGE_2. OT receptors are present in high concentrations also in human pregnant decidua, where OT has been shown to stimulate phospholipase-C activity and increase the mobilization of arachidonic acid (25) and prostaglandin E_2 production (26). OT therefore has a dual effect in labor; it stimulates contractions through myometrial receptors and causes the release of $PGF_{2\alpha}$ through decidual receptors (26). The released $PGF_{2\alpha}$ diffuses into the adjacent myometrium and causes contractions and enhances the action of other oxytocics (27). The enhancement was observed at considerably lower concentrations than the direct oxytocic effects of $PGF_{2\alpha}$. The authors suggested that $PGF_{2\alpha}$ transformed unexcitable Ca^{++} channels into excitable ones. Such a mechanism, if present also in human uterus, would reinforce and magnify the direct stimulus provided by oxytocin and explain the marked reduction with advancing labor in the dose of oxytocin required to maintain labor.

OXYTOCIN AND THE PROPAGATION OF CONTRACTIONS

The recruitment of great numbers of cells to contract simultaneously and the synchronization of contractions over large areas are essential for uterine contractions to become effective and labor to progress. This can be achieved by increasing the concentration of circulating oxytocin or increasing the numbers of OT receptors. It can be achieved also by improving cell-to-cell coupling, which permits impulses to propagate longer distances. Gap junctions provide low-resistance coupling between cells and thus serve to multiply the responses to direct stimuli (28). Rapid propagation of impulses and synchronization of contractions is of particular importance in multitocous species like the rat and rabbit, in which a directional force is required to propel the fetuses toward the cervix and overcome the resistance of the cervix. In the human uterus, their role may be of less importance since the anatomical configuration of the uterus and the distribution of myometrial OT receptors provide the directional force required to dilate the cervix (Fig. 8).

We have shown that in the rat synchronous activation of the entire length of the uterine horn is required for labor to progress (6). Strong laborlike contractions cannot effect the expulsion of fetuses as long as the contractions remain local and are not rapidly propagated along the horn. Oxytocin cannot transform an asynchronous uterus into a synchronized one. This transformation is dependent on the steroid hormones; it is inhibited by progesterone and promoted by estrogen (6) and is probably mediated by the effects of the sex steroids on gap-junction formation as described in Chapter 3 and reference 28.

OT Receptors and Gap Junctions

Gap-junction formation and OT-receptor formation are temporally closely correlated in the rat, suggesting a common regulatory mechanism. Chan et al. (29) have

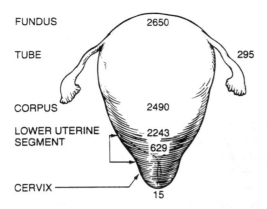

FUNDUS   2650

TUBE   295

CORPUS   2490

LOWER UTERINE SEGMENT   2243   629

CERVIX   15

Fig. 8. Distribution of myometrial OT receptors in the pregnant human uterus at term. (Values are fmol/mg DNA, means for 3 uteri removed for medical reasons.) (From Fuchs A-R, Fuchs F, Physiology of parturition, in: Gabbe S, Niebyl J, Simpson JL, eds, Obstetrics, normal and problem pregnancies, 1st ed, 1985:337, courtesy of Churchill Livingstone.)

recently shown that the two processes could be temporally dissociated by means of a continuous infusion of naproxen, a prostaglandin-synthesis inhibitor, given from day 20 of gestation onward. This treatment prevented the increase in OT-receptor levels in the entire uterus, usually observed on day 23, while the gap-junction numbers in the longitudinal muscle layer increased to normal levels. All treated rats failed to give birth on day 23, but delivered late on day 24, when OT-receptor levels had risen to control values. The rise in OT receptors is thus essential for the onset of spontaneous labor, and gap junctions play a permissive but not a primary role.

The naproxen-induced alterations in the timing of the appearance of gap junctions and OT receptors are likely to be indirect, mediated by a naproxen-induced delay in luteolysis and the normal decline in plasma progesterone (30), which is a prerequisite for the onset of labor in rats (6).

Garfield and Hayashi (31) have investigated the occurrence of gap junctions in samples of human pregnant myometrium obtained at cesarean section. Before the onset of labor few or no gap junctions were found, but in samples taken at various stages of labor gap junctions were present in 80% of the patients. Because gap junctions appear in human pregnant myometrium only during labor they, like PGs, probably play a permissive rather than primary role in the mechanism of labor in women, providing for the progressive synchronization of contractions in advanced labor. Because of the high concentration of OT receptors in human myometrium, large numbers of myometrial cells are stimulated simultaneously in response to oxytocin pulses, resulting in synchronized contractions even in the absence of gap junctions. Because the concentration of OT receptors is higher in the upper segment than in the lower segment (16), oxytocin has the ability to provide the directional force needed to efface and dilate the cervix even in the absence of gap junctions.

SUMMARY

Figure 9 is a diagrammatic representation of the factors involved in the activation of human myometrium in labor. Oxytocin receptors, prostaglandin synthesis, and gap-junction formation are the three main factors controlling myometrial function during labor in women. The primary maternal signal for the onset of labor is oxytocin, which is secreted in pulses of increasing frequency. The high levels of circulating estrogen and the increasing distention of the myometrium at term increase the formation of OT receptors, so that the low-amplitude pulses of OT are able to stimulate the myometrium to contract. OT receptors in the decidua also are increased, and the decidua begins to produce prostaglandin $F_{2\alpha}$, in response to OT; the released $PGF_{2\alpha}$ diffuses into the adjacent myometrium and potentiates the OT-induced contractions. Various factors excreted by the maturing fetus: OT, AVP, PAF, growth factors, possibly cortisol, and, in the presence of infection, various cytokines, stimulate PGE production in the amnion cells. PGE_2 concentration in the amniotic fluid rises and some PGE_2 passes through the membranes. In spite of extensive degradation in the chorion, some PGE_2 probably reaches the decidua and myometrium, causing further enhancement of OT action. Gap-junction formation in the myometrium increases under the influence of estrogens and distention and possibly the prostaglandins or other arachidonic acid metabolites released from the decidua. Their presence in myometrial cells results in a further potentiation and synchronization of the OT- and $PGF_{2\alpha}$- induced contractions. The corpus and fundus are more muscular and possess higher concentrations of OT receptors than the lower segment and, therefore, exert greater force and slowly pull the lower segment up, thereby effacing the cervix and gradually causing the cervix to dilate. Pressure on the cervical pole of the membranes and the internal os of the cervix increases.

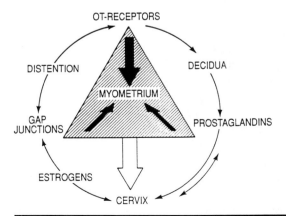

Fig. 9. Diagram summarizing the main factors in uterine contractility.

Tissues in these areas are especially sensitive to traumatic stimuli and begin to release prostaglandins in large amounts (32–34). These diffuse into the endocervix and cause rapid collagen remodeling and cervical ripening. Labor has now reached an irreversible phase where only positive and reinforcing feedback mechanisms are in operation.

REFERENCES

1. Liggins GC, Fairclough RJ, Grieves SA, Kendall JZ, Knox BS. The mechanisms of initiation of parturition in the ewe. Rec Prog Horm Res 1973;29:111-49.
2. Fuchs A-R. The role of oxytocin in human parturition. In: Martini L, James VH, eds. Endocrinology of pregnancy: current topics in experimental endocrinology. New York: Academic Press, 1983:251-65.
3. Fuchs A-R. The role of oxytocin in parturition. In: Huszar G, ed. Biochemistry of the human uterus. Boca Raton, FL: CRC Press, 1986:163-84.
4. Fuchs A-R. Oxytocin in animal parturition. In: Amico J, Robinson AG, eds. Oxytocin: clinical and laboratory studies. Excerpta Medica, Intl Congr Ser 666. New York: Elsevier, 1985:207-35.
5. Fuchs F. Role of maternal and fetal oxytocin in human parturition. In: Amico J, Robinson AG, eds. Oxytocin: clinical and laboratory studies. Excerpta Medica, Intl Congr Ser 666. New York: Elsevier, 1985:236-55.
6. Fuchs A-R. Hormonal control of myometrial function during pregnancy and parturition. Acta Endocr (Copenh) 1978;89(suppl):1-70.
7. Casey ML, MacDonald PC. The initiation of labor in women: regulation of phospholipid and arachidonic acid metabolism and of prostaglandin production. Sem Perinatol 1986;10:270-5.
8. MacDonald PC. Overview—analysis of factors associated with term and preterm labor [Abstract]. Symposium on Uterine Contractility. Serono Symposia, USA, St. Louis, MO, 1990.
9. Fuchs A-R, Romero R, Parra M, et al. Pulsatile release of oxytocin: significant increase in spontaneous labor. Am J Obstet Gynecol 1990 (in press).
10. Morris M, Steven SW, Adamo MR. Plasma oxytocin during pregnancy and lactation in the cynomolgus monkey. Biol Reprod 1980;23:782-7.
11. Rodbard D, Huston J Jr, Munson PJ. BASRIA RIA data processing basic programs. Vanderbilt Medical Center, Dept Radiol and Radiol Sci/Dept Endocrinol, 1980.
12. Knaus H. Zur Physiologie des Corpus Luteum III–IV. Mitteilung. Arch Gynäk 1929;138:201-16.
13. Caldeyro-Barcia R, Theobald GW. Sensitivity of the pregnant human myometrium to oxytocin. Am J Obstet Gynecol 1968;102:1181-2.
14. Kofler E, Husslein P, Langer M, Fuchs A-R, Fuchs F. Die Bedeutung der Oxytocinempfindlichkeit für den spontanen Wehenbeginn beim Menschen. Geburtsh u Frauenheilk 1983;43:995-1000.
15. Soloff MS. "Minireview": regulation of oxytocin action at the receptor level. Life Sci 1979;25:1453-60.
16. Fuchs A-R, Fuchs F, Husslein P, Soloff MS. Oxytocin receptors in pregnant human uterus. Am J Obstet Gynecol 1984;150:734-41.
17. Caldeyro-Barcia R, Poseiro JJ. Oxytocin and contractility of the pregnant human uterus. Ann NY Acad Sci 1959;75:813-30.

18. Nickerson M. Receptor occupancy and tissue response. Nature 1956;178:697-8.
19. Fuchs A-R, Periyasamy S, Alexandrova M, Soloff MS. Correlation between oxytocin receptor concentration and responsiveness to oxytocin in pregnant rat myometrium. Effect of ovarian steroids. Endocrinology 1983;113:742-9.
20. Leavitt WW, Okulicz WC, McCracken JA, Schramm W, Robidoux WF. Rapid recovery of nuclear estrogen receptor and oxytocin receptor in the ovine uterus following progesterone withdrawal. Biochem 1985;22:687-91.
21. Fuchs A-R, Periyasamy S, Soloff MS. Systemic and local regulation of oxytocin receptors in the rat uterus. Can J Biochem Cell Biol 1983;61:614-24.
22. Andersen LF, Lyndrup J, Akerlund M, Melin P. Oxytocin receptor blockade: a new principle in the treatment of preterm labor. J Perinatol 1989;6:196-9.
23. Gamissans O, Balasch J. Prostaglandin synthetase inhibitors in the treatment of preterm birth. In: Fuchs F, Stubblefield PG, eds. Preterm birth: causes, prevention and management. New York: Macmillan, 1984:223-4.
24 Keirse MJNC. Endogenous prostaglandins in human parturition. In: Keirse MJNC, Anderson AB, Bennebroek M, Gravenhorst J, eds. Human parturition, Boerhaave Series, vol 15. Leiden: Leiden Univ Press, 1979:101-42.
25. Schrey MP, Read AM, Steer PJ. OT and AVP stimulate inositol phosphate production in human gestational myometrium and decidua cells. Biosci Rep 1986;6:613-9.
26. Fuchs A-R, Fuchs F, Husslein P, Soloff MA, Fernstrom MJ. Oxytocin receptors and human parturition: a dual role for oxytocin in the initiation of labor. Science 1982;215:1396-8.
27. Coleman HA, Parkington H. Induction of prolonged excitability in myometrium of pregnant guinea pig by $PGF_{\alpha2}$. J Physiol (Lond)1988;399:33-47.
28. Garfield R. Propagation and modulation of contractility [Abstract]. Symposium on Uterine Contractility: Mechanisms of Control. Serono Symposia, USA, St. Louis, MO, 1990.
29. Chan WY, Berezin I, Daniel EE. Effects of inhibition of prostaglandin synthesis on uterine oxytocin receptor concentration and myometrial gap junction density in parturient rats. Biol Reprod 1988;39:1117-28.
30. Fuchs A-R, Smitasiri Y, Chantharaksri U. The effect of indomethacin on uterine contractility and luteal regression in pregnant rats at term. J Reprod Fertil 1976;48:321-36.
31. Garfield RE, Hayashi RH. Appearance of gap junctions in the myometrium of women during labor. Am J Obstet Gynecol 1981;140:254-60.
32. Mitchell MD, Keirse MJNC, Anderson ABM, Turnbull AC. Evidence for a local control of prostaglandins within the pregnant human uterus. Br J Obstet Gynaecol 1977;84:35-8.
33. Keirse MJNC, Thiery M, Parewigck W, Mitchell MD. Chronic stimulation of prostaglandin synthesis during cervical ripening before the onset of labor. Prostaglandins 1983;25:671-82.
34. Fuchs A-R, Goeschen K, Rasmussen AB, Rehnstrom JV. Cervical ripening by endocervical and extra-amniotic PGE_2. Prostaglandins 1984;28:217-27.

14

Oxytocin Binding and Mode of Action

Melvyn S. Soloff

Department of Biochemistry, Medical College of Ohio, Toledo

E quation of the endocrine status of an organism with circulating concentrations of hormones does not appear to be appropriate for oxytocin, at least with respect to the responsiveness of uterine smooth muscle to the peptide. The sensitivity of the myometrium to oxytocin (OT) changes considerably in the course of pregnancy and during the estrous cycle, when OT concentrations in the blood show little change or are declining (1–5). Although any link in the chain of events occurring between receptor occupancy and uterine contractions can potentially alter sensitivity to oxytocin, modulation of OT-receptor concentrations appears to be a pivotal step. Uterine receptors for this hormone are upregulated by estrogen and downregulated by progesterone, likely accounting for the changes in receptor concentrations during pregnancy and the estrous/menstrual cycle (6–12). Continued infusion of oxytocin also may lead to downregulation of cognate myometrial receptors (13–15), but the physiological relevance of this phenomenon is not clear. Certain divalent metal cations modify OT-receptor interactions in an acute manner (16), but the physiological significance of this type of regulation also remains to be established.

Increases in the concentration of decidual OT receptors also occur during pregnancy, possibly accounting for OT stimulation of decidual $PGF_{2\alpha}$ release at term (17). The endometrium may be the major target of oxytocin during the estrous cycle, as OT-stimulated $PGF_{2\alpha}$ release may initiate luteolysis in some species (12, 13, 18). During lactation, when blood levels of oxytocin are elevated because of nipple stimulation, the low concentrations of OT receptors in the uterus relative to the mammary gland may explain the unresponsiveness of both endometrium and myometrium to oxytocin when the mammary gland is responsive. The changing sensitivity of the myometrium to vasopressin (19–22) also suggests that regulation of vasopressin receptor levels may occur. To understand neurohypophysial hor-

Acknowledgments: Studies from this laboratory were supported by grant HD-8406 from the National Institutes of Health.

mone actions on the reproductive tract, therefore, it is important to study regulation of receptor levels as well as events mediating neurohypophysial hormone-receptor interaction. The eventual purification and characterization of oxytocin receptors should make both goals possible.

OXYTOCIN BINDING SITES

Binding sites for [³H]oxytocin have been demonstrated in myometrial plasma membrane fractions in several species. Separate lines of evidence, reviewed elsewhere (23, 24), have indicated that the binding sites are associated with receptor function. Half-maximal binding to uterine membranes occurred with 1- to 2-nM peptide, consistent with the dose of oxytocin causing half-maximal responses in vitro. A half-maximal response in vivo, however, can be produced with substantially lower concentrations of oxytocin. Binding to myometrial sites was specific for a number of oxytocin analogs, and the affinity of each analog was generally proportional to its uterotonic potency. Binding also was target-tissue and target-cell specific. Agents causing increases in oxytocin binding, such as estrogen treatment or the addition of specific metal ions, favored an increased myometrial response and/or sensitivity to oxytocin. Progesterone administration inhibited the estrogen-induced effects, both on the concentration of myometrial oxytocin receptors and myometrial sensitivity to oxytocin. Occupancy of binding sites by oxytocin or analogs corresponded to putative effector function, such as inhibition of $(Ca^{++} + Mg^{++})$ATPase activity of rat myometrial plasma membranes.

An ¹²⁵I-labeled oxytocin antagonist (25), ¹²⁵I-[(1-β-mercapto-β,β-cyclopenta methylenepropionic acid)2-O-methyltyrosine,4-threonine,8-ornithine,9-tyrosylamino] vasotocin, that binds specifically to oxytocin target cells (25–27) has been used to quantitate oxytocin receptors in the past three years. Oxytocin is inactivated, both biologically and as a ligand, when it is iodinated at the 2-tyrosyl residue (28, 29). However, O-methylation of the 2-tyrosine of the antagonist prevents iodination at this position. Monoiodination of the 9-tyrosylamide residue of the antagonist actually resulted in an increased affinity for receptor sites (25, 27). In membranes from mammary gland of the lactating rat, monoiodinated antagonist had an affinity about 150 times greater than the noniodinated form (27). Although the iodinated antagonist offers great promise under conditions where the amount of membranes is limiting or receptor concentrations are relatively low and in autoradiographic studies, it should be noted that the ability of a number of nonradioactive oxytocin analogues to compete with labeled antagonist did not precisely correspond in rank order to their ability to inhibit [³H]oxytocin binding by rat mammary gland membranes (27). In particular, the apparent Kd of arginine vasopressin binding was about 4 times smaller than that of oxytocin when measured with the antagonist, but about 4 times greater than that of oxytocin relative to [³H]oxytocin binding. Despite the differences, however, the iodinated antagonist has little affinity for vasopressin receptors in the kidney medulla (V_2 receptors) and liver (V_1 receptors) (28) and offers great promise in supplanting the lower specific activity tritiated hormone.

VASOPRESSIN BINDING SITES IN THE MYOMETRIUM

Vasopressin is more potent than oxytocin in stimulating myometrial contractions in nonpregnant women (19–21) and in women during the first trimester of pregnancy (22). The greater motility of the uterus that occurs during menstruation might be due to vasopressin because inhibition of vasopressin release by water-loading reduced uterine contractions (30). Uterine activity could then be reestablished by IV administration of vasopressin, but not oxytocin. Because of the greater sensitivity of the myometrium to oxytocin in the later stages of pregnancy (2), the question arises as to whether there is a single neurohypophysial hormone-receptor population that shifts specificity from vasopressin to oxytocin in later stages of gestation or whether there are separate vasopressin and oxytocin receptors, the relative concentrations of which change during pregnancy.

Consistent with its high uterotonic potency in the nonpregnant uterus, vasopressin was as effective as oxytocin in inhibiting the binding of [^{3}H]oxytocin to fundus and corpus plasma membrane preparations (31). Guillon and coworkers (32) suggested that there are separate receptors for vasopressin and oxytocin in the myometrium of nonpregnant women. The concentration of high-affinity [^{3}H]vasopressin binding sites was about six-times that of high-affinity [^{3}H]oxytocin binding sites. In addition, the order of potency of analogs inhibiting [^{3}H]oxytocin binding was different from that inhibiting [^{3}H]vasopressin binding. Because the ligand specificity of myometrial vasopressin receptors was primarily of the V_1 subtype, which is characteristic of vascular smooth muscle, it is possible that vascular contamination of the membrane preparation contributed to vasopressin binding.

Maggi and coworkers (33) similarly provided evidence for separate populations of oxytocin and V_1 vasopressin receptors in rabbit myometrium. At the time of parturition, a 17-fold increase in oxytocin binding sites was seen, while the number of vasopressin binding sites was unchanged. The greater sensitivity of the myometrium to vasopressin in the nonpregnant uterus may be due to a greater number of vasopressin than oxytocin receptors. During pregnancy, the shift in sensitivity of the myometrium to oxytocin may be due to the upregulation of receptors for oxytocin but not for vasopressin. Until separate myometrial oxytocin and vasopressin receptors are isolated physically, however, we can only speculate on the mechanisms responsible for changing sensitivities of the myometrium to the two peptides during pregnancy.

CHARACTERIZATION OF OXYTOCIN BINDING SITES

Solubilization of Oxytocin Receptors

A fraction of the binding sites of membranes from either uterine myometrium from pregnant rats or involuted mammary gland from rats was solubilized with the zwitterionic detergent 3-[(3-cholamidopropyl)dimethylammonio]-2-hydroxy-1-propane sulfonate (CHAPSO) (34). Further solubilization of binding activity did not occur on repeated extraction of membranes. The low yield of extractable binding activity could be due to the association of receptors with relatively insoluble proteins, such as actomyosin filaments that are anchored on the cytoplasmic surface of smooth-muscle cells (35). Indeed, relaxation of contractile filaments in crude membrane fractions from lactating rat mammary gland resulted in a substantial increase in the amount of oxytocin receptor solubilized (Soloff, unpublished).

The bindings of [^{3}H]oxytocin in CHAPSO extracts of rat mammary gland and intact plasma membranes were similar or identical (34). Several oxytocin analogs inhibited [^{3}H]oxytocin binding in the same rank order in both preparations. Both solubilized and intact membrane preparations also required Mg^{++} for [^{3}H]oxytocin binding. The concentration of binding sites in solubilized extracts of uterine myometrium taken from rats in labor was considerably greater than extracts taken several days before labor, corroborating results with intact membranes (8). These findings suggest that the marked rise in receptor concentration near the end of gestation is not due to the unmasking of cryptic receptor sites because solubilization would be expected to expose hidden binding sites. The binding of [^{3}H]oxytocin to CHAPSO solubilized extracts from intestinal smooth muscle, which is not a target for oxytocin, was negligible.

Molecular Size of Oxytocin Receptors

Sizes of intact membrane receptors for oxytocin in rat myometrium and mammary gland were estimated by radiation inactivation studies (36). Exposure of membranes to increasing doses of ^{60}Co radiation resulted in the inactivation of binding activity. From the rate of loss of binding, the functional sizes of oxytocin receptors in mammary gland of the lactating rat and rat myometrial membranes were both estimated to be about 58,000 D (36).

Molecular size estimates also have been made by photoaffinity-labeling studies. Fahrenholz's laboratory used an analog of tritiated 1-deamino-[8-lysine]vasopressin, containing a photoreactive azidophenylamidino group at the side chain of 8-Lys, to covalently label myometrial oxytocin receptors from near-term guinea pigs (37). Electrophoretic analyses in denaturing SDS-polyacrylamide gels showed specific labeling of a protein with an apparent mol wt of 78,000 ± 5,000. A second band with an apparent mol wt of 43,000 ± 4,000 was found in lesser amounts. The mol wt of oxytocin receptors from the regressed mammary gland of the rat was estimated to be 65,000 ± 3,000 when the same photoaffinity ligand was used (38). Cross-linking of the ligand to vasopressin receptors was ruled out by use of an oxytocin-receptor-specific agonist. This peptide competed with [^{3}H]vasopressin binding sites on mammary membranes but did not inhibit binding of vasopressin to membranes from liver and kidney. Presumably, therefore, [^{3}H]vasopressin was bound to oxytocin receptors on mammary membranes.

We have employed two-step affinity chromatography to obtain an enriched fraction of oxytocin receptors from the mammary gland of the lactating rat (Soloff et al., unpublished). Oxytocin was immobilized to agarose by conjugating the carboxyl-terminal of the free acid form of oxytocin to aminohexyl Sepharose with water soluble carbodiimide. Oxytocin binding activity was adsorbed to the column and the putative receptor was eluted with pH 4.5 buffer. The eluted material was then adsorbed to WGL-Sepharose and, following rinsing, eluted with N-acetylglucosamine. Specific binding activity was not adsorbed to Concanavalin A-Sepharose. The apparent mol wt of the purified receptor was about 65,000 on SDS-polyacrylamide gel electrophoresis, consistent with the size of the ^{125}I-labeled antagonist-receptor complex resulting from coupling the antagonist and membrane receptor and with a water-soluble derivative of succinylimidosuberate before solubilization with SDS and with the results of Müller et al (38).

Gel filtration of CHAPSO-solubilized extracts of rat myometrium indicated that the native receptor exists in a larger molecular weight form (34). A more detailed analysis of the native receptor from the mammary gland of the lactating rat showed that it coeluted with bacterial β-galactosidase, indicating an apparent Stoke's radius of about 68.4 Å (Soloff, unpublished). A smaller form, corresponding to an apparent Stoke's radius of about 30.5 Å also was seen. The relative sizes of the native and putative subunits of the oxytocin receptor are comparable to those shown with glycine (39) and $GABA_A$ (40) receptors, both of which form ligand-gated ion channels. There are no indications at the present time, however, whether oxytocin receptors in contractile cells comprise a ligand-gated channel, belong to the seven transmembrane family of G-protein coupled receptors, or represent unique structures.

Information About the Receptor Gained from the Use of Oxytocin Analogs/Antagonists

The iodinated oxytocin antagonist cited above, with an iodinated tyrosyl amide replacing the carboxyl-terminal glycinamide, had a pA_2^* of 7.7 when tested on rat uterus in vitro, indicating an apparent Kd of about 20 nM (25). The apparent Kd of the antagonist estimated from binding to uterine plasma membranes from estrogen-treated rats was 48 pM. Although the basis of the discrepancy in estimated Kd values from the bioassay and binding studies is not clear, the carboxyl-terminal glycinamide of oxytocin does not appear to be required for interaction with receptor sites. Yet, this residue is required for agonist activity (41), suggesting that the carboxyl-terminal residues of oxytocin are important for intrinsic activity. The same conclusions have been reached regarding the structure of vasopressin agonists and antagonists (42). The significance of these findings may become more apparent once the structures of neurohypophysial hormone receptors are understood.

COUPLING BETWEEN OT-RECEPTOR OCCUPANCY AND CELL CONTRACTION

An understanding of the mechanisms of OT action has been slow to develop, in comparison to what is known about the actions of many other hormones. There is little question that calcium is involved in mediating the contractile response to

---

*pA_2 is the negative log of the molar concentration of antagonist reducing the response of $2\times$ units of agonist to that of $1\times$, administered before antagonist.

oxytocin. It still is not clear, however, whether the source of activator calcium is intracellular, extracellular, or a combination of both. There is some evidence to suggest that voltage-sensitive calcium channels are involved, while other studies indicate that oxytocin is effective in depolarized myometrium. There also is evidence, both pro and con, for the involvement of polyphosphoinositides and G-proteins. These studies are summarized in the following section.

Ca++

OT-induced contractions of rat myometrium were shown to be dependent upon extracellular Ca^{++}, even after depolarization of the myometrial plasma membrane with KCl (43). In contrast, other studies have shown that uterine contractions were prevented, presumably by inhibition of voltage-sensitive Ca^{++} gating, with calcium-channel blockers (44, 45). Other studies have suggested that the actions of oxytocin were mediated by a distinct population of membrane Ca^{++} channels. OT- but not acetylcholine-induced contractions of rat myometrium were seen when Ca^{++} in the medium was replaced with Mg^{++} (46). Whether one or the other channel type is voltage-sensitive was not established.

Injection of size-fractionated poly(A^+) RNA from bovine endometrium into *Xenopus laevis* oocytes resulted in oscillating currents in response to the addition of oxytocin to the bathing medium after voltage clamping (47). The response appeared to be specific, as it was inhibited by an oxytocin antagonist. These data are consistent with the effects of oxytocin being mediated by receptor-regulated calcium gating.

Other studies have suggested that oxytocin also mobilizes Ca^{++} from intracellular stores. In one of the most recent studies demonstrating this point, Anwer and Sanborn measured intracellular free Ca^{++} concentrations directly in myometrial cells loaded with fura-2 (48). Replacement of extracellular Ca^{++} with EGTA resulted in a 57% reduction in the intracellular free Ca^{++} transient induced by oxytocin. Presumably the remaining 43% arises from intracellular sources.

(Ca++ + Mg++)ATPase

The Ca^{++} concentration gradient maintained by cells results from the extrusion of Ca^{++} by a high-affinity Ca^{++} pump (49). This process involves hydrolysis of ATP by calcium-and magnesium-dependent ATPase activity—$(Ca^{++} + Mg^{++})$ATPase—as demonstrated with several different cell types (50).

OT-inhibited $(Ca^{++} + Mg^{++})$ATPase activity in myometrial plasma membrane fractions from estrogen-treated rabbits (51). Characterization of this activity in rat myometrial plasma membrane indicated that activity was linked to occupancy of OT-receptor site (52): Half-maximal inhibition of activity occurred with 1-nM oxytocin, corresponding approximately with the apparent Kd of OT binding. Several oxytocin analogs inhibited ATPase activity in proportion to their affinity for myometrial receptor sites and their uterotonic potencies. OT-inhibited $(Ca^{++} + Mg^{++})$ATPase activity also was target-tissue specific, being present on fat cell membranes that contain OT receptors, but absent on rat duodenal membranes that lack receptors. Myometrial $(Ca^{++} + Mg^{++})$ATPase activity was stimulated by estrogen, and the effects of estrogen were opposed by progesterone treatment. At the beginning of labor in the rat, when plasma estrogen/progesterone concentration ratios are the greatest, OT inhibition of $(Ca^{++} + Mg^{++})$ATPase activity was 10,000 times greater than on day 18 (53). This increase likely is the result of estrogen-induced increases in both OT-receptor concentration and $(Ca^{++} + Mg^{++})$ATPase activity. $(Ca^{++} + Mg^{++})$ATPase activity in sarcolemma from human pregnant myometrium also was inhibited by oxytocin (54). The ATPase was similar to the Ca^{++}-extrusion ATPase of erythrocyte membranes with respect to its high affinity for Ca^{++}, inhibition by vanadate, and dependency on calmodulin.

Hormone-inhibited $(Ca^{++} + Mg^{++})$ATPase activities on plasma membrane fractions have now been demonstrated using several hormones and their target cells (55–57). Regulation of Ca^{++} efflux appears to be one of several mechanisms for elevating intracellular free calcium ion concentrations in liver cells in response to vasopressin stimulation (58, 59), and it is possible that the actions of oxytocin on calcium levels may likewise occur at several sites.

Phosphoinositol Metabolism

Several studies have suggested that the effects of oxytocin on the myometrium involve polyphosphoinositide hydrolysis. Oxytocin caused the rapid formation of inositol trisphosphate by guinea pig myometrial strips (60) and increased the production of inositol phosphates by human gestational myometrium (61). Vasopressin, however, was more effective than oxytocin in the human uterus (61), despite the fact that oxytocin is far more potent in causing uterine contractions at parturition, when the samples were taken. Elevation of inositol trisphosphate increases intracellular free Ca^{++} concentrations from stores in smooth endoplasmic reticulum by interaction with inositol trisphosphate receptors (62, 63). Consistent with these results, the addition of inositol trisphosphate to the microsomal fraction of homogenates of myometrium from near-term pregnant cows caused the release of Ca^{++} into the medium (64).

Oxytocin also has been shown to stimulate the formation of inositol phosphates in mammary tissue slices (27, 65). Like human gestational myometrium (61), rat mammary tissue inositol phosphates were increased by lower concentrations of arginine vasopressin than oxytocin. These results raise the question of whether the stimulation of inositol phosphate formation by oxytocin is the result of occupancy of vasopressin receptors, rather than OT receptors (27). Indeed, vasopressin receptors were demonstrated in mammary tissue by binding studies with [^{3}H]vasopressin (27). Vasopressin stimulates inositol phosphate formation in a number of different cell types (63, 64, 66–69), including cells derived from a mammary tumor (70, 71). Vasopressin also stimulates the formation of inositol phosphates in vascular tissue (72–74), which may comprise a significant portion of mammary gland and myometrial samples. Marc, et al. (75) subsequently showed that the effects of oxytocin on guinea pig myometrial strips appeared to be mediated by oxytocin receptors, as vasopressin was less effective than oxytocin in stimulating the accumulation of inositol phosphates. An oxytocin analog lacking vasopressor activity also stimulated uterine phosphoinositol metabolism. These studies point out the importance of using oxytocin and vasopressin analogs to demonstrate a correspondence between uterotonic potency and stimulation of phosphoinositol formation.

Possible Involvement of a G-Protein

GTP-binding proteins (G-proteins) have been implicated in the coupling of hormone receptors to adenylate cyclase and of photoreceptors to cGMP phosphodiesterase (76). In addition, G-proteins are involved in the regulation of phosphoinositol turnover by a phosphatidylinositol-specific phospholipase C, presumably by coupling hormone receptors to the enzyme. Anwer and Sanborn (48) found that pretreatment of rat myometrial cells in culture with pertussis toxin, which prevents some types of G-protein actions, partially inhibited oxytocin-induced transients in intracellular free calcium, as measured by fura-2 fluorescence. The inhibition with pertussis toxin was greater when extracellular calcium concentrations were reduced. These data were interpreted to indicate that oxytocin-induced mobilization of calcium from intracellular, but not from extracellular, sources is mediated by a pertussis-toxin-sensitive mechanism, consistent with G-protein involvement of oxytocin action.

In contrast to these findings, OT-stimulated generation of inositol trisphosphate by intact guinea pig myometrium and uterine contractions were insensitive to pertussis toxin, under conditions where the expression of G_i was totally prevented (75). Guanine nucleotides reduce the affinity of G-protein coupled receptor sites for agonist, as shown with several cell types and agonists (77–81). Consistent with the findings of Marc et al. (75) the nonhydrolyzable GTP analogs, guanosine-5'-O-(3-thio-triphosphate (GTPγS) and guanylyl-imidodiphosphate (Gpp(NH)p), in concentrations between 1 and 250 μM, had no effect on the binding of [³H]oxytocin to plasma membranes from the rat myometrium (Soloff, unpublished). In membrane preparations from the mammary gland of the lactating rat, 250-μM GTPγS reduced the concentration of OT binding sites by about 25%, while not affecting the affinity for the hormone (82). It is not clear whether OT receptors of the myometrium and mammary gland differ in their coupling to G-proteins or whether there is a second population of receptor sites in the mammary gland that is coupled to G-protein. Vasopressin receptors are present in mammary gland (78) in concentrations that correspond to about 25% of those of OT receptors, and it is possible that the reduction in mammary binding sites for [³H]oxytocin with GTPγS might be due to an effect on the vasopressin receptor population and not on oxytocin receptors.

REFERENCES

1. Caldeyro-Barcia R, Sereno J. The response of the human uterus to oxytocin throughout pregnancy. In: Caldeyro-Barcia R, Heller H, eds. Oxytocin. Oxford: Pergamon Press, 1961:177-202.

2. Schneider W, Stumpf C. Über den einfluss des sexual cyclus auf hypophysen-hinterlappenextrakt-auswertungen nach der methode von P. Holton. Arch Int Pharmacodyn 1953;94:406-15.
3. Flatters M. Über die Vorzüge der Verwendung von Ratten-Uteri im Proöstrus zur Auswertung von Oxytocin. Arch Exp Path Pharmakol 1954;221:171-6.
4. Guerne JM, Stutinsky F. Étude in vivo des variations de la sensibilité à l'ocytocine de l'utérus de la ratte cyclique. J Physiol (Paris) 1961;53:357-8.
5. Chan WY, O'Connell M, Pomeroy SR. Effects of the estrous cycle on the sensitivity of rat uterus to oxytocin and desamino-oxytocin. Endocrinology 1963;72:279-82.
6. Soloff MS. Uterine receptors for oxytocin: effects of estrogens. Biochem Biophys Res Commun 1975;65:205-12.
7. Nissenson R, Flouret G, Hechter O. Opposing effects of estradiol and progesterone on oxytocin receptors in rabbit uterus. Proc Natl Acad Sci USA 1978;75:2044-8.
8. Soloff MS, Alexandrova M, Fernström MJ. Oxytocin receptors: triggers for parturition and lactation? Science 1979;204:1313-5.
9. Alexandrova M, Soloff MS. Oxytocin receptors and parturition, I. Control of oxytocin receptor concentration in the rat myometrium at term. Endocrinology 1980;106:730-5.
10. Fuchs A-R, Periyasamy S, Alexandrova M, Soloff MS. Correlation between oxytocin receptor concentration and responsiveness to oxytocin in pregnant rat myometrium. Effect of ovarian steroids. Endocrinology 1983;113:742-9.
11. Soloff MS, Fernström MA, Periyasamy S, Soloff S, Baldwin S, Wieder M. Regulation of oxytocin receptor concentration in rat uterine explants by estrogen and progester-one. Can J Biochem Cell Biol 1983;61:625-30.
12. Roberts JS, McCracken JA, Gavagan JE, Soloff MS. Oxytocin-stimulated release of prostaglandin $F_{2\alpha}$ from ovine endometrium in vitro: correlation with estrous cycle and oxytocin-receptor binding. Endocrinology 1976;99:1107-14.
13. Flint APF, Sheldrick EL. Continuous infusion of oxytocin prevents induction of uterine oxytocin receptor and blocks luteal regression in cyclic ewes, J Reprod Fertil 1985;75:623-31.
14. Engstrøm T, Atke A, Vilhardt H. Receptor binding characteristics and contractile responsiveness of the myometrium following prolonged infusion of bradykinin and oxytocin in rats. J Endocrinol 1988;118:81-5.
15. Eiler H, Armstrong-Backus CS, Lyke WA. Desensitization of rabbit myometrium to oxytocin and prostaglandin $F_{2\alpha}$. Am J Physiol 1989;257:E20-6.
16. Soloff MS, Grzonka Z. Effect of manganese on relative affinities of receptor for oxytocin analogues. Binding studies with rat myometrial and mammary gland membranes. J Biol Chem 1986;254:3899-906.
17. Fuchs A-R, Fuchs F, Husslein P, Soloff MS. Oxytocin receptors in the human uterus during pregnancy and parturition. Am J Obstet Gynecol 1984;150:734-41.
18. Soloff MS, Fields MJ. Changes in uterine oxytocin receptor concentrations throughout the estrous cycle of the cow. Biol Reprod 1989;40:283-7.
19. Joelsson I, Ingelman-Sundberg A, Sandberg F. The in vivo effect of oxytocin and vasopressin on the nonpregnant human uterus. Br J Obstet Gynaecol 1966;73:832-6.
20. Coutinho EM, Lopes ACV. Response of the nonpregnant uterus to vasopressin as an index of ovarian function. Am J Obstet Gynecol 1968;102:479-89.
21. Bengtsson LP. Effect of progesterone upon the in vivo response of the human

myometrium to oxytocin and vasopressin. Acta Obstet Gynecol Scand 1970;49 (suppl 6):19-25.

22. Embrey MP, Moir JC. A comparison of the oxytocic effects of synthetic vasopressin and oxytocin. Br J Obstet Gynaecol 1967;74:648-52.

23. Soloff MS. Regulation of oxytocin action at the receptor level. Life Sci 1979;25: 1453-60.

24. Soloff MS. Oxytocin receptors and mechanisms of oxytocin action. In: Amico JA, Robinson AG, eds. Oxytocin: clinical and laboratory studies. Amsterdam: Elsevier, 1985:259-76.

25. Elands J, Barberis C, Jard S, et al. ^{125}I-labelled d(CH$_2$)$_5$[Tyr(Me)^2,Thr^4,Tyr^9]OVT: a selective oxytocin receptor ligand. Eur J Pharmacol 1987;147:197-207.

26. Johnson AE, Ball GF, Coirini H, Harbaugh CR, McEwen BS, Insel TR. Time course of the estradiol-dependent induction of oxytocin receptor binding in the ventromedial hypothalamic nucleus of the rat. Endocrinology 1989;125:1414-9.

27. Soloff MS, Fernström MA, Fernström MJ. Vasopressin and oxytocin receptors on plasma membranes from rat mammary gland. Demonstration of vasopressin receptors by stimulation of inositol phosphate formation, and oxytocin receptors by binding of a specific ^{125}I-labeled oxytocin antagonist, d(CH$_2$)$_5$^{1}[Tyr(Me)^2,Thr^4,Tyr-NH$_2$^{9}]OVT. Biochem Cell Biol 1988;67:152-62.

28. Morgat JL, Hung LT, Cardinaud R, et al. Peptidic hormone interactions at the molecular level—preparation of highly labelled ^{3}H oxytocin. J Labelled Compd 1970;6:276-84.

29. Flouret G, Terada S, Yang F, Nakagawa SH, Nakahara T, Hechter O. Iodinated neurohypophysial hormones as potential ligands for receptor binding and intermediates in synthesis of tritiated hormones. Biochemistry 1977;16:2119-24.

30. Cobo E, Cifuentes R, de Villamizar M. Inhibition of menstrual uterine motility during water diuresis. Am J Obstet Gynecol 1978;132:313-20.

31. Fuchs A-R, Fuchs F, Soloff MS. Oxytocin receptors in nonpregnant human uterus. J Clin Endocrinol Metab 1985;60:37-41.

32. Guillon G, Balestre MN, Roberts JM, Bottari SP. Oxytocin and vasopressin: distinct receptors in myometrium. J Clin Endocrinol Metab 1987;64:1129-35.

33. Maggi M, Genazzani AD, Giannini S, et al. Vasopressin and oxytocin receptors in vagina, myometrium and oviduct of rabbits. Endocrinology 1988;122:2970-80.

34. Soloff MS, Fernström MA. Solubilization and properties of oxytocin receptors in rat mammary gland membranes. Endocrinology 1987;120:2474-82.

35. Small JV. Contractile units in vertebrate smooth muscle cells. Nature 1974;249: 324-27.

36. Soloff MS, Beauregard G, Potier M. Determination of the functional size of oxytocin receptors in plasma membranes from mammary gland and uterine myometrium of the rat by radiation inactivation. Endocrinology 1988;122:1769-72.

37. Fahrenholz F, Hackenberg M, Müller M. Identification of a myometrial oxytocin receptor protein. Eur J Biochem 1988;174:81-5.

38. Müller M, Soloff MS, Fahrenholz F. Photoaffinity labelling of the oxytocin receptor in plasma membranes from rat mammary gland. FEBS Lett 1989;242:333-6.

39. Grenningloh G, Rienitz A, Schmitt B, et al.The strychnine-binding subunit of the glycine receptor shows homology with nicotinic acetylcholine receptors. Nature 1987;328:215-20.

40. Schofield PR, Darlison MG, Fujita N, et al. Sequence and functional expression of the GABA$_A$ receptor shows a ligand-gated receptor super-family. Nature 1987;328:221-7.

41. Berde B, Boissonnas RA. Basic pharmacological properties of synthetic analogues and homologues of the neurohypophysial hormones. In: Berde B, ed. Handbook of experimental pharmacology, vol. 23. Neurohypophysial hormones and similar polypeptides. New York: Springer-Verlag, 1968:802-70.

42. Manning M, Olma A, Klis W, et al.Carboxy terminus of vasopressin required for activity but not binding. Nature 1984;308:652-3.

43. Marshall JM. Effects of neurohypophysial hormones on the myometrium. In: Greep RO, Astwood EB, Knobil E, Sawyer WH, Geiger SR, eds.The pituitary gland and its neuroendocrine control, part 1, Handbook of physiology, sec 7: Endocrinology, vol. 4. Washington, DC: American Physiological Society, 1974:469-92.

44. Forman A, Gandrup P, Andersson KE, Ulmsten U. Effects of nifedipine on oxytocin- and prostaglandin F$_{2\alpha}$-induced activity in the postpartum uterus. Am J Obstet Gynecol 1982;144:665-70.

45. Csapo AI, Puri CP, Tarro S, Henzl MR. Deactivation of the uterus during normal and premature labor by the calcium antagonist nicardipine. Am J Obstet Gynecol 1982;142:483-91.

46. Sakai K, Yamaguchi T, Morita S, Uchida M. Agonist-induced contraction of rat myometrium in Ca-free solution containing Mn. Gen Pharmacol 1983;14:391-400.

47. Morley SD, Meyerhof W, Schwarz J, Richter D. Functional expression of the oxytocin receptor in *Xenopus laevis* oocytes primed with mRNA from bovine endometrium. J Mol Endocrinol 1988;1:77-81.

48. Anwer K, Sanborn BM. Changes in intracellular free calcium in isolated myometrial cells: role of extracellular and intracellular calcium and possible involvement of guanine nucleotide-sensitive proteins. Endocrinology 1989;124:17-23.

49. Schatzmann HJ, Vincenzi FF. Calcium movements across the membrane of human red cells. J Physiol (Lond) 1969;201:369-95.

50. Pershadsingh HA, McDonald JM. A high affinity calcium-stimulated magnesium-dependent adenosine triphosphatase in rat adipocyte plasma membranes. J Biol Chem 1980;255:4087-93.

51. Åkerman KEO, Wikström MKF. (Ca^{2+} + Mg^{2+})-stimulated ATPase activity of rabbit myometrium plasma membrane is blocked by oxytocin. FEBS Lett 1979;97:283-7.

52. Soloff MS, Sweet P. Oxytocin inhibition of (Ca^{2+} + Mg^{2+})ATPase activity in rat myometrial plasma membranes. J Biol Chem 1982;257:10687-93.

53. Huszar G. Cellular regulation of myometrial contractility and essentials of tocolytic therapy. In: Huszar G, ed. The physiology and biochemistry of the uterus in pregnancy and labor. Boca Raton, FL: CRC Press, 1986:107-26.

54. Popescu LM, Nutu O, Panoiu C. Oxytocin contracts the human uterus at term by inhibiting the myometrial Ca^{2+}-extrusion pump. Biosci Rep 1985;5:21-8.

55. Pershadsingh HA, McDonald JM. Direct addition of insulin inhibits a high affinity Ca^{2+}-ATPase in isolated adipocyte plasma membranes. Nature 1979;281:495-7.

56. Yamaguchi M. Effect of calcitonin on Ca-ATPase activity of plasma membrane in liver of rats. Endocrinol Jpn 1979;26:605-9.

57. Lin S-H, Wallace MA, Fain JN. Regulation of Ca^{2+}-Mg^{2+}-ATPase activity in hepatocyte plasma membranes by vasopressin and phenylephrine. Endocrinology 1983;113:2268-75.

58. Monck JR, Reynolds EE, Thomas AP, Williamson JR. Novel kinetics of single cell Ca^{2+} transients in stimulated hepatocytes and A10 cells measured using fura-2 and fluorescent videomicroscopy. J Biol Chem 1988;263:4569-75.

59. Rooney TA, Sass EJ, Thomas AP. Characterization of cytosolic calcium oscillations induced by phenylephrine and vasopressin in single fura-2-loaded hepatocytes. J Biol Chem 1989;264:17131-41.

60. Marc S, Lieber D, Harbon S. Carbachol and oxytocin stimulate the generation of inositol phosphates in the guinea pig myometrium. FEBS Lett 1986;201:9-14.

61. Schrey MP, Cornford PA, Read AM, Steer PJ. A role for phosphoinositide hydrolysis in human uterine smooth muscle during parturition. Am J Obstet Gynecol1988;159: 964-70.

62. Streb H, Bayerdorffer E, Hasse W, Irvine RF, Schulz I. Effect of inositol-1,4,5-trisphosphate on isolated subcellular fractions of rat pancreas. J Membr Biol 1984;81:241-53.

63. Spät A, Fabiato A, Rubin RP. Binding of inositol trisphosphate by a liver microsomal fraction. Biochem J 1986;233:929-32.

64. Carsten ME, Miller JD. Ca^{2+} release by inositol trisphosphate from Ca^{2+}-transporting microsomes derived from uterine sarcoplasmic reticulum. Biochem Biophys Res Commun 1985;130:1027-31.

65. Zhao X, Gorewit RC. Inositol-phosphate response to oxytocin-stimulation in dispersed bovine mammary cells. Neuropeptides 1987;10:227-33.

66. Tolbert MEM, White AC, Aspry K, Cutts J, Fain JN. Stimulation by vasopressin and a-catecholamines of phosphatidylinositol formation in isolated rat liver parenchymal cells. J Biol Chem 1980;255:1938-44.

67. Kirk CJ, Michell RH. Phosphatidylinositol metabolism in rat hepatocytes stimulated by vasopressin. Biochem J 1981;194:155-65.

68. Bhalla T, Enyedi P, Spät A, Antoni FA. Pressor-type vasopressin receptors in the adrenal cortex: properties of binding, effects on phosphoinositide metabolism and aldosterone secretion. Endocrinology 1985;117:421-3.

69. Woodcock EA, McLeod JK, Johnston CI. Vasopressin stimulates phosphatidylinositol turnover and aldosterone synthesis in rat adrenal glomerulosa cells: comparison with angiotensin II. Endocrinology 1986;118:2432-6.

70. Koreh K, Monaco ME. The relationship of hormone-sensitive and hormone-insensitive phosphatidylinositol to phosphatidylinositol 4,5-bisphosphate in the WRK-1 cell. J Biol Chem 1986;261:88-91.

71. Kirk CJ, Guillon G, Balestre M-N, Jard S. Stimulation by vasopressin and other agonists, of inositol-lipid breakdown and inositol phosphate accumulation in WRK1 cells. Biochem J 1986;240:197-204.

72. Nabika T, Velletri PA, Lovenberg W, Beaven MA. Increase in cytosolic calcium and phosphoinositide metabolism induced by angiotensin II and [Arg]vasopressin in vascular smooth muscle cells. J Biol Chem 1985;260:4661-70.

73. Aiyar N, Nambi P, Stassen FL, Crooke ST. Vascular vasopressin receptors mediate phosphatidylinositol turnover and calcium efflux in an established smooth muscle cell line. Life Sci 1986;39:37-45.

74. Fox AW, Friedman PA, Abel PW. Vasopressin receptor mediated contraction and [^{3}H]inositol metabolisms in rat tail artery. Eur J Pharmacol 1987;135:1-10.

75. Marc S, Leiber D, Harbon S. Fluoroaluminates mimic muscarinic- and oxytocin-

receptor-mediated generation of inositol phosphates and contraction in the intact guinea-pig myometrium. Biochem J 1988;255:705-13.

76. Casey PJ, Gilman AG. G protein involvement in receptor-effector coupling. J Biol Chem 1988;263:2577-80.

77. Fischer JB, Schonbrunn A. The bombesin receptor is coupled to a guanine nucleotide-binding protein which is insensitive to pertussis and cholera toxins. J Biol Chem 1988;263:2808-16.

78. Goodman RR, Cooper MJ, Gavish M, Snyder SH. Guanine nucleotide and cation regulation of the binding of [^{3}H]cyclohexyladenosine and [^{3}H]diethylphenylxanthine to adenosine A_1 receptors in brain membranes. Mol Pharmacol 1982;21:329-35.

79. Koch BD, Schonbrunn A. The somatostatin receptor is directly coupled to adenylate cyclase in GH_4C_1 pituitary cell membranes. Endocrinology 1984;114:1784-90.

80. Hinkle PM, Kinsella PA. Regulation of thyrotropin-releasing hormone binding by monovalent cations and guanyl nucleotides. J Biol Chem 1984;259:3445-9.

81. U'Prichard DC, Snyder SH. Guanyl nucleotide influences of ^{3}H-ligand binding to α-noradrenergic receptors in calf brain membranes. J Biol Chem 1978;253:3444-9.

82. Soloff MS. Oxytocin receptors in the uterus. In: Carsten ME, Miller JD, eds. Uterine function: molecular and cellular aspects. New York: Plenum, 1990 (in press).

15

The Regulation of Arachidonic Acid Metabolism in Pregnancy

M. D. Mitchell and S. Lundin-Schiller

Department of Obstetrics and Gynecology, University of Utah School of Medicine, Salt Lake City

A n increase in the rate of prostaglandin biosynthesis by intrauterine tissues is important in the events leading to parturition in women. It has been shown that amnion obtained after labor has a higher rate of prostaglandin biosynthesis than amnion obtained before labor (1–3). Furthermore, the arachidonic acid content of amnion taken after labor is decreased (4, 5). In order to study the regulation of arachidonic acid metabolism in amnion, a method for establishing primary cultures of human amnion was developed by Okita et al. (6). The cells in culture were shown to be morphologically similar to the cells in amnion tissue and to have similar enzymatic activities and lipid composition. This culture technique has been used in the majority of studies discussed here.

Amnion prostaglandin production can be regulated essentially at three places in the biosynthetic pathway: (*a*) release of substrate [phospholipase A_2, phospholipase C, diacyl- and monoacylglycerol lipases; (*b*) conversion of substrate to intermediate prostaglandins (fatty acid cyclo-oxygenase [synonymous with prostaglandin endoperoxide synthase]); and (*c*) conversion of intermediate prostaglandins to primary prostaglandins (e.g., prostaglandin endoperoxide E-isomerase and prostaglandin endoperoxide F-reductase). Increased free intracellular calcium and activation of protein kinase C and protein kinase A appear to be important in regulating the prostaglandin biosynthetic pathway in amnion. As seen in Figure 1, raising intracellular calcium levels by treatment of amnion cells with ionomycin, a calcium ionophore, increases prostaglandin E_2 production in a dose-dependent manner. Raising free intracellular calcium likely stimulates release of arachidonic acid by activation of the calcium-dependent phospholipases A_2 and C in amnion (7, 8). The importance of calcium in the extracellular environment for amnion prostaglandin biosynthesis has been described (9). Figure 2 shows the effects of activation of protein kinase C by the phorbol esters, phorbol 12,13-dibutyrate (PDBu) and phorbol 12-myristate 13-acetate (PMA). Activation of protein kinase C results in stimulation of amnion cell PGE_2 biosynthesis. Studies

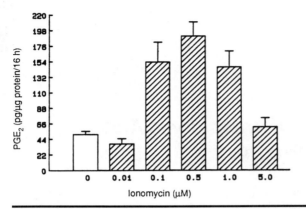

Fig. 1. The effects of ionomycin on PGE_2 production by amnion cells. (Mean ± SEM; n = 4.)

by Zakar and Olson suggest that this stimulation is due both to increasing de novo synthesis of fatty acid cyclo-oxygenase and to stimulation of the release of arachidonic acid (10). Catecholamines and β-adrenergic agonists have been shown to increase prostaglandin production by amnion cells (5, 11). β-adrenergic receptors are coupled to adenylate cyclase by a G-protein (G_s), which after the agonist binds the receptor, activates adenylate cyclase resulting in increased levels of cyclic 3'5'-adenosine monophosphate (cAMP). Moore et al. have shown that amnion contains cAMP-dependent kinase activity and cAMP-enhanced phosphoproteins (12).

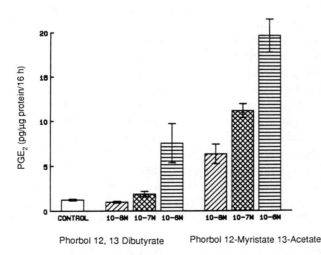

Fig. 2. The effects of phorbol esters on PGE_2 production by amnion cells. (Mean ± SEM; n = 4.)

Many studies have been conducted in an effort to understand the physiological modulators of amnion arachidonic acid metabolism. Amnion is an avascular tissue but is in direct contact with amniotic fluid on one side and chorion laeve on the other. Substances that regulate amnion prostaglandin biosynthesis, therefore, likely emanate from the fetus via amniotic fluid or the chorion laeve. Substances in amniotic fluid and factors secreted by chorion cells have been shown to alter amnion prostaglandin production and, in some cases, have been demonstrated to act via the above-mentioned second messengers. We briefly review our findings in relation to the information available in this area.

DEFINED SUBSTANCES IN AMNIOTIC FLUID

Epidermal growth factor (EGF) and transforming growth factor alpha (TGFα) have both been shown to stimulate amnion cell prostaglandin production (Fig. 3) (13, 14). EGF/TGFα levels as measured by radioreceptor assay increase in amniotic fluid during labor (15). EGF stimulate amnion cells at least in part by the induction of fatty acid cyclo-oxygenase protein (16). Additionally, platelet-activating factor (PAF), a substance originally described to be released from basophils, has been found in amniotic fluid. PAF found in amniotic fluid is associated with lamellar bodies that are released from the fetal lung, and the concentration of PAF in amniotic fluid increases during the later stages of gestation (17). It is thought that PAF increases free cytosolic calcium levels in amnion, thereby activating phospholipases to release arachidonic acid and thus stimulating amnion PGE_2 production.

Moore et al. have demonstrated that oxytocin stimulates prostaglandin production in amnion cells by activation of phosphatidylinositol turnover resulting in increased free intracellular calcium and protein kinase C activity (18). Preliminary studies in our laboratory are consistent with these findings (see Fig. 4). Oxytocin has also been shown to increase decidual prostaglandin production, and this effect is significantly greater in tissues taken from women who have labored

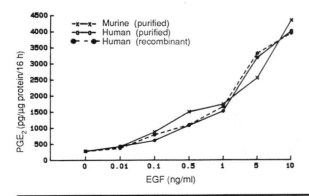

Fig. 3. The effects of epidermal growth factor from various sources on PGE_2 production by amnion cells.

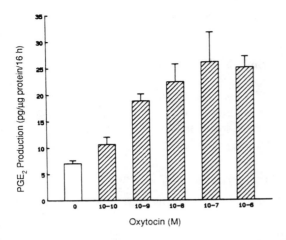

Fig. 4.   The effects of increasing concentrations by oxytocin on PGE_2 production by amnion cells. (Mean ± SEM; n = 4.)

(19). These data suggest oxytocin may be important in regulating intrauterine prostaglandin production at term.

Prior to labor, there is an increase in fetal cortisol levels. Glucocorticoids inhibit prostaglandin formation in most cell types, presumably by the induction of lipocortins. This would seem to be counterproductive to the labor process. Recent studies from two groups demonstrate the presence of several members of the lipocortin family in amnion and chorion and further that there are changes in the properties of these proteins with labor (20, 21). Interestingly, we have shown that dexamethasone stimulates amnion cell prostaglandin production (Fig. 5), while

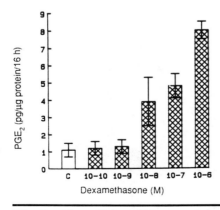

Fig. 5.   The effects of dexamethasone at various concentrations on PGE_2 production by amnion cells. (Mean ± SEM; n = 4.)

also stimulating lipocortin formation (22). Studies by Smieja and Olson (23) indicating that dexamethasone may increase fatty acid cyclo-oxygenase protein in amnion cells are consistent with our findings.

Endothelins are a family of proteins with vasoconstrictor properties and are produced by vascular endothelium (24). Endothelin 1 has been shown to stimulate myometrial contractions and to activate phospholipases A_2 and C (25–27). Recent studies have revealed that endothelin 1 is present in amniotic fluid and induces prostaglandin formation by myometrial cells in vitro (28). The concentrations of endothelin 1 in amniotic fluid do not change with gestational age. We have demonstrated that endothelin 1 inhibits amnion cell PGE_2 biosynthesis (Fig. 6). This is somewhat paradoxical given its ability to induce phosphatidylinositol turnover in endothelial cells and its action on myometrial cells. Excitingly, we have recently found that amnion synthesizes endothelin 1 (and probably endothelin 2). Production of endothelin 1 by amnion can be stimulated by the cytokines interleukin 1β (IL-1β) and tumor necrosis factor (TNF), but preliminary evidence suggests, not consistently by interleukin 6. Preliminary data suggest that EGF and phorbol esters also stimulate amnion endothelin 1 production (Fig 7).

In collaboration with R. Romero, we have proposed (29) that inflammatory mediators produced by the host (mother or fetus) in response to bacterial infection stimulate intrauterine tissues (amnion, chorion, and decidua) to produce prostaglandins. In response to bacteria, activated macrophages invade the intrauterine tissues and amniotic fluid and produce such inflammatory mediators as IL-1β and TNF. It has been shown that concentrations of IL-1 and TNF are increased in the amniotic fluid of patients with intra-amniotic infection (30, 31). Furthermore, we have demonstrated that these substances as well as bacterial endotoxin stimulate prostaglandin production by cultured amnion and decidual cells (30–33) (e.g., Fig. 8).

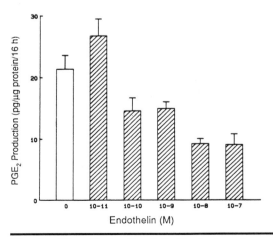

Fig. 6. The effects of endothelin-1 at various concentrations on PGE_2 production by amnion cells. (Mean ± SEM; n = 4.)

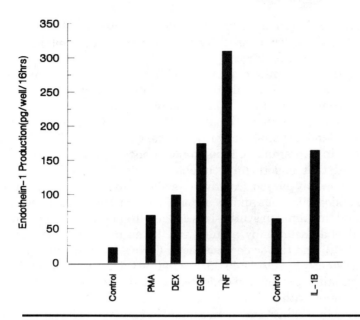

Fig. 7. The effects of various agents on endothelin 1 production by amnion cells. (PMA-phorbol-12–myristate-13–acetate, 10^{-7}M; DEX = dexamethasone, 10^{-6}M; EGF = epidermal growth factor, 10 ng/ml; TNF = tumor necrosis factor, 100 ng/ml; IL-1β = interleukin 1β, 10 ng/ml.)

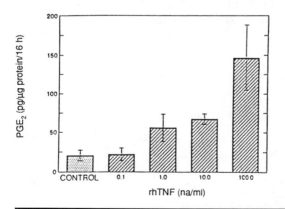

Fig. 8. The effects of tumor necrosis factor on PGE$_2$ production by amnion cells. (Mean ± SEM; n = 4.)

NONCHARACTERIZED SUBSTANCES IN AMNIOTIC FLUID

Several as yet uncharacterized substances in amniotic fluid have also been shown to alter amnion prostaglandin production. Mitchell et al. have reported that amniotic fluid increases PGE_2 production by amnion cells in a dose-dependent manner (34). At term, amniotic fluid is comprised of the products of fetal urination. Fetal urine stimulates both prostaglandin endoperoxide synthase activity and amnion cell PGE_2 synthesis in vitro (Fig. 9) (35, 36).

Antiphospholipase proteins have been detected in amniotic fluid and intrauterine tissues. These could presumably decrease availability of substrate for conversion to prostaglandins. Two proteins isolated from amniotic fluid obtained at term before labor inhibit arachidonic acid release and PGF synthesis in human endometrial cells (37). The molecular weights of these two proteins are reported to be 150,000–160,000 D and 70,000–80,000 D. The activity of these substances is reduced significantly in labor (38). Furthermore, Liggins and Wilson reported that conditioned media from chorions taken at term prior to labor inhibit phospholipase A_2 activity (39). This antiphospholipase activity is thought to be due to the 70,000–80,000 D protein isolated from amniotic fluid.

Recent studies to evaluate the effects of whole amniotic fluid from different gestational ages and fractions of amniotic fluid on amnion cell PGE_2 production reveal that whole amniotic fluid stimulates amnion cell PGE_2 production (40). However, stimulation by "term before labor" (NIL) and "term labor" amniotic fluid is significantly greater than stimulation by amniotic fluid obtained at 17–19 weeks' gestation (Fig. 10). Fractionation of the amniotic fluid from the three groups revealed multiple discernible peaks of stimulatory activity in each group (Fig. 11). The majority of peaks had retention times that were similar among the three groups, and peak stimulatory activities were greater in term NIL and term labor samples than in 17–19 week samples.

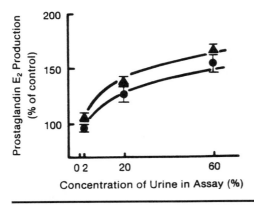

Fig. 9.   The effects of human urine on the activity of prostaglandin endoperoxide synthase from bovine seminal vesicle.

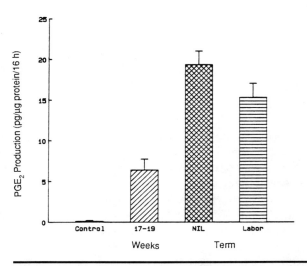

Fig. 10. The effects of whole amniotic fluid from 17–19 weeks' gestation, NIL, and term labor on PGE_2 production by amnion cells. (Mean ± SEM; n = 4.)

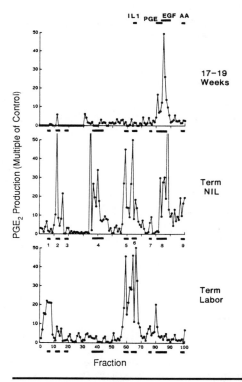

Fig. 11. The effects of fractions of amniotic fluid on PGE_2 production by amnion cells.

DEFINED SUBSTANCES FROM CHORION

Chorion cells have been shown to secrete a number of protein hormones. Corticotropin-releasing hormone (CRH) is one of these hormones that has stimulatory effects on amnion cell prostaglandin production (41, 42) (Fig. 12). Components of the renin-angiotensin system have been identified in chorionic cells, and it is thought that the renin and prorenin found in amniotic fluid is produced by the chorion (43–46). Prorenin and renin plasma levels increase dramatically early in pregnancy and remain elevated until delivery (47). Likewise, amniotic fluid has been shown to have high levels of both prorenin and renin, reported to be as much as 30 times higher than maternal plasma at term (48). Chorionic prorenin and renin may also contribute to the elevated levels of these hormones in plasma. As yet, the function of prorenin and renin and other components of the system in amniotic fluid and chorion is unknown. However, it has been shown in isolated human placental cotyledons perfused in vitro that angiotensin II injections into the fetal circulation result in increased PGE and 6-oxo-prostaglandin F1α release into the fetal circulation (49). Others have shown higher levels of active renin in the fetal artery, vein, and chorionic tissue in pregnancy-induced hypertension patients (50). These data suggest a role for intrauterine renin-angiotensin system in the control of placental blood flow. Other studies have shown that in perfused fetal membranes lowering the osmolarity of the perfusate results in increased renin release, suggesting a role for renin in the control of volume and electrolyte balance of amniotic fluid (51). We have found that renin (0.1–1.0 U/ml) will stimulate amnion cell PGE_2 production.

Chorion is also a steriodogenic tissue and it has been shown that the ability for chorion to produce progesterone from pregnenolone is reduced in tissues taken

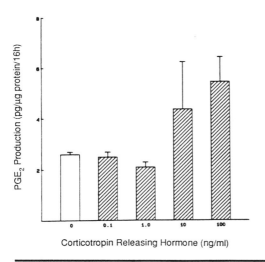

Fig. 12. The effects of corticotropin-releasing hormone at various concentrations on PGE_2 production by amnion cells. (Mean ± SEM; n = 4.)

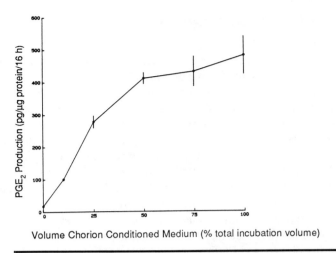

Volume Chorion Conditioned Medium (% total incubation volume)

Fig. 13. The effects of chorion conditioned media at various concentrations on PGE_2 by amnion cells. (Mean ± SEM; n = 4.)

after labor (52). This may lead to a local progesterone withdrawal, thus removing the prostaglandin synthesis inhibition of progesterone.

NONCHARACTERIZED SUBSTANCES FROM CHORION

In collaboration with William Gibb, we have demonstrated that chorion secretes uncharacterized factors that regulate amnion cell prostaglandin biosynthesis (Figs. 13–15) (53). This chorion-derived activity stimulates amnion cell PGE_2 production in a time- and dose-dependent manner. The activity in chorion conditioned

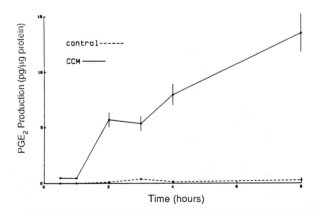

Time (hours)

Fig. 14. Time-course of action of chorion conditioned media on PGE_2 production by amnion cells. (Mean ± SEM; n = 4.)

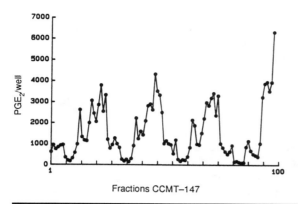

Fig. 15. The effects of fractions of chorion condition media on PGE$_2$ production by amnion cells.

medium (CCM) is in large part due to a heat labile protein of mol wt >30,000 as determined by anisotropic ultrafiltration. Treatment of the chorion with heat or protease effectively eliminates stimulatory activity. Additionally, the mRNA translation inhibitor, cycloheximide, at 1 and 10 µg/ml inhibited the amnion cell response to the chorion-derived activity. The activity is directed substantially to a point in the prostaglandin biosynthetic pathway after substrate release. Present data do not exclude the possibility of an action on prostaglandin endoperoxide E-isomerase, and studies are ongoing to address this point. A prostaglandin stimulatory factor emanating from the chorion laeve would be of distinct importance in the regulation of amnion and possibly decidual prostaglandin production.

FINAL COMMENT

The regulation of amnion prostaglandin biosynthesis appears to result from a complex interplay of several stimulatory and inhibitory substances that may be increased or decreased near term. The actions of these substances are at multiple levels in the prostaglandin biosynthetic pathway. A number of these substances are produced by the fetus or the chorion laeve and may play a role in the control of membrane rupture, cervical ripening, and uterine contractions at the time of parturition. Further study of these substances, their effects on intrauterine prostaglandin production and what regulates their transfer to the myometrium (54) is crucial to the complete understanding of the events leading to parturition in women.

REFERENCES

1. Mitchell MD. Prostaglandins at parturition and in the neonatal infant. Biochem Soc Trans 1980;8:659-62.
2. Okazaki T, Casey ML, Okita JR, MacDonald PC, Johnston JM. Initiation of human

parturition, XII. Biosynthesis and metabolism of prostaglandins in human fetal membranes and uterine decidua. Am J Obstet Gynecol 1981;139:373-81.

3. Olson DM, Skinner K, Challis JRG. Prostaglandin output in relation to parturition by cells dispersed from human intrauterine tissues. J Clin Endocrinol Metab 1983;57: 694-9.

4. Okita JR, MacDonald PC, Johnston JM. Mobilization of arachidonic acid from specific glycerophospholipids of human fetal membranes during early labor. J Biol Chem 1982;257:14029-34.

5. Bleasdale JE, Johnston JM. Prostaglandins and human parturition: regulation of arachidonic acid metabolism. In: Scarpelli EM, Cosmi EV, eds. Reviews in perinatal medicine, vol 5. New York: Alan Liss, 1985:151-91.

6. Okita JR, Sagawa N, Casey ML, Snyder JM. A comparison of human amnion tissue and amnion cells in primary culture by morphological and biochemical criteria. In Vitro 1983;19:117-26.

7. Okazaki T, Okita JR, MacDonald PC, et al. Initiation of human parturition, X. Substrate specificity of phospholipase A_2 in human fetal membranes. Am J Obstet Gynecol 1978;130:432-8.

8. DiRenzo GC, Johnston JM, Okazaki T, et al. Phosphatidylinositol-specific phospholipase C in fetal membranes and uterine decidua. J Clin Invest 1981;67:847-56.

9. Olson DM, Opavsky MA, Challis JRG. Prostaglandin synthesis by human amnion is dependent upon extracellular calcium. Can J Physiol Pharmacol 1983;61:1089-92.

10. Zakar T, Olson DM. Stimulation of human amnion prostaglandin E_2 production by activators of protein kinase-C. J Clin Endocrinol Metab 1988;67:915-23.

11. Warrick C, Skinner K, Mitchell BF, Challis JRG. Relationship between cyclic adenosine monophosphate and prostaglandin output by dispersed cells from human amnion and decidua. Am J Obstet Gynecol 1985;153:66-71.

12. Moore JJ, Suster MA, Moore RM. Cyclic 3', 5'-adenosine monophosphate-dependent kinase and phosphoproteins in human amnion. Proc Soc Exp Biol Med 1988;189: 84-93.

13. Mitchell MD. Epidermal growth factor actions on arachidonic acid metabolism in human amnion cells. Biochim Biophys Acta 1987;928:240-2.

14. Mitchell MD. Actions of transforming growth factors on amnion cell prostaglandin biosynthesis. Prostaglandins, Leukotrienes, and EFA 1988;33:157-8.

15. Romero R, Wu YK, Oyarzun E, Hobbins JC, Mitchell MD. A potential role for epidermal growth factor/α-transforming growth factor in human parturition. Eur J Obstet Gynecol Reprod Biol 1989;33: 55-60.

16. Casey ML, Korte K, MacDonald PC. Epidermal growth factor stimulation of prostaglandin E_2 biosynthesis in amnion cells. Induction of prostaglandin H_2 synthase. J Biol Chem 1988;263:7846-54.

17. Angle M, Maki N, Johnston JM. Bioactive metabolites of glycerophospholipid metabolism in relation to parturition. In: McNellis D, Challis JRG, MacDonald PC, Nathanielsz PW, Roberts JM, eds. The onset of labor: cellular and integrative mechanisms. Ithaca, NY: Perinatology Press, 1988:125-38.

18. Moore JJ, Dubyak GR, Moore RM, Kooy DV. Oxytocin activates the inositol-phospholipid-protein kinase-C system and stimulates prostaglandin production in human amnion cells. Endocrinology 1988;123:1771-7.

19. Wilson T, Liggins GC, Whittaker DJ. Oxytocin stimulates the release of arachidonic

acid and prostaglandin F2α from human decidual cells. Prostaglandins 1988;35(5): 771-80.

20. Gibb W, Lavoie JC. Immunological demonstration of lipocortins I and II in human intrauterine tissues at term [Abstract]. In: Proc 35th annu meet Soc Gynecol Invest. Baltimore, 1988:374.

21. Everson WV, Hirth J, Brockman DE, Myatt L. Changes in lipocortins in human fetal membranes at parturition [Abstract]. In: Proc 37th annu meet Soc Gynecol Invest. St. Louis, 1990:200.

22. Mitchell MD, Lytton FD, Varticovski L. Paradoxical stimulation of both lipocortin and prostaglandin production in human amnion cells by dexamethasone. Biochem Biophys Res Commun 1988;151:137-41.

23. Smieja Z, Olson DM. Dexamethasone and 12-0-tetradecanoylphorbol 13-acetate (TPA) stimulate prostaglandin H synthase activity in cultured human amnion cells [Abstract]. In: Proc 36th annu meet Soc Gynecol Invest. San Diego, 1989:146.

24. Masaki T. The discovery, the present state, and the future prospects of endothelin. J Cardiovasc Pharmacol 1989;13:S1-4.

25. Kozuka M, Ito T, Hirose S, Takahashi K, Hagiwara H. Endothelin induces two types of contractions of rat uterus: phasic contractions by way of voltage-dependent calcium channels and developing contractions through a second type of calcium channels. Biochem Biophys Res Commun 1989;159:317-23.

26. Resink TJ, Scott-Burden T, Buhler FR. Activation of phospholipase A_2 by endothelin in cultured vascular smooth muscle cells. Biochem Biophys Res Commun 1989;158: 279-86.

27. Resink TJ, Scott-Burden T, Buhler FR. Endothelin stimulates phospholipase C in cultured vascular smooth muscle cells. Biochem Biophys Res Commun 1988;157: 1360-8.

28. Romero R, Avila C, Mitchell MD. Endothelin-1 in human parturition [Abstract]. In: Proc 37th annu meet Soc Gynecol Invest. St. Louis, 1990:351.

29. Romero R, Mazor M, Wu YK, Sirtori M, Oyarzun E, Mitchell MD, Hobbins JC. Infection in the pathogenesis of preterm labor. In: Creasy RK, Warshaw JB, eds. Seminars in perinatology; vol 12. Philadelphia: Grune & Stratton, 1988:262-79.

30. Romero R, Manogue KR, Mitchell MD, et al. Infection and labor, IV. Cachetin-tumor necrosis factor in the amniotic fluid of women with intraamniotic infection and preterm labor. Am J Obstet Gynecol 1989;161:336-41.

31. Romero R, Brody DT, Oyarzun E, et al. Infection and labor, III. Interleukin-1: a signal for the onset of parturition. Am J Obstet Gynecol 1989;160:1117-23.

32. Romero R, Hobbins JC, Mitchell MD. Endotoxin stimulates prostaglandin E_2 production by human amnion. Obstet Gynecol 1988;71:227-8.

33. Mitchell MD. Prostaglandin biosynthesis by human decidual cells in primary monolayer culture: effects of inflammatory mediators [Abstract]. In: Proc 36th annu meet Soc Gynecol Invest. San Diego, 1989:300.

34. Mitchell MD, MacDonald PC, Casey ML. Stimulation of PGE_2 synthesis in human amnion cells maintained in monolayer culture by a substance(s) in amniotic fluid. Prostaglandins, Leukotrienes, Med 1984;15:399-407.

35. Strickland DM, Saeed SA, Casey ML, Mitchell MD. Stimulation of prostaglandin biosynthesis by urine of the human fetus may serve as a trigger for parturition. Science 1983;220:521-2.

36. Casey ML, MacDonald PC, Mitchell MD. Stimulation of prostaglandin E_2 production in amnion cells in culture by a substance(s) in human fetal and adult urine. Biochem Biophys Res Commun 1983;114:1056-63.

37. Wilson T, Liggins GC, Aimer GP, Skinner SJM. Partial purification and characterization of two compounds from amniotic fluid which inhibit phospholipase activity in human endometrial cells. Biochem Biophys Res Commun 1985;131:22-9.

38. Wilson T, Liggins CC, Joe L. Purification and characterization of uterine phospholipase inhibitor that loses activity after labor onset in women. Am J Obstet Gynecol 1989;160:602-6.

39. Liggins GC, Wilson T. Isolation of an inhibitor of phospholipase A_2 from human chorion [Abstract]. In: Proc meet Int Union Physiol Sci. Vancouver Island, 1986:40.

40. Dowling DD, Romero R, Mitchell MD, Lundin-Schiller S. Isolation of multiple substances in amniotic fluid that regulate amnion prostaglandin E_2 production: the effects of gestational age and labor [Abstract]. In: Proc 36th annu meet Soc Gynecol Invest. San Diego, 1989:414.

41. Jones SA, Challis JRG. Local stimulation of prostaglandin production by corticotropin releasing hormone in human fetal membranes and placenta. Biochem Biophys Res Commun 1989;159:192-9.

42. Mitchell MD, Romero R, Gibb W, Harris AN, Dowling D, Schiller SL. The regulation of prostaglandin biosynthesis during human labor. In: Belfort P, Pinotti JA, Eskes TKAB, eds. Pregnancy and labor. Carnforth: Parthenon, 1989:11-8.

43. Poisner AM, Wood GW, Poisner R, Inagami T. Localization of renin in trophoblasts in human chorion laeve at term pregnancy. Endocrinology 1981;109:1150-5.

44. Egan DA, Grzegorczyk V, Tricarico KA, Ruetic A, Holleman WH, Marcotte PA. Human placental chorionic renin: production, purification, and characterization. Biochim Biophys Acta 1988;965:68-75.

45. Pinet F, Corvol M-T, Bourguignon J, Corvol P. Isolation and characterization of renin-producing human chorionic cells in culture. J Clin Endrocrinol Metab 1988;67:1211-20.

46. Lenz T, Sealey JE, August P, James GD, Laragh JH. Tissue levels of active and total renin, angiotensinogen, human chorionic gonadotropin, estradiol, and progesterone in human placentas from different methods of delivery. J Clin Endocrinol Metab 1989;69:31-7.

47. Sealey JE, Wilson M, Morganti AA, Zervoudakis I, Laragh JH. Changes in active and inactive renin throughout normal pregnancy. Clin Exp Hyper [A] 1982;A4 (11, 12):2373-84.

48. Skinner SL, Cran EJ, Gibson R, Taylor R, Walters WAW, Catt KJ. Angiotensins I and II, active and inactive renin, renin substrate, renin activity, and angiotensinase in human liquor amnii and plasma. Am J Obstet Gynecol 1975;121:626-30.

49. Glance DG, Elder MG, Myatt L. Prostaglandin production and stimulation by angiotensin II in the isolated perfused human placental cotyledon. Am J Obstet Gynecol 1985;151:387-91.

50. Brar HS, Kjos SL, Dougherty W, Do Y-S, Tam HB, Hsueh WA. Increased feto-placental active renin production in pregnancy-induced hypertension. Am J Obstet Gynecol 1987;157:363-7.

51. Cooke SF, Craven DJ, Symonds EM. Osmolarity changes can enhance the release of renin from human chorion. Am J Obstet Gynecol 1985;151:819-21.

52. Mitchell BF, Challis JRG. Estrogen and progesterone metabolism in human fetal membranes. In: Mitchell BF, ed. The physiology and biochemistry of human fetal membranes. Ithaca, NY: Perinatology Press, 1988:5-28.

53. Lundin-Schiller S, Gibb W, Mitchell MD. Characterization of a substance(s) secreted by chorion laeve that stimulates amnion PGE_2 production [Abstract]. In: Proc 70th annu meet Endocr Soc. New Orleans, 1988:581.

54. Nakla S, Skinner K, Mitchell BF, Challis JRG. Changes in prostaglandin transfer across human fetal membranes obtained after spontaneous labor. Am J Obstet Gynecol 1986;155:1337-41.

16

Mode of Action of Prostaglandins in Myometrial Cells

Frank Hertelendy and Miklós Molnár

Department of Obstetrics and Gynecology, St. Louis University Medical School and St. Mary's Health Center, St. Louis, Missouri

T he primary prostaglandins, $PGF_{2\alpha}$ and PGE_2, and possibly other metabolites of arachidonic acid (AA), represent key links in the chain of events leading to parturition in the human and other mammalian species (1–4). There is also abundant evidence that $PGF_{2\alpha}$ and PGE_2 are essential for oviposition in birds (5, 6), and recent evidence supports the involvement of these prostaglandins in oviposition and parturition in reptiles (7). Thus prostaglandins appear to be an important component of a highly conserved mechanism. Yet despite such experimental evidence supporting a role of prostaglandins in uterine function, relatively little is known about the mode of action of these powerful substances.

It is generally accepted that prostaglandins, like other uterotonins, bind to specific receptors on the plasmalemma, initiating a chain of biochemical reactions leading to myometrial contraction. Although an increase in intracellular free calcium ion concentration ($[Ca^{++}]_i$) is viewed as the principal common denominator in the action of myometrial agonists, contractile responses to a given dose of uterotonins may also be influenced by endocrine factors, mainly sex steroids. For example, it is known that the oxytocin response evolves gradually with the progression of gestation in the human and precipitously in the rat, rabbit, and other mammals, shortly before parturition when the progesterone:estrogen ratio declines. This observation has been attributed to an increase in myometrial oxytocin receptor concentration under the influence of a rise in estrogen:progesterone (8).

The physiological role of prostaglandins in parturition has been supported largely by a documented increase in their production by uterine and fetal tissues at term. This, in turn, is believed to be regulated also by steroid hormones, with estrogen promoting and progesterone suppressing the production of prostaglan-

Acknowledgments: This work was supported in part by grants from NIH (HD-09763), NSF (INT-8421360), and the Kerényi Prenatal Research Fund. M. Molnár is the recipient of a fellowship from the Lalor Foundation.

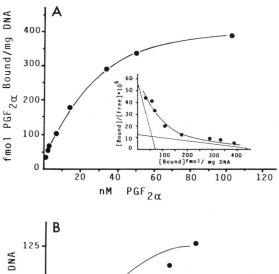

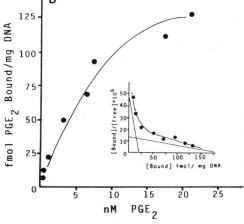

Fig. 1. Specific binding of $PGF_{2\alpha}$ (A) and PGE_2 (B) in rat myometrial membrane enriched fraction. Particulate fraction (0.2-mg protein) from pooled myometrial tissue from 19- to 21-day pregnant rats was incubated at 37°C in 0.2 ml vol for 60 min with increasing amounts of [^{3}H]PG. Nonspecific binding of radiolabel was determined in the presence of 100-fold excess of unlabeled PG and was subtracted from total binding values. Inset shows Scatchard plot constructed from data. Apparent Kd's of 1.3 nM and 35.4 nM were obtained for the high- and low-affinity $PGF_{2\alpha}$ binding sites, respectively, with the corresponding maximal binding values (B_{max}) of $PGF_{2\alpha}$ (70 and 460 fmol/mg DNA). The corresponding values for PGE_2 were 0.45 nM and 12 nM for Kd_1 and Kd_2, and 21 and 168 fmol/mg DNA for B_{max} and $B_{max\,2}$. (From Molnár M, Hertelendy F, $PGF_{2\alpha}$ and PGE_2 binding to rat myometrium during gestation, parturition, and postpartum, Am J Physiol 1990;258:E740–70.)

dins. It has also been frequently observed that much larger doses of prostaglandins are required to terminate pregnancy at midtrimester than at term (9). However, attempts to demonstrate an increase in prostaglandin receptors that could be correlated with changes in sex steroid levels have not been successful (10, 11).

CONCENTRATION OF PROSTAGLANDIN RECEPTORS AROUND THE TIME OF PARTURITION

We have recently reexamined the question of whether the concentration of pros-taglandin receptors increases around the time of parturition. We used crude myometrial membrane preparations (12) from pregnant rats during the last few days of gestation, at parturition, and during the postpartum period. We found that in pooled myometrial preparations both [^{3}H]PGF$_{2\alpha}$ and [^{3}H]PGE$_2$ were taken up in a specific, time- and concentration-dependent, manner. Scatchard analysis revealed high- and low-affinity binding sites for PGF$_{2\alpha}$ and PGE$_2$ (Fig. 1). The affinity of both binding sites for PGF$_{2\alpha}$ and the Kd of the low-affinity site of PGE$_2$ remained essentially the same during gestation and postpartum, and were similar to the binding affinities of nonpregnant rat myometrial preparations (Table 1).

Curiously, there was a 10-fold increase in the Kd value of the high-affinity PGE$_2$ binding site for day 21 of gestation compared to 1 day postpartum. Although the maximal binding capacity (B$_{max}$) of both low- and high-affinity sites for PGF$_{2\alpha}$ as well as PGE$_2$ tended to be higher at parturition, significant increments were observed only after parturition: 12–24 h after in the case of PGF$_{2\alpha}$ and 3 days postpartum in the case of PGE$_2$. Concomitantly with these changes, plasma and amniotic fluid levels of prostanoids increased up to 40-fold (Table 2), whereas

Table 1. Apparent dissociation constants (Kd) for PGF$_{2\alpha}$ and PGE$_2$ binding in rat myometrial membrane preparation before, during, and after parturition.

	PGF$_{2\alpha}$ (nM)		PGE$_2$ (nM)	
	Kd$_1$	Kd$_2$	Kd$_1$	Kd$_2$
Gestation				
17 days	2.8 ± 0.05	19.5 ± 0.87	$0.26 \pm 0.05^*$	20.0 ± 1.40
21 days	2.7 ± 0.06	18.9 ± 0.95	$0.13 \pm 0.01^*$	15.8 ± 2.90
Paturition	2.6 ± 0.24	20.3 ± 4.67	$0.45 \pm 0.03^*$	10.9 ± 0.90
Postpartum				
12 h	3.0 ± 0.25	18.4 ± 0.50	$0.51 \pm 0.10^*$	15.3 ± 2.20
1 day	2.5 ± 0.35	12.9 ± 1.78	1.36 ± 0.10	18.2 ± 3.90
3 days	—	—	1.48 ± 0.16	11.7 ± 0.50
Nonpregnant	3.1 ± 0.71	17.9 ± 2.10	1.12 ± 0.11	8.0 ± 1.50

Note: Values are the mean ± SEM of four separate experiments, using pooled myometrial preparations from groups of rats at the indicated times of gestation and postpartum, as well as from nonpregnant animals.

*P < 0.01 compared to nonpregnant myometrium.

Table 2. Prostanoid levels in uterine venous plasma (PL) and in the amniotic fluid (AF) during gestation.

Gestation Period/ Preparation	$PGF_{2\alpha}$	PGE_2	PGF_M	TXB_2	6-keto PGF_1
Day 16					
PL	0.18 ± 0.04	—	0.06 ± 0.02	0.31 ± 0.08	0.09 ± 0.01
AF	0.32 ± 0.04	1.90 ± 0.39	0.42 ± 0.09	0.45 ± 0.13	0.08 ± 0.01
Day 19					
PL	0.61 ± 0.09	—	0.56 ± 0.14	0.35 ± 0.05	0.08 ± 0.02
AF	0.58 ± 0.06	0.81 ± 0.06	0.28 ± 0.04	0.59 ± 0.12	0.15 ± 0.02
Day 20					
PL	$0.76 \pm 0.09^{**}$	—	$1.95 \pm 0.18^{**}$	0.32 ± 0.07	0.08 ± 0.05
AF	$1.55 \pm 0.15^{**}$	1.36 ± 0.09	—	$1.48 \pm 0.15^{*}$	—
Day 21					
PL	$1.38 \pm 0.29^{**}$	—	$2.32 \pm 0.27^{**}$	0.24 ± 0.04	0.22 ± 0.05
AF	$4.73 \pm 0.74^{**}$	$6.07 \pm 1.40^{*}$	$2.51 \pm 0.62^{*}$	$4.11 \pm 1.16^{*}$	$0.76 \pm 0.14^{**}$
During parturition					
PL	$2.60 \pm 0.46^{**}$	—	$2.05 \pm 0.48^{*}$	0.64 ± 0.19	$0.33 \pm 0.10^{*}$
Day 3 postpartum					
PL	0.05 ± 0.01	—	ND	0.04 ± 0.01	ND

Note: Concentrations are expressed in ng/ml ± SEM; ND = nondetectable; PGF_M = 13,14-dihydro-15 keto-PGF_2.
$^{*}P < 0.05.$ $^{**}P < 0.01$ compared to day 16.

uterine venous plasma progesterone decreased from 269 ± 33 ng/ml at day 16 to 24 ± 1 at day 21 and 15 ± 1 during parturition, raising the estrogen:progesterone ratio 25-fold. Furthermore, postpartal prostanoid levels decreased drastically at the time when PG-receptor concentrations increased, exposing an inverse relationship between uterine PG production and available myometrial binding sites. We therefore considered the possibility that the high endogenous levels of $PGF_{2\alpha}$ and PGE_2 preceding parturition may reduce the concentration of unoccupied receptors, thereby masking the measurable increase of B_{max}.

We chose three experimental approaches to test this possibility. First, we raised endogenous levels of $PGF_{2\alpha}$ and PGE_2 by injecting 1 μg of either $PGF_{2\alpha}$ or PGE_2 into one uterine horn 30 min before excision of both horns. When binding capacity was assessed in membrane preparations derived from PG-treated and the untreated contralateral uterine horns, we observed a significant decrease in the binding capacity of both low- and high-affinity receptors in PG-treated preparations (Fig. 2).

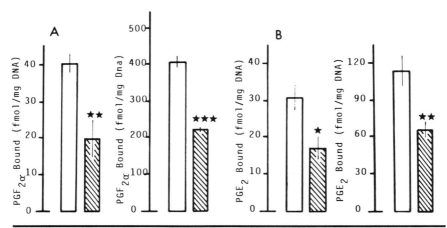

Fig. 2. Effect of intrauterine administration of $PGF_{2\alpha}$ or PGE_2 (1 µg/rat) on subsequent in vitro uptake of $[^3H]PGF_{2\alpha}$ and $[^3H]PGE_2$. Rats (n = 4/group) were laparotomized under Nembutal anesthesia within 24-h postpartum and PGs were injected (1 ml) into one uterine horn, with the contralateral horn receiving 1% ethanol in saline (1 ml). After 30 min, the animals received an overdose of Nembutal, and both uterine horns were excised and myometrial membranes prepared. Open bars show specific uptake of $[^3H]PGF_{2\alpha}$ and $[^3H]PGE_2$ in crude myometrial membrane fraction of vehicle-treated horns, whereas hatched bars show the same in PG-treated uterine horns. (*P < 0.05; **P < 0.025; ***P < 0.01 by paired t-test.) (From Molnár M, Hertelendy F, $PGF_{2\alpha}$ and PGE_2 binding to rat myometrium during gestation, parturition, and postpartum, Am J Physiol 1990;258:E740–70.)

In the second approach, endogenous PG levels were suppressed by chronic treatment of 15-day pregnant rats with indomethacin (2×2 mg/day for 4 days) and PG binding to myometrial preparation was compared on day 20 of gestation to vehicle-treated controls. Such treatment with indomethacin, which has been shown to "upregulate" PGE receptors in rat liver membranes (13) caused a 2- to 3-fold increase in both $PGF_{2\alpha}$ and PGE_2 binding (Fig. 3).

Fetal membranes are major contributors to uterine production of PGs (3, 4), and uterine stretch has also been shown to promote PG release (14). In our third experimental approach, we eliminated these factors by unilateral fetectomy, removing both fetuses and placentas on day 14 of pregnancy from the experimental side, leaving the contralateral horn intact. Groups of animals were killed on day 20, during delivery, 12 h, 1 day, and 5 days postpartum, and $PGF_{2\alpha}$ and PGE_2 binding was compared to the intact, contralateral myometrium. We found a 2- to 3-fold increase in the specific binding of $PGF_{2\alpha}$ to both high- and low-affinity receptors at parturition in the fetectomized myometrial membrane preparation compared to the contralateral pregnant myometrium (Fig. 4). By 12-h postpartum, PGE_2 binding

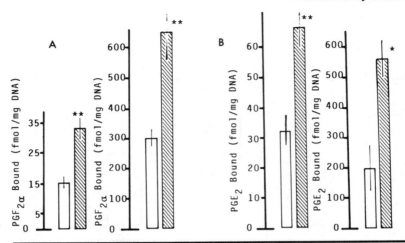

Fig. 3. Effect of indomethacin treatment on the maximal binding capacities of high- and low-binding sites for $PGF_{2\alpha}$ (A) and PGE_2 (B). The open bars represent control rats, and the hatched bars represent indomethacin-treated rats (2 mg/Kg b.w. twice a day for 4 days). (N = 4 ± SEM; *P < 0.05; **P < 0.01 by Student's t-test.)(From Molnár M, Hertelendy F, $PGF_{2\alpha}$ and PGE_2 binding to rat myometrium during gestation, parturition, and postpartum, Am J Physiol 1990;258:E740–70.)

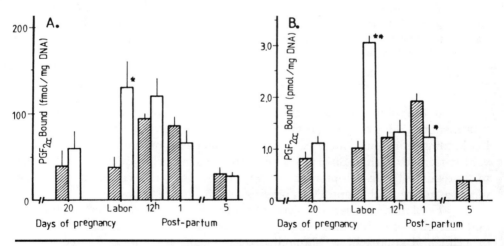

Fig. 4. Effect of fetectomy on high- (A) and low-affinity (B) binding of $PGF_{2\alpha}$ in rat myometrial membrane preparation. The hatched bars represent the maximal binding capacity of $PGF_{2\alpha}$ receptors in the pregnant uterine horns. The open bars show the binding capacity of the fetectomized horns, from which the fetoplacental units were removed. Results are mean ± SEM of four different experiments done in duplicate. Statistical analysis of data was performed using paired t-test. (*P < 0.05; **P < 0.01 when compared with contralateral pregnant horns.) (From Molnár M, Hertelendy F, $PGF_{2\alpha}$ and PGE_2 binding to rat myometrium during gestation, parturition, and postpartum, Am J Physiol 1990;258:E740–70.)

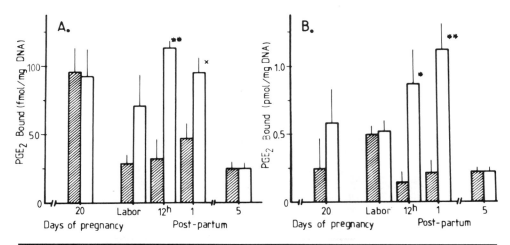

Fig. 5. Effect of fetectomy on high- (*A*) and low-affinity (*B*) binding of PGE$_2$ in rat myometrial membrane preparation. The hatched bars represent pregnant horns, and the open bars represent fetectomized horns. Results are mean ± SEM of four different experiments done in duplicate. (*P < 0.05; **P < 0.01 by paired t-test.) (From Molnár M, Hertelendy F, PGF$_{2\alpha}$ and PGE$_2$ binding to rat myometrium during gestation, parturition, and postpartum, Am J Physiol 1990;258:E740–70.)

in fetectomized myometrial preparation increased significantly and remained higher until 1-day postpartum compared to intact uteri (Fig. 5).

These results suggest that the concentration of both PGF$_{2\alpha}$ and PGE$_2$ binding sites increase around the time of parturition. However, the quantitation by conventional receptor binding techniques are obscured by a striking increase in endogenous levels of prostaglandins, which may form stable, slowly dissociating complexes with their receptors. Final answers await the structural identification of PG receptors and their quantitation, using tools of molecular biology.

The significant increase in estrogen:progesterone ratio in uterine venous blood preceding these changes provide circumstantial evidence for a possible control of PG receptors by female sex steroids. Combined with the well-documented influence on PG synthesis, estrogen and progesterone may provide the underlying mechanism for the action of prostaglandins.

POSTRECEPTOR ACTION OF PGF$_{2\alpha}$: COMPARISON WITH OXYTOCIN

Experiments with Permeabilized Cells

Many types of cells, permeabilized for example with digitonin or saponin, have been used successfully to study various aspects in the transduction of hormone- or drug-generated signals (15). In the present studies we used digitonin to permeabilize

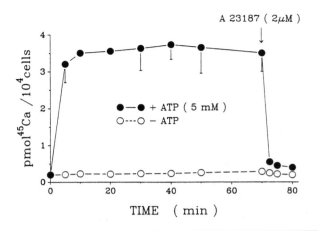

Fig. 6. Time-course of ^{45}Ca uptake by digitonin-treated human myometrial cells during incubation in a buffer containing 20-mM PIPES, 140-mM KCl, 3-mM NaCl, 6-mM MgCl$_2$, 0.1% BSA, 5-μCi ^{45}Ca, 5-μg/ml ruthenium red, pH 7.0. Note that addition of A23187 at the time indicated by the arrow released essentially all of the accumulated ^{45}Ca.

cultured human myometrial cells (HMC), in order to evaluate the action of PGF$_{2\alpha}$ and compare this to those elicited by oxytocin and inositol 1,4,5-trisphosphate (IP$_3$). In the presence of ATP, these cells rapidly accumulate ^{45}Ca, reaching equilibrium within 10 min (Fig. 6). Following ^{45}Ca-loading in a buffer approximating intracellular ionic composition, the cells were exposed to agonists, and at designated times, aliquots were removed and rapidly filtered and washed on Millipore filters. The ^{45}Ca retained in the cells, as measured by scintillation counting, is expressed as the fraction of total releasable ^{45}Ca that is obtained after the addition of 2μM A23187, which removes all but a small portion of ^{45}Ca remaining after the stimulatory (or placebo) period. These cells are also well suited to study the effects of nucleotides, such as GTP analogs, as well as inositol phosphates and other substances that would otherwise not permeate the cell membrane.

Exposure of digitonized HMC to 100-nM PGF$_{2\alpha}$ resulted in a rapid, biphasic release of ^{45}Ca compared to untreated controls (Fig. 7A). The first phase peaked at 1 min and the second at 5 min, after which the rate of ^{45}Ca efflux declined. A very similar pattern was observed following stimulation with oxytocin (Fig. 7B). When ^{45}Ca efflux was measured at 1 and 5 min after the addition of these uterotonic agonists, dose-related responses were obtained (Fig. 8). Maximal effects with oxytocin were obtained at 10 nM, releasing about one third of the total releasable ^{45}Ca, whereas PGF$_{2\alpha}$ produced its maximal responses at 0.1–1 μM, releasing about 25% and 40% in 1 and 5 min, respectively. It has been reported that the IP$_3$-sensitive Ca^{++} pool represents about one-third of total releasable extramitochondrial Ca^{++} (16). Morever, we have found that no ^{45}Ca could be re-

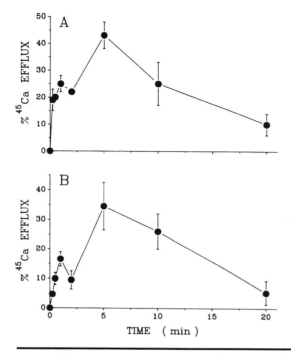

Fig. 7. Kinetics of PGF$_{2\alpha}$-induced ^{45}Ca efflux. Human myometrial cells were preloaded with ^{45}Ca (5 µCi) in the presence of ATP and ruthenium red for 30 min and then stimulated with 100-nM PGF$_{2\alpha}$ (panel A) or 10-nM oxytocin (panel B). Values are expressed as percent of total releasable calcium and represent mean ± SEM of six experiments.

leased by either PGF$_{2\alpha}$ or oxytocin when ^{45}Ca loading was performed in the presence of vanadate, which inhibits the uptake of ^{45}Ca by sarcoplasmic reticulum. Taken together, these observations have indicated that both PGF$_{2\alpha}$ and oxytocin mobilize intracellular Ca^{++} via the messenger molecule IP$_3$. However, a series of subsequent experiments have caused us to rule out this mechanism with respect to the action of PGF$_{2\alpha}$, and confirm it with respect to the action of oxytocin. First, we stimulated ^{45}Ca-labeled digitonized cells with PGF$_{2\alpha}$, oxytocin, and IP$_3$ in the presence and absence of 2-Nitro-4-carboxyphenyl N,N-diphenyl-carbamate (NCDC), a serine esterase inhibitor that has been shown to inhibit phosphoinositide-specific phospholipase C (17) and measured the release of ^{45}Ca. As shown in Fig. 9, NCDC significantly suppressed the action of oxytocin (which has been proposed to act by activating phospholipase C), but had no effect on ^{45}Ca efflux stimulated by PGF$_{2\alpha}$ or IP$_3$.

It has been reported that prostaglandins (18), as well as IP$_3$ (19) can stimulate Ca^{++} release from a microsomal fraction of bovine myometrial homogenate. To find out whether PGF$_{2\alpha}$ releases Ca^{++} from an IP$_3$-sensitive pool,

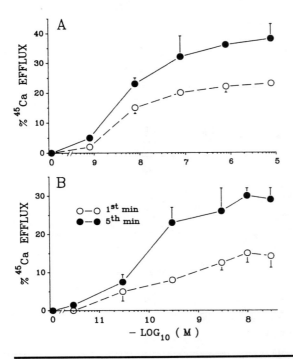

Fig. 8. Dose responses of $PGF_{2\alpha}$- (*A*) and oxytocin-stimulated (*B*) ^{45}Ca efflux from ^{45}Ca-loaded human myometrial cells after 1 and 5 min of stimulation. Results are mean ± SEM of three experiments.

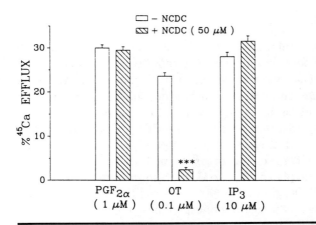

Fig. 9. Effect of NCDC on $PGF_{2\alpha}$-, oxytocin (OT)-, and inositol 1,4,5-trisphosphate (IP_3)-promoted ^{45}Ca efflux. Cells were exposed to NCDC 15 min before the addition of agonists.

we exposed digitonized HMC to heparin, which has been reported to inhibit IP_3-promoted Ca^{++} release in vascular and tracheal smooth-muscle cells (20, 21). The results of such an experiment clearly show that heparin inhibited ^{45}Ca efflux in response to oxytocin and IP_3, but it had no effect on the action of $PGF_{2\alpha}$ (Fig. 10). Thus, we may conclude that in permeabilized cells, both $PGF_{2\alpha}$ and oxytocin, as well as IP_3, one of the products of phospholipase C activation, cause a rapid release of Ca^{++} from nonmitochondrial compartments. However, unlike the action of oxytocin, $PGF_{2\alpha}$-supported ^{45}Ca efflux does not involve the activation of phospholipase C.

Experiments with Intact Cells

In fura 2-loaded HMC, basal $[Ca^{++}]_i$ was found to be 150 nM, whether or not the suspending medium contained calcium. In the presence of 1-mM extracellular Ca^{++}, both $PGF_{2\alpha}$ and oxytocin caused a rapid and dose-dependent increase in $[Ca^{++}]_i$ (Fig. 11). The relative magnitude of this rise was similar to that recently reported for these uterotonins by Mackenzie et al. (22). However, omission of Ca^{++} from the medium abolished Ca transients in HMC exposed to $PGF_{2\alpha}$, even at concentrations that maximally stimulated $[Ca^{++}]_i$ at 1-mM $[Ca^{++}]_{ex}$. On the other hand, the potency of oxytocin remained unchanged ($EC_{50} \approx 1$ nM), even though the absolute increase in $[Ca^{++}]_i$ was markedly reduced. These observations are consistent with those reported for rat myometrial cells (23). By raising $PGF_{2\alpha}$ levels above 1 μM, we were able to observe an increase in $[Ca^{++}]_i$ to a maximum of 295 nM with an EC_{50} of ≈ 2 μM.

To obtain more direct information on the possible involvement of IP_3 in the regulation of $[Ca^{++}]_i$ by $PGF_{2\alpha}$, we incubated confluent HMC cultures for 24–48 h with [^3H]myoinositol and measured the production of [^3H]inositol phosphates after separation by chromatography (24). $PGF_{2\alpha}$ at 10- to 100-nM concentration, which

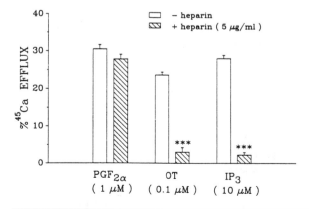

Fig. 10. Effect of heparin on $PGF_{2\alpha}$-, oxytocin (OT)-, and IP_3-stimulated ^{45}Ca efflux. Heparin was added to the cell suspension 15 min before the introduction of agonists.

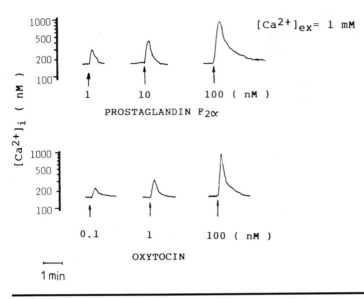

Fig. 11. Dose-dependent elevation of $[Ca^{++}]_i$ by $PGF_{2\alpha}$ and oxytocin in fura-2-loaded human myometrial cells. A representative tracing from several similar experiments is shown.

maximally raised $[Ca^{++}]_i$ in calcium-containing medium, had no effect on inositol phosphates. However, at 1- to 10-μM concentrations, $PGF_{2\alpha}$ caused an up to 50% increase, with IP_3 levels peaking within 30 sec. In Ca-free medium, $PGF_{2\alpha}$ was ineffective. Oxytocin, on the other hand, stimulated inositol lipid turnover in the concentration range that was effective in raising $[Ca^{++}]_i$ and was independent of extracellular Ca^{++}.

Pertussis toxin has been shown in a number of cell types to inhibit G-protein-mediated cellular events such as agonist-promoted phosphoinositide hydrolysis and Ca^{++} mobilization. When HMC cultures were pretreated with pertussis toxin, the oxytocin- but not $PGF_{2\alpha}$-induced increase in $[Ca^{++}]_i$ or inositol phosphate accumulation was significantly suppressed. Moreover, treatment of cells with the protein kinase C-activating phorbol ester, TPA, inhibited in a dose-related manner oxytocin-promoted production of inositol phosphates in HMC prelabeled for 24 h with $[^3H]$myoinositol. The same concentrations of TPA had no effect on responses provoked by $PGF_{2\alpha}$ (10 μM).

These experiments are supportive of our studies using permeabilized cells. By using several approaches, we found that the action of $PGF_{2\alpha}$ on raising $[Ca^{++}]_i$ is unlikely to be linked to inositol lipid breakdown. Even though at much higher concentrations (1–10 μM), $PGF_{2\alpha}$ stimulated inositol phosphate generation, the process required extracellular Ca^{++} and was not the result of a G-protein-coupled signal-transducing mechanism. The way in which $PGF_{2\alpha}$ promotes inositol lipid breakdown remains uncertain. It is conceivable, however, that at high, pharmacological doses, $PGF_{2\alpha}$ diffuses into the cell, reaching concentrations sufficient to mobilize intracellular Ca^{++}, as it does in permeabilized cells, possibly by its ionophoretic property (18). Combined with receptor-mediated Ca^{++} influx, $[Ca^{++}]_i$ may reach levels that could activate phospholipase C, generating IP_3 and diacylglycerol (DAG). Alternately, changes in membrane fluidity brought about by high concentrations of $PGF_{2\alpha}$ (25) may render the phosphoinositides more accessible to phospholipase C. It is our belief, however, that these mechanisms do not come into play at concentrations of $PGF_{2\alpha}$ that the myometrial cells normally encounter.

COMPARISON OF $PGF_{2\alpha}$ AND OXYTOCIN ACTION ON ARACHIDONIC ACID RELEASE

It has been often proposed that $PGF_{2\alpha}$-triggered uterine contractions may be sustained by an "autocatalytic" process involving the Ca^{++}-dependent activation of phospholipase A_2, the release of AA, and its conversion to prostanoids. $PGF_{2\alpha}$ derived in such a way may promote Ca^{++} mobilization, raising $[Ca^{++}]_i$, or by diffusing to neighboring cells it could enhance Ca^{++} influx via a receptor-mediated process. Whereas oxytocin, by raising $[Ca^{++}]_i$, could activate a similar pathway, it can also generate DAG by stimulating inositol lipid breakdown, providing the immediate precursor for AA release by DAG and monoacylglycerol lipases. Accordingly, confluent monolayers of HMC were labeled with [^{3}H]AA for 24–48 h and then stimulated with $PGF_{2\alpha}$ (100 nM) or oxytocin (10 nM). At frequent intervals, up to 20 min, the reaction was stopped, the lipids were extracted, and the major phospholipids as well as the free arachidonate were separated by radio-TLC. Phospholipids and arachidonate were identified by cochromatography with authentic reference standards, and the radioactivity was determined.

As illustrated in Figure 12, $PGF_{2\alpha}$ caused a rapid increase in free [^{3}H]AA and a corresponding decrease in the labeling of phosphatidyl-ethanolamine (PE). Both changes were statistically significant after 60 sec. Importantly, the radioactivity in phosphoinositides (PI) or DAG did not change during the 20 min incubation. (The figure illustrates only 1- and 5-min time-points.) In contrast, oxytocin provoked a rapid increase (maximum at 30 sec) in DAG, which then gradually declined, corresponding to an increase in phosphatidic acid (PA). Oxytocin also increased significantly free [^{3}H]AA, reaching maximal values within 5 min. At the same time, the AA content of PI decreased transiently, as well as the labeling of PE. After 5-min incubation, [^{3}H]AA levels rapidly declined, and both PE and PI returned to control values indicative of reesterification of lysophospholipids. Interestingly, oxytocin also stimulated the deacylation of phosphatidylcholine (PC), as shown by the sustained and significant decrease in the radioactivity of this phospholipid.

These results add support to our notion that $PGF_{2\alpha}$-induced changes in phospholipid turnover are mainly the result of increased Ca^{++} influx and the activation of phospholipase A_2, which preferentially hydrolyzes PE in HMC as has also been found in human amnion cells (3), providing AA, the common precursor of both

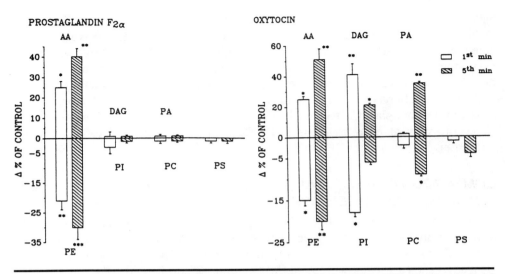

Fig. 12. Effects of $PGF_{2\alpha}$ (100 nM) and oxytocin (100 nM) on phospholipid metabolism in [^{3}H]AA-labeled human myometrial cells. Values are expressed as percent change compared to unstimulated control incubations. The results are mean ± SEM of three experiments. (AA = arachidonic acid; DAG = diacylglycerol; PA = phosphatidic acid; PE = phosphatidyl-ethanolamine; PC = phosphatidylcholine; PS = phosphatidylserine; $^*P < 0.05$; $^{**}P < 0.01$; $^{***}P < 0.001$ by ANOVA and Newman-Keul's test for equal n.)

contractile and relaxant metabolites. The immediate response to oxytocin is the breakdown of inositol lipids generating DAG, which is phosphorylated to PA or deacylated, releasing AA. This is complemented by the activation of PLA_2 acting on both PE and PC. The end result of both mechanisms is the provision of AA for PG synthesis and the maintenance of uterine activity that is essential for parturition.

CONCLUSIONS

The physiological role attributed to prostaglandins in the regulation of myometrial function is supported by the present observations. Confirming earlier studies, evidence has been presented for a high-affinity, specific, and stable association of $PGF_{2\alpha}$ and PGE_2 with a myometrial cell membrane preparation. New evidence indicates that the concentration of $PGF_{2\alpha}$ and PGE_2 receptors increase with approaching parturition, but the simultaneous, dramatic increase in uterine production of these prostaglandins handicaps conventional assay techniques. Although these results should be confirmed with species other than the pregnant rat, it seems reasonable to suggest, nonetheless, that along with enhanced synthesis of prostaglandins, a marked increase in their receptor concentrations contributes to the initiation and completion of parturition.

With regard to the postreceptor action of the uterotonic prostaglandins, our studies in cultured human myometrial cells have demonstrated that $PGF_{2\alpha}$ raises $[Ca^{++}]_i$ by a mechanism that is independent of the G-protein-coupled inositol lipid cycle that seems to be the pathway of action of oxytocin. Furthermore, a rise in $[Ca^{++}]_i$ activates on one hand the contractile mechanism and on the other phospholipase A_2, providing the precursor AA for further synthesis of eicosanoids. Such an "autocatalytic" process may be an important factor for sustained myometrial contraction. Other factors, such as oxytocin, gap junctions, and relaxin may play equally important roles in the regulation of myometrial functions.

REFERENCES

1. MacDonald PC, Porter JC, Schwartz BE, Johnston JM. Initiation of parturition in the human female. Semin Perinatol 1978;2:273-86.
2. Liggins GC. Endocrinology of parturition. In: Novy MJ, Resko JA, eds. Fetal endocrinology of parturition. New York: Academic Press, 1981:211-37.
3. Bleasdale JE, Johnston JM. Prostaglandins and human parturition: regulation of arachidonic acid mobilization. Rev Perinatal Med 1985;5:151-91.
4. Challis JRG, Olson DM. In: Knobil E, Neill J, et al., eds. The physiology of parturition. New York: Raven Press, 1988:2177-216.
5. Hertelendy F. Prostaglandins in avian endocrinology. In: Epple A, Stetson MH, eds. Avian endocrinology. New York: Academic Press, 1980:455-80.
6. Hertelendy F. Regulation of oviposition. In: MacDonald PC, Porter J, eds. Rpt of the 4th Ross Conf Obstet Res. Columbus, Ohio: Ross Laboratories, 1983:79-83.
7. Guillette LJ Jr. Prostaglandins and reproduction in reptiles. In: Epple A, et al., eds. Proc XIth Int Symp Comp Endocrinol. New York: Liss, 1990 (in press).
8. Alexandrova M, Soloff MS. Oxytocin receptors and parturition, I. Control of oxytocin receptor concentration in the myometrium at term. Endocrinology 1980;106:730-5.
9. Calder A. The clinical use of prostaglandins for early and late abortion. In: Hillier K, ed. Eicosanoids and reproduction. Lancaster: MTP, 1987:184-94.
10. Fukai H, Den K, Sakamoto H, Kodaira H, Uchida F, Takagi S. Study of oxytocin receptor, II. Oxytocin and prostaglandin $F_{2\alpha}$ receptors in human myometria and amnion-decidua complex during pregnancy and labor. Endocrinol Jpn 1984;31:565-70.
11. Giannopoulos G, Jackson K, Kredentser J, Tulchinsky D. Prostaglandin E and $F_{2\alpha}$ receptors in human myometrium during the menstrual cycle and in pregnancy and labor. Am J Obstet Gynecol 1985;153:904-10.
12. Lintner F, Tóth M, Hertelendy F. Copurification of prostaglandin $F_{2\alpha}$ receptors with rat uterine plasma membranes. Experientia 1983;39:1102-3.
13. Rice MG, McRae JR, Storm DR, Robertson RP. Up-regulation of hepatic prostaglandin E receptors in vivo induced by prostaglandin synthesis inhibitors. Am J Physiol 1981;241:E291-7.
14. Kloeck FK, Jung H. In vitro release of prostaglandins from the human myometrium under the influence of stretching. Am J Obstet Gynecol 1973;115:1066-9.
15. Wolf BA, Comens PG, Ackerman KE, Sherman WR, McDaniel ML. The digitonin-permeabilized pancreatic islet model. Effect of myoinositol 1,4,5-trisphosphate. Biochem J 1985;227:965-9.
16. Taylor CW, Putney JW Jr. Phosphoinositides and calcium signaling. In: Cheung WY, ed. Calcium and cell function, vol 7. New York: Academic Press, 1987:1-38.

17. Walenga R, Vanderhoek JY, Feinstein MB. Serine esterase inhibitors block stimulus-induced mobilization of arachidonic acid and phosphatidyl-inositide-specific phospholipase C activity in platelets. J Biol Chem 1980;255:6024-7.

18. Carsten ME, Miller JD. Effects of prostaglandins and oxytocin on calcium release from uterine microsomal fraction. J Biol Chem 1977;252:1576-81.

19. Carsten ME, Miller JD. Ca^{++} release by inositol trisphosphate from Ca^{++} transporting microsomes derived from uterine sarcoplasmic reticulum. Biochem Biophys Res Commun 1985;130:1027-31.

20. Kobayashi S, Somlyo AV, Somlyo AP. Heparin inhibits the inositol 1,4,5-trisphosphate-dependent, but not the independent, calcium release induced by guanine nucleotide in vascular smooth muscle. Biochem Biophys Res Commun 1988;153:625-31.

21. Chopra LC, Twort CHC, Ward JPT, Cameron IR. Effects of heparin on inositol 1,4,5-trisphosphate and guanosine 5'-0-(3-thiotriphosphate) induced calcium release in cultured smooth muscle cells from rabbit trachea. Biochem Biophys Res Commun 1989;163:262-8.

22. Mackenzie LW, Word RA, Casey ML, Stull JT. Myosin light chain phosphorylation in human myometrial smooth muscle cells. Am J Physiol 1990;258:C92-8.

23. Khursheed A, Sanborn BM. Changes in intracellular free calcium in isolated myometrial cells: role of extracellular and intracellular calcium and possible involvement of guanine nucleotide-sensitive proteins. Endocrinology 1989;124:17-23.

24. Berridge MJ, Irvine RF. Inositol trisphosphate, a novel second messenger in cellular signal transduction. Nature 1984;312:315-21.

25. Deliconstantinos G, Fotiou S. Effect of prostaglandins E_2 and $F_{2\alpha}$ on membrane calcium binding, Ca^{++}/Mg^{++}-ATPase activity and membrane fluidity in rat myometrial plasma membranes. J Endocrinol 1986;110:395-404.

26. Molnár M, Hertelendy F. $PGF_{2\alpha}$ and PGE_2 binding to rat myometrium during gestation, parturition, and postpartum. Am J Physiol 1990;258:E740-70.

17

Relaxin Promotes Diverse Physiological Processes in the Pregnant Rat

O. D. Sherwood, S. J. Downing, M. Lao Guico-Lamm, and J.-J. Hwang

Department of Physiology and Biophysics and College of Medicine, University of Illinois at Urbana-Champaign

In 1926 F. L. Hisaw discovered relaxin when he found that the injection of serum from pregnant guinea pigs or rabbits into virgin guinea pigs shortly after estrus promoted a noticeable relaxation of the pubic ligament (1). Relaxin is produced in the female reproductive tract, and the highest levels are produced during pregnancy. The source of relaxin, however, varies among species. For example, in pigs, rabbits, and guinea pigs, it is the corpora lutea, placenta, and uterus, respectively (2). Progress toward the isolation of relaxin was slow, and interest in relaxin was generally low for 50 years following its discovery. There was, however, a surge of research on relaxin from the late 1940s through the 1950s. Although impure porcine relaxin was used, pioneering discoveries concerning the biological effects of relaxin on the female reproductive tract of estrogen-pretreated nonpregnant animals were made during that period. Relaxin was found to promote softening of the cervix in estrogen-primed cattle, inhibit spontaneous contractions of the uterine myometrium in estrogen-primed guinea pigs, promote growth of the uterus in estrogen-primed rats, and promote growth and lobulation of the mammary glands in rats primed with estrogen plus progesterone (2). These biological effects, since confirmed with highly purified relaxin, provided valuable insight concerning probable physiological roles of relaxin during pregnancy. In the mid-1970s, relaxin preparations of well-documented high purity began to be described. Since 1974, highly purified relaxin has been obtained from the pig, rat, shark, horse, rabbit, and whale (2, 3). The availability of these hormone preparations triggered a resurgence of research on the chemistry and physiology of relaxin that has been sustained for 15 years.

Acknowledgments: The authors are grateful to J. Sherwood for typing and helping with the editing of this manuscript and to the School of Life Sciences Artist Service for help in preparation of the illustrations.

In 1979 Sherwood and coworkers isolated relaxin from the ovaries of pregnant rats (4), and since then, they have studied the secretion and physiological effects of relaxin in that species. There are both strategic and practical reasons for employing the rat as an experimental animal for the study of the physiology of relaxin during pregnancy. A great deal is known concerning reproductive physiology in the pregnant rat; therefore, new discoveries can be integrated with existing information to provide a comprehensive understanding of the physiology of relaxin. There is presently no reason to believe that findings concerning the biological effects of relaxin in the pregnant rat do not apply to other mammalian species. Relaxin is produced within the ovaries of pregnant rats; therefore, the source of relaxin is readily removed during pregnancy. Porcine relaxin, which is the only relaxin available in large quantities, is biologically active in the rat. The pregnant rat has a short gestation period and is relatively inexpensive. This chapter summarizes recent studies of relaxin in the pregnant rat. Following brief descriptions of its chemistry and secretion, findings concerning the physiological effects of relaxin in the pregnant rat are presented in more detail.

CHEMISTRY OF RAT RELAXIN

Relaxin has superficial structural features that are similar to those of insulin (see Fig. 1). The two hormones are comprised of A and B chains of similar length, and they contain disulfide bridges that have the same disposition. The similarities in their superficial structural features led to the postulation that relaxin and insulin evolved from a common ancestral gene. If that is the case, considerable evolutionary divergence occurred between the two hormones. There is only about 20% homology in the amino acid sequences of rat relaxin and rat insulin, and the homology is largely attributable to the identical disposition of the half-cystine residues involved in disulfide bridge formation and adjacent glycine residues important for chain folding (see Fig. 1). There is no evidence that relaxin and insulin share either immunological determinants or biological effects.

There is striking variation in the primary structure of relaxin among species (2). The amino acid sequence homology between rat relaxin and porcine

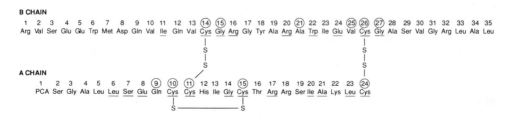

Fig. 1. Covalent structure of rat relaxin (see reference 5). Numbers of residues that are identical in rat relaxin and rat insulin (see reference 6) are circled. Residues that are identical in rat relaxin and porcine relaxin are underlined.

relaxin, for example, is slightly less than 40%, and the invariant positions are largely confined to the half-cystine residues and adjacent glycine residues (see Fig. 1). There are experimental implications to the extraordinary divergence of relaxin's structure among species. A homologous radioimmunoassay is advisable when rigorous studies of the secretion of relaxin in a given species are to be conducted. When studies of the physiological effects of relaxin are to be conducted in a given species, relaxin obtained from that species should be used when possible.

SECRETION OF RELAXIN IN THE PREGNANT RAT

A homologous rat relaxin radioimmunoassay (7) has been used to study the production and secretion of relaxin and their control. The corpora lutea produce both relaxin and progesterone during the second half of the approximately 23-day gestation period. A portion of the relaxin accumulates in small, membrane-bound granules until 2 or 3 days before birth, when the luteal cells degranulate and ovarian relaxin content declines rapidly to low levels (2). (See Fig. 2.)

Luteal cells also secrete relaxin actively throughout the second half of pregnancy. The regulation of the release of relaxin from day 10 to day 20 differs from its regulation during the 3 days immediately before birth, which are desig-

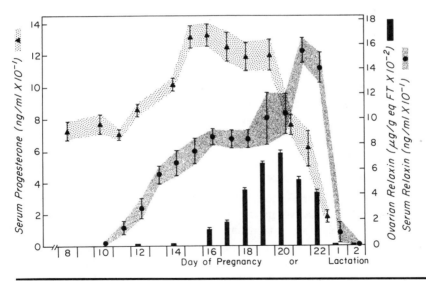

Fig. 2. Mean relaxin immunoactivity levels (±SE) in extracts of ovaries and relaxin and progesterone immunoactivity levels in peripheral sera. (From Pepe GJ, Rothchild I, A comparative study of serum progesterone levels in pregnancy and in various types of pseudopregnancy in the rat, Endocrinology 1974;95: 275–9, and Sherwood OD, Downing SJ, Golos TG, Gordon WL, Tarbell MK, Influence of light-dark cycle on antepartum serum relaxin and progesterone immunoactivity levels and on birth in the rat, Endocrinology 1983;113:997–1003, with permission.)

nated the antepartum period. During the first period, relaxin becomes detectable in the serum by day 10, rises rapidly to 40–80 ng/ml by day 14, and remains relatively constant until day 20 (see Fig. 2). During this period, relaxin synthesis, relaxin secretion, and progesterone secretion are promoted by placental luteotropic factor(s) that act(s) in concert with estrogen and inhibited by a pituitary suppressive factor (2). The chemical nature of these factors remains unknown. From day 20 until birth, there is a surge in serum relaxin to maximal levels that generally range from 120–220 ng/ml, and this surge in relaxin is followed by a rapid decline throughout the approximately 24 h after birth (8, 10). This antepartum relaxin surge coincides temporally with the marked decline in serum progesterone levels required for delivery in the rat. The antepartum elevation of relaxin levels in the peripheral blood appears attributable to relaxin released during the rapid degranulation of luteal cells that occurs at luteolysis. There is evidence the putative luteolytic process associated with the antepartum surge in relaxin occurs at 24-h intervals and that its timing is linked to the photoperiod and influenced by the conceptuses (2).

Delivery in the rat normally lasts about 90 min. During delivery relaxin immunoactivity levels in the peripheral serum surge markedly (see Fig. 3). Mean maximal levels of relaxin during delivery were found to be greater than 150 ng/ml and generally as high as those in the antepartum surge (2, 10). The physiological significance, if any, of the brief surge in serum relaxin levels during delivery is not known. It is clear, however, that the ovary is influenced by events taking place during delivery. Mean relaxin levels decline to less than 5 ng/ml by 24 h after delivery.

The ovaries secrete increasing quantities of estrogen during the second half of rat pregnancy (11). This estrogen may contribute to relaxin's actions. Available evidence indicates that relaxin's effects upon the female reproductive tract are augmented by or dependent upon estrogen (2).

PHYSIOLOGICAL ROLES OF RELAXIN IN THE PREGNANT RAT
Influence of Relaxin on Delivery

Although it has long been postulated that relaxin is vital during pregnancy and/or at parturition, the putative physiological roles of relaxin have, until recently, received little experimental attention. Initial experiments in the 1950s that involved ovariectomized rodents and hormone replacement therapy with crude porcine relaxin and ovarian steroids provided early indications that progesterone, but not relaxin, is essential for the maintenance of pregnancy, whereas relaxin in combination with estrogen is essential for normal delivery (12–15). Since 1985, Sherwood and coworkers conducted several studies that examined the physiological role of relaxin during pregnancy in the rat (16–24). Advances in the last 15 years gave those studies advantages over earlier work; the availability of highly purified relaxin, knowledge of the secretory profile of relaxin during pregnancy, and development of hybridoma methodology made it possible to determine the effects of relaxin under physiological conditions that closely mimic those of normal rat

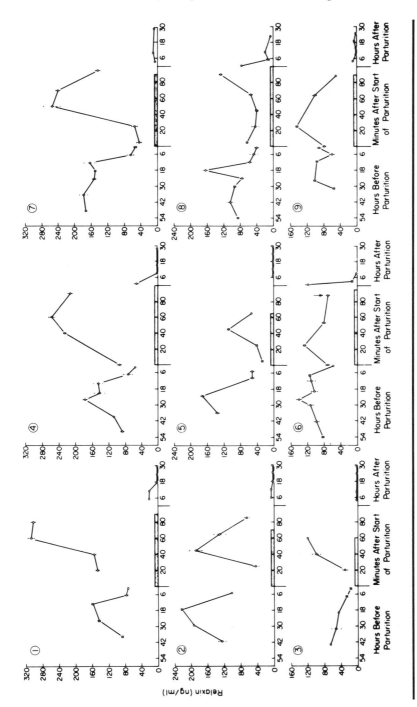

Fig. 3. Mean relaxin immunoactivity levels (±SE) in peripheral sera during late pregnancy, delivery, and postpartum. The duration of delivery is indicated with stippling above the abscissas. (From Sherwood OD, Crnekovic VE, Development of a homologous radioimmunoassay for rat relaxin, Endocrinology 1979; 104:893–7, with permission.)

pregnancy. With the initial study, Downing and Sherwood (16) examined the influence of relaxin on the length of gestation, duration of labor and delivery, and fetal survival. Rats were ovariectomized on day 9, and throughout the remainder of pregnancy, they were given progesterone plus estrogen and/or highly purified porcine relaxin in doses selected to provide serum levels similar to those observed in intact pregnant rats (see Fig. 4). Ovariectomized rats given hormone replacement therapy with progesterone plus estrogen, or progesterone plus relaxin, exhibited prolonged gestation, prolonged labor, and reduced fetal survival. In contrast, ovariectomized rats given relaxin in combination with progesterone and estrogen exhibited birth parameters that did not differ from intact controls.

The ovariectomized pregnant rat provided strong evidence that relaxin in combination with estrogen is required for normal birth. Nevertheless, there are limitations to that experimental model. A principal limitation is the inability to accurately restore blood levels of known ovarian hormones to their normal physiological patterns following ovariectomy. Additionally, there may be ovarian hormones other than relaxin, progesterone, and estrogen that have important physiological effects on pregnancy and parturition, and blood levels of these hormones are reduced or eliminated after ovariectomy. Finally, the use of porcine relaxin to

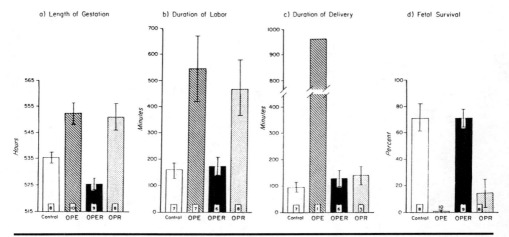

Fig. 4. The influence of hormone replacement therapy with porcine relaxin and estrogen throughout the second half of pregnancy on birth in rats. Pregnant rats were ovariectomized on day 9 and given progesterone, P, implants, plus one of the following injection regimens: estrogen, E (group OPE), E and highly purified porcine relaxin, R (group OPER), or porcine relaxin (group OPR). The P implants were removed on the evening of day 21 to mimic the decline in serum P levels that occurs at luteolysis. (Mean ± SE are for the numbers of animals shown at the base of each bar.) (From Downing SJ, Sherwood OD, The physiological role of relaxin in the pregnant rat, I, The influence of relaxin on parturition, Endocrinology 1985;116:1200–5, with permission.)

mimic the effects of rat relaxin can be criticized, since porcine relaxin demonstrates only 40% amino acid sequence homology with that of rat relaxin (5). A more specific and less invasive approach toward the study of the influence of relaxin in the pregnant rat is to neutralize the biological actions of endogenous relaxin in intact animals. Lao Guico-Lamm et al. (21) developed a monoclonal antibody, designated MCA1, that not only binds rat relaxin with high specificity and high affinity but also neutralizes rat relaxin's biological activity in vivo. Passive immunization with highly purified MCA1 was done throughout the last 10 days of gestation to determine the influence of endogenous relaxin on delivery in the intact pregnant rat (22). Unanesthetized rats were injected once daily (days 12–22) via tail vein with 5-mg MCA1, 5 mg of monoclonal antibody for fluorescein (MCAF, monoclonal antibody control), or phosphate-buffered saline (PBS, vehicle control). Animals were observed continuously for birth from 2100 h on day 22 until 1200 h on day 24. Mother rats were then autopsied to determine if fetuses and/or placentae were retained in utero.

The administration of monoclonal antibody per se did not influence birth. There were no differences between PBS and MCAF controls with any of the birth parameters (see Fig. 5). In contrast, neutralization of endogenous relaxin with MCA1 did influence birth; only the time of onset of straining did not differ from

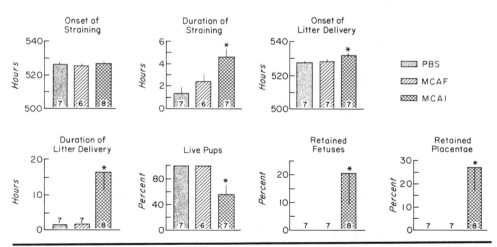

Fig. 5. Influence of neutralization of endogenous relaxin throughout the second half of pregnancy on birth in rats. Each bar represents the mean (±SE), and the number of animals is shown at the base of (or above) each bar. Asterisks denote mean values of MCA1-treated rats that differ (P < 0.05) from those in PBS- and MCAF-treated control rats. (From Lao Guico-Lamm M, Sherwood OD, Monoclonal antibodies specific for rat relaxin, II, Passive immunization with monoclonal antibodies throughout the second half of pregnancy disrupts birth in intact rats, Endocrinology 1988;123:2479–85, with permission.)

controls. The onset of litter delivery was somewhat delayed relative to controls, and this appears to be due to the prolonged duration of straining. The duration of litter delivery in MCA1-treated rats was approximately 12-fold longer than in controls, and the incidence of live pups at birth was approximately 50% that of controls. About 20% of the fetuses and placentae were retained in utero on day 24. Passive immunization of relaxin had no apparent influence on normal ovarian function; the time of occurrence of functional luteolysis in MCA1-treated and control animals were in close agreement (22).

The prolonged duration of straining and litter delivery, reduced incidence of live pups, and increased incidence of retained fetuses and placentae in MCA1-treated rats (Fig. 5) are consistent with, but not as severe as, the disturbances of birth observed in ovariectomized steroid-treated rats in the absence of relaxin (Fig. 4). It is possible that the MCA1 did not completely neutralize endogenous relaxin's bioactivity in intact pregnant rats. Alternatively, the hormone milieu in ovariectomized steroid-treated pregnant rats may have been far from physiological, thereby causing severe disturbances of birth that were not simply attributable to a lack of relaxin. Consistent with this possibility, Cheah and Sherwood (20) recently demonstrated that estrogen produces dose-dependent deleterious effects on birth in the absence of relaxin in ovariectomized pregnant rats.

Whereas passive immunization of endogenous relaxin throughout the second half of gestation established that relaxin is essential for normal delivery in the rat, it provided no insight concerning the period(s) during the second half of pregnancy when relaxin is required. Hwang et al. (24) examined the possibility that relaxin may be important during the 3 days before birth when the antepartum surge in relaxin occurs (Fig. 2). Unanesthetized rats were injected once daily (days 20–22) via tail vein with either 10-mg MCA1 or PBS-vehicle control. The dose of MCA1 was twice that previously used to neutralize relaxin during the last 10 days of gestation (22), since serum relaxin levels during the antepartum period are nearly double those during most of the second half of pregnancy. Rats were observed continuously for birth and maternal behavior from 2100 h on day 22 until day 2 postpartum.

Passive immunization of relaxin during the antepartum period had deleterious effects upon birth, but they were not as severe as those that followed passive immunization of relaxin throughout the second half of pregnancy (see Fig. 6). The onset of straining, duration of straining, and onset of litter delivery in MCA1-treated rats did not differ significantly from those in PBS-treated controls. The mean duration of litter delivery was approximately 5-fold longer than that in controls. There was no significant difference in the incidence of live pups between MCA1-treated and PBS-treated controls at birth, and neither fetuses nor placentae were retained in utero in either treatment group. With MCA1-treated rats, there was a marked reduction in the incidence of live pups by day 2 postpartum, and this was, at least in part, attributable to abnormal postpartum maternal behavior. Of the 7 MCA1-treated rats, 4 rats either ate their young or ignored them. This study provided strong evidence that endogenous relaxin is needed during the antepartum period in the rat for normal litter delivery and high postpartum pup survival.

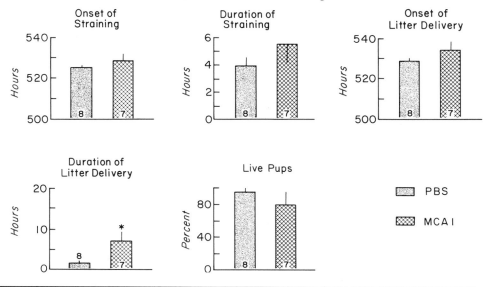

Fig. 6. Influence of neutralization of endogenous relaxin during the antepartum period on birth in rats. Each bar represents the mean (±SE), and the number of animals is shown at the base of (or above) each bar. Asterisk denotes mean value of MCA1-treated rats that differs (P < 0.05) from that of PBS-treated control rats. (From Hwang J-J, Shanks RD, Sherwood OD, Monoclonal antibodies specific for rat relaxin, IV, Passive immunization with monoclonal antibodies during the antepartum period reduces cervical growth and extensibility, disrupts birth, and reduces pup survival in intact rats, Endocrinology 1989;125:260–6, with permission.)

Influence of Relaxin on the Cervix

Efforts to understand the mechanism(s) whereby relaxin deficiency during the second half of pregnancy disrupts birth have been targeted principally on the cervix for two main reasons. First, it has been known for more than 25 years that porcine relaxin promotes estrogen-dependent growth and softening of the cervix in nonpregnant rats (2). In the pregnant rat, there is a close temporal association between the progressive increases in cervical weight and softening that occur from day 12 until term (2, 24) and elevated levels of both relaxin and estrogen in the serum (see Fig. 7). Second, the observations that labor and delivery were prolonged, pup survival was low, and fetuses and placentae were retained in utero following prolonged relaxin deficiency (16, 22) are consistent with the view that the cervix failed to grow or to become as soft in these rats as in intact controls.

The influence of relaxin on the growth and softening of the cervix was examined in both ovariectomized rats given hormone replacement therapy (18, 19) and in intact rats in which endogenous relaxin was neutralized with monoclonal antibody MCA1 (23, 24). Cervices were removed at 1200 h on day 22, about 14 h

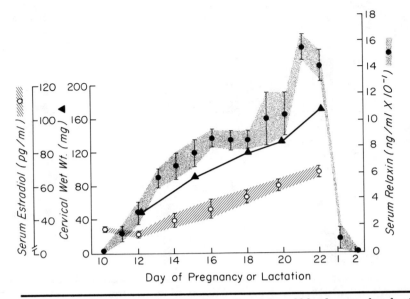

Fig. 7. Mean (±SE) cervical weight and peripheral blood serum levels of relaxin and estrogen during the second half of pregnancy in rats. (From Sherwood OD, Crnekovic VE, Development of a homologous radioimmunoassay for rat relaxin, Endocrinology 1979;104:893–7; Taya K, Greenwald GS, In vivo and in vitro ovarian steroidogenesis in the pregnant rat, Biol Reprod 1981;25:683–91; and Hwang J-J, Shanks RD, Sherwood OD, Monoclonal antibodies specific for rat relaxin, IV, Passive immunization with monoclonal antibodies during the antepartum period reduces cervical growth and extensibility, disrupts birth, and reduces pup survival in intact rats, Endocrinology 1989;125:260–6, with permission.)

before delivery normally occurs. The cervices were weighed and the degree of cervical softening was determined by measuring the tension generated with extension of intact cervices. A 1-mm extension was applied to each cervix at 30-min intervals until a total of 8 mm extension was applied. The tension generated with extension was used as an indication of the degree of softness of the tissue; the more tension generated with extension, the harder the cervix. These experiments demonstrated that relaxin plays a major role in promoting both the growth and extensibility of the cervix during pregnancy. The effects of neutralization of endogenous relaxin throughout the second half of pregnancy and during the 3-day antepartum period on cervical growth and extensibility are shown in Figure 8. Cervical weights were lower in MCA1-treated rats than in control rats, and they were lowest in animals where endogenous relaxin was neutralized throughout the second half of pregnancy. Tension generated on extension of cervices obtained from MCA1-treated rats was greater than the tension generated on extension of cervices

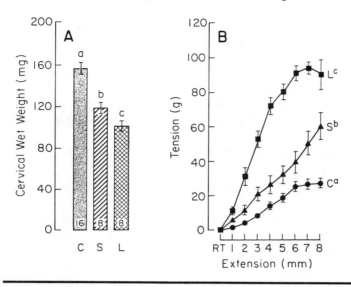

Fig. 8. Influence of neutralization of endogenous relaxin on the weight and extensibility of the rat cervix. *A*: Mean (±SE) wet weight of cervices obtained from PBS-treated controls, C, and rats treated with MCA1 either throughout the second half of pregnancy (long treatment, L) or during the 3-day antepartum period (short treatment, S). *B*: Mean (±SE) tension at extension of cervices of the three groups for eight successive 1-mm extensions at 30-min intervals. Different superscripts denote significant differences among groups (P < 0.05). There were 16 animals in the control group and 8 in each MCA1-treated group. (RT = resting tension.) (From Hwang J-J, Sherwood OD, Monoclonal antibodies specific for rat relaxin, III, Passive immunization with monoclonal antibodies throughout the second half of pregnancy reduces cervical growth and extensibility in intact rats, Endocrinology 1988;123:2486–90, and Hwang J-J, Shanks RD, Sherwood OD, Monoclonal antibodies specific for rat relaxin, IV, Passive immunization with monoclonal antibodies during the antepartum period reduces cervical growth and extensibility, disrupts birth, and reduces pup survival in intact rats, Endocrinology 1989;125:260–6, with permission.)

obtained from control rats, and it was greatest in rats where endogenous relaxin was neutralized throughout the second half of pregnancy.

These studies of the influence of relaxin on the cervix in the pregnant rat provide compelling evidence that relaxin's beneficial effects upon birth are attributable, at least in part, to its effects upon the cervix. With those treatments, where the rat cervices had little, if any, access to relaxin, growth and extensibility of the cervix were lowest, and birth disruptions were most profound. The observation that passive immunization of endogenous relaxin during the antepartum period inhibits growth and extensibility of the cervix and disrupts birth less profoundly than does deprivation of relaxin throughout the second half of pregnancy may be interpreted to infer that endogenous relaxin plays a role throughout the second half of pregnancy in promoting the cervical modifications required for normal birth.

The mechanism(s) whereby relaxin promotes growth and softening of the cervix is poorly understood. It is known that relaxin promotes an increase in collagen solubility, a decrease in collagen concentration, and an increase in glycosaminoglycan's content in the cervices of steroid-treated pregnant rats; these effects of relaxin may contribute to the growth and/or softening of the cervix (19).

Influence of Relaxin on Uterine Contractility

For more than 30 years, numerous studies demonstrated that relaxin renders the uterus quiescent in nonpregnant rats (2), and Downing and Sherwood (17) provided evidence supporting the long-held view that relaxin restrains uterine contractile activity during the second half of rat pregnancy. In pregnant rats, the frequency of uterine contractions diminishes throughout the second half of pregnancy, when relaxin levels in the blood are elevated. When rats were ovariectomized on day 9 and given replacement therapy with progesterone and estrogen, the frequency of intrauterine pressure cycles was considerably greater than that of intact controls; whereas when replacement therapy consisted of progesterone, estrogen, and relaxin, the frequency of intrauterine pressure cycles declined to levels that did not differ from those of intact controls (see Fig. 9).

The physiological significance, if any, of relaxin's apparent restraining effects upon uterine contractile activity during the second half of pregnancy re-

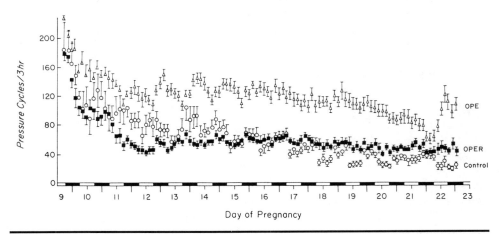

Fig. 9. Mean frequency (±SE) of intrauterine pressure cycles in intact pregnant rats (control), ovariectomized pregnant rats treated with progesterone and estrogen (OPE), and ovariectomized pregnant rats treated with progesterone, estrogen, and highly purified porcine relaxin (OPER). Means are from 25 or more rats. (From Downing SJ, Sherwood OD, The physiological role of relaxin in the pregnant rat, II, The influence of relaxin on uterine contractile activity, Endocrinology 1985;116:1206–14, with permission.)

mains to be established. Relaxin may contribute during this period to the safety and growth of the fetuses (2, 25). Although neutralization of endogenous relaxin throughout the second half of pregnancy did not influence the number of live fetuses, fetal weights, or placental weights on day 22, uterine activity was not measured in that study (23), and it is possible that small amounts of "unneutralized" relaxin reduced uterine contractility.

Does the antepartum surge in serum relaxin levels have important effects upon uterine contractility? More than 10 years ago, it was postulated (25) that the antepartum surge in relaxin may provide a mechanism that protects the fetuses and placentae during the antepartum period of progesterone withdrawal. According to this hypothesis, relaxin may act directly on the uterus to restrain contractile activity until overridden by contractile agents, such as oxytocin and prostaglandins, or other mechanisms that bring about the strong, highly coordinated uterine contractions that occur at delivery (17). Recent reports led to the postulation of a second and indirect mechanism whereby relaxin may influence the timing of delivery by acting centrally to suppress oxytocin secretion (26, 27). Inconsistent with the hypotheses that relaxin influences the timing of birth through either direct or indirect effects on uterine contractility during the antepartum period are the findings that neutralization of endogenous relaxin either throughout the second half of pregnancy (22) or during the antepartum period (24) did not influence the time of onset of labor. Also making it difficult to understand a putative inhibitory effect of relaxin on oxytocin secretion is the knowledge that serum relaxin surges to extremely high levels during delivery, when oxytocin levels in the rat are also elevated (7, 27). Whereas the importance of relaxin's effects on uterine contractility are not presently apparent, such effects cannot be ruled out. It is possible that the severe disturbances of birth that follow relaxin deprivation during the second half of pregnancy (16, 20, 22) are attributable in part to abnormal uterine contractility.

In addition to its quiescent effects on myometrial contractility, numerous studies demonstrated that porcine relaxin promotes general metabolic effects on the nonpregnant rat uterus (increased uterine water content, wet weight, glycogen content, and protein content) that are similar to changes that occur in the uterine composition during the second half of pregnancy (2). That endogenous rat relaxin plays a major role in promoting these changes during the second half of gestation remains to be demonstrated; neutralization of endogenous relaxin throughout the second half of pregnancy did not influence uterine weights on day 22 (23).

Influence of Relaxin on the Mammary Glands

Since the mid 1940s, sporadic reports indicated that the administration of porcine relaxin, in combination with ovarian steroids, promoted growth and differentiation of the mammary glands in nonpregnant rats (2). Hwang et al. (24) recently demonstrated that endogenous relaxin may have important effects upon the mammary glands in pregnant rats. Following neutralization of endogenous relaxin with MCA1 during the antepartum period, there was a marked reduction in the incidence of live pups by day 2 postpartum (see Fig. 10). Although the reduction in pup survival in MCA1-treated animals was attributable in part to atypical mater-

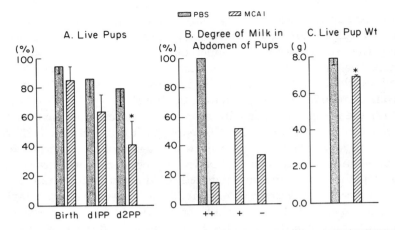

Fig. 10. Influence of neutralization of endogenous relaxin during the antepartum period on postpartum pup survival and growth in rats. Mean (±SE) incidence of live pups (A) in PBS-treated control (n = 8) and MCA1-treated rats (n = 7). The degree of milk in the abdomen of pups (B) and the mean (±SE) live pup weight on day 2 postpartum (day 2 pp) (C) in the litters of PBS-treated controls (n = 76) and MCA1-treated rats (n = 39). Three scores (-, +, ++) designate absence of, little, and abundant milk in the abdomen, respectively. Asterisk denotes significant difference (P < 0.05) from control value. (From Hwang J-J, Shanks RD, Sherwood OD, Monoclonal antibodies specific for rat relaxin, IV, Passive immunization with monoclonal antibodies during the antepartum period reduces cervical growth and extensibility, disrupts birth, and reduces pup survival in intact rats, Endocrinology 1989;125:260–6, with permission.)

nal behavior, there was evidence that surviving pups whose mothers showed apparent normal behavior did not receive normal nourishment: the amount of milk observed in the abdomen and body weights were low. New findings by Hwang et al. (unpublished) may account for these observations. Following passive immunization of endogenous relaxin throughout the second half of pregnancy, the mammary nipples of MCA1-treated rats were less developed than those of PBS-control rats.

SUMMARY

It is not established that relaxin is an essential hormone in the pregnant rat. Whereas relaxin does not appear to be required for either maintenance of pregnancy or growth of the fetuses, relaxin is required for rapid and safe delivery of the pups. The mechanism(s) whereby relaxin facilitates birth is not well understood, but there is strong evidence that it does so to a large extent by promoting both growth and softening of the cervix. There is evidence that relaxin also inhibits the frequency of spontaneous uterine contractions during the second half of pregnancy, but the physiological significance of relaxin's effects upon uterine contractility, if any, remains to be determined. Finally, the long-held but untested hypothesis that relaxin has important effects upon development and/or function of the mammary glands in pregnant rats has received support.

Do relaxin's effects upon diverse processes during pregnancy apply to other mammalian species? Although sweeping statements concerning the physiological role of relaxin in pregnant mammals cannot be made, studies of the role of relaxin in pregnant pigs are consistent with those in the rat; relaxin is required for normal delivery (28) and promotes growth and softening of the cervix (29). These findings in two species encourage the view that relaxin may have similar vitally important roles in other mammalian species.

REFERENCES

1. Hisaw FL. Experimental relaxation of the pubic ligament of the guinea pig. Proc Soc Exp Biol Med 1926;23:661-3.
2. Sherwood OD. Relaxin. In: Knobil E, Neill J, eds. The physiology of reproduction. New York: Raven Press, 1988:585-673.
3. Schwabe C, Bullesbach EE, Heyn H, Yoshioka M. Cetacean relaxin. Isolation and sequence of relaxins from *Balaenoptera acutorostrata* and *Balaenoptera edeni*. J Biol Chem 1989;940-3.
4. Sherwood OD. Purification and characterization of rat relaxin. Endocrinology 1979;104:886-92.
5. John MJ, Borjesson BW, Walsh JR, Niall HD. Limited sequence homology between porcine and rat relaxins: implications for physiological studies. Endocrinology 1981;108:726-9.
6. Lomedico P, Rosenthal N, Efstratiadis A, Gilbert W, Kolodner R, Tizard R. The structure and evolution of the two nonallelic rat preproinsulin genes. Cell 1979;18:545-58.
7. Sherwood OD, Crnekovic VE. Development of a homologous radioimmunoassay for rat relaxin. Endocrinology 1979;104:893-7.
8. Sherwood OD, Crnekovic VE, Gordon WL, Rutherford JE. Radioimmunoassay of relaxin throughout pregnancy and during parturition in the rat. Endocrinology 1980;107:691-8.
9. Pepe GJ, Rothchild I. A comparative study of serum progesterone levels in pregnancy and in various types of pseudopregnancy in the rat. Endocrinology 1974;95:275-9.
10. Sherwood OD, Downing SJ, Golos TG, Gordon WL, Tarbell MK. Influence of light-dark cycle on antepartum serum relaxin and progesterone immunoactivity levels and on birth in the rat. Endocrinology 1983;113:997-1003.
11. Taya K, Greenwald GS. In vivo and in vitro ovarian steroidogenesis in the pregnant rat. Biol Reprod 1981;25:683-91.
12. Smithberg M, Runner M. The induction and maintenance of pregnancy in prepuberal mice. J Exp Zool 1956;133:441-57.
13. Hall K. The effect of relaxin extracts, progesterone and oestradiol on maintenance of pregnancy, parturition, and rearing of young after ovariectomy in mice. J Endocrinol 1957;15:108-17.
14. Kroc RL, Steinetz BG, Beach VL. The effects of estrogens, progestagens, and relaxin in pregnant and nonpregnant laboratory rodents. Ann NY Acad Sci 1959;75:942-80.

15. Steinetz BG, Beach VL, Kroc RL. The physiology of relaxin in laboratory animals. In: Lloyd CW, ed. Recent progress in the endocrinology of reproduction. New York: Academic Press, 1959:389-423.

16. Downing SJ, Sherwood OD. The physiological role of relaxin in the pregnant rat, I. The influence of relaxin on parturition. Endocrinology 1985;116:1200-5.

17. Downing SJ, Sherwood OD. The physiological role of relaxin in the pregnant rat, II. The influence of relaxin on uterine contractile activity. Endocrinology 1985;116: 1206-14.

18. Downing SJ, Sherwood OD. The physiological role of relaxin in the pregnant rat, III. The influence of relaxin on cervical extensibility. Endocrinology 1985;116:1215-20.

19. Downing SJ, Sherwood OD. The physiological role of relaxin in the pregnant rat, IV. The influence of relaxin on cervical collagen and glycosaminoglycans. Endocrinology 1986;118:471-9.

20. Cheah SH, Sherwood OD. Effect of preparturient 17β-estradiol and relaxin on parturition and pup survival in the rat. Endocrinology 1988;122:1958-63.

21. Lao Guico-Lamm M, Voss EW, Sherwood OD. Monoclonal antibodies specific for rat relaxin, I. Production and characterization of monoclonal antibodies that neutralize rat relaxin's bioactivity in vivo. Endocrinology 1988;123:2472-8.

22. Lao Guico-Lamm M, Sherwood OD. Monoclonal antibodies specific for rat relaxin, II. Passive immunization with monoclonal antibodies throughout the second half of pregnancy disrupts birth in intact rats. Endocrinology 1988;123:2479-85.

23. Hwang J-J, Sherwood OD. Monoclonal antibodies specific for rat relaxin, III. Passive immunization with monoclonal antibodies throughout the second half of pregnancy reduces cervical growth and extensibility in intact rats. Endocrinology 1988;123: 2486-90.

24. Hwang J-J, Shanks RD, Sherwood OD. Monoclonal antibodies specific for rat relaxin, IV. Passive immunization with monoclonal antibodies during the antepartum period reduces cervical growth and extensibility, disrupts birth, and reduces pup survival in intact rats. Endocrinology 1989;125:260-6.

25. Porter DG. The myometrium and the relaxin enigma. Anim Reprod Sci 1979;2:77-96.

26. Summerlee JAS, O'Byrne KT, Paisley AC, Breeze MF, Porter DG. Relaxin affects the central control of oxytocin release. Nature 1984;309:372-4.

27. Jones SA, Summerlee AJS. Relaxin acts centrally to inhibit oxytocin release during parturition: an effect that is reversed by naloxone. J Endocrinol 1986;111:99-102.

28. Nara BS, Welk FA, Rutherford JE, Sherwood OD, First NL. Effect of relaxin on parturition and frequency of live births in pigs. J Reprod Fertil 1982;66:359-65.

29. O'Day MB, Winn RJ, Easter RA, Dziuk PJ, Sherwood OD. Hormonal control of the cervix in pregnant gilts, II. Relaxin promotes changes in the physical properties of the cervix in ovariectomized hormone-treated pregnant gilts. Endocrinology 1989;125:3004-10.

18

Sensory and Autonomic Innervation of the Female Reproductive Tract: Some Characteristics and Functional Roles

Harold H. Traurig[1] and Raymond E. Papka[2]

[1]Department of Anatomy and Neurobiology, University of Kentucky College of Medicine, Lexington, and [2]Department of Anatomical Sciences, College of Medicine, University of Oklahoma Health Sciences Center, Oklahoma City

T he innervation of the female reproductive system by nor-adrenergic (NA) and cholinergic (ACH) nerves has been extensively reviewed (1). Autonomic nerves are accompanied by afferent fibers originating from neurons in lumbosacral dorsal root ganglia (DRG). It is now well established that most peripheral and central neurons and their processes contain chemical markers for peptides that may serve transmitter functions (2). Thus, markers for substance P (SP), cholecystokinin (CCK), calcitonin gene-related peptide (CGRP), neurokinin A (NKA), galanin (GAL), vasoactive intestinal polypeptide (VIP), neuropeptide Y (NPY), and other peptides have been localized in nerves and/or coexist with NA or ACH in some autonomic nerves innervating a number of organ systems, including the female reproductive organs (2–8). Whether these peptides participate in classic neurotransmitter mechanisms, serve as trophic factors, or participate in local effector responses remains to be elucidated (2, 9). Further, actions of female reproductive organ nerves are modified by the hormonal milieu (10–13). Thus, in a general sense, the innervation of the female reproductive system consists of subsets of interacting, sex steroid-sensitive autonomic and afferent neurons characterized by combinations of codings for NA, ACH, and/or peptides. Coded terminals innervate specific peripheral targets mediating myometrial contraction, sensation, blood flow, autonomic transmission, and other visceral reflexes related to reproductive processes and behavior. This chapter summarizes salient data characterizing the distributions and functional implications of subclasses of peripheral autonomic and

Acknowledgments: Original studies by R. E. Papka and H. H. Traurig reported here were supported by NIH grants #1-R01-NS22526 and BRSG-RR05374; Alumni Research Grant and Presbyterian Health Foundation, University of Oklahoma.

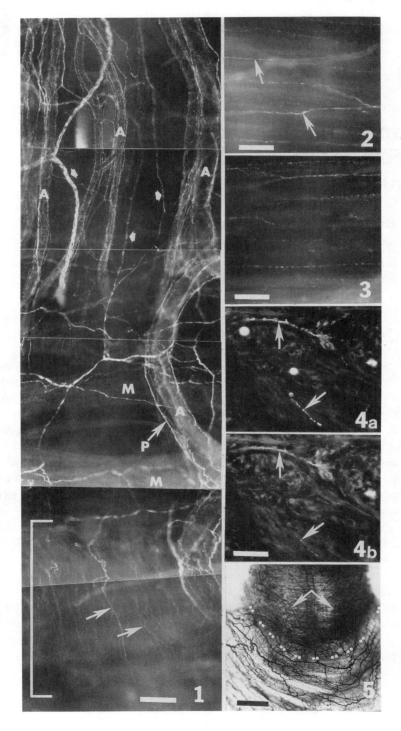

◀ **Figs. 1–5. 1:** Montage of whole mount of mesometrium (M) showing radial arterioles (A) as they emanate from rat uterine artery (out of view at top of figure), course through mesometrium, and approach the uterine wall (large, white bracket). Many nerves immunostained (I) for protein gene product 9.5 (PGP), a marker for nerve fibers (48), follow peri- (A) or paravascular (P) courses, while others (arrowheads) travel free in mesometrium. Numerous PGP-I fibers enter the substance of the uterine wall (arrows). Calibration bar (CB = 200 μ.)

2: Whole mount of rat uterine myometrium showing PGP-I nerves (arrows, other fibers out of focal plane) coursing parallel to, and intimately with, myometrial smooth-muscle fascicles, suggesting a functional relationship. (CB = 100 μ.)

3: Similar to preparation in Figure 2, except immunostained for synapsin I (SY). SY is a protein associated with synaptic vesicles; SY-I distinguishes nerve terminals containing synaptic vesicles from preterminal fibers of passage (49). SY-I terminals course parallel to, and intimately with, myometrial smooth-muscle fascicles, suggesting a functional relationship. (CB = 100 μ.)

4: Same cryostat section of rat uterus doubly immunostained for the neuro-peptides CGRP (*a*) and SP (*b*). Many uterine nerves (arrows) costore CGRP + SP. (CB = 100 μ.)

5: Whole mount of rat cervix-vagina junction (white dots) stained for acetylcho-linesterase, an indirect marker for cholinergic (ACH) nerves. Dense plexuses of ACH nerves ramify in vaginal wall (below dots) and in portio vaginalis of cervix, which protrudes into the vaginal lumen (arrows). (CB = 500 μ.)

sensory neurons innervating female reproductive organs, with emphasis on uterus and cervix.

EXTRINSIC INNERVATION OF THE FEMALE REPRODUCTIVE SYSTEM

The origins and courses of nerves innervating the female reproductive system are similar in most species, and detailed descriptions are available for the rat (14, 15). Generally, for all classes of afferent and efferent nerves, the innervation densities (see Fig. 5) are highest in cervix and proximal vagina followed by oviduct and uterine horns (corpus uteri) (see Figs. 2 and 3). There is a modest distribution of nerves to the ovary, principally associated with the stroma and vasculature. Post-ganglionic autonomic nerves emanate from inferior mesenteric (IMG), lumbosacral paravertebral, and paracervical ganglia (PG), the latter located in the adventitia at the vaginal-cervical junction. Preganglionic input originates in spinal cord and fibers follow pre- and paravertebral plexuses to IMG. Postganglionic fibers follow paired hypogastric nerves, which join the hypogastric plexus and distribute with postganglionic branches of PG. Preganglionic fibers to PG originate from L_6–S_1 cord levels in rat and follow the pelvic nerves to PG (14–17). PG and IMG postganglionic fibers follow blood vessels (see Fig. 1) distributing to uterus (see Figs. 2 and 3), cervix (see Fig. 5), vagina, and other pelvic viscera. Pelvic and pudendal nerves also innervate perineal skeletal muscle, skin, and external genitalia (16, 17). Afferent nerves arising predominantly from DRG neurons T_{13} and L_1 innervate ovary, oviduct, and rostral uterine horn while L_6 and S_1 DRG provide afferent fibers to vagina, cervix, and caudal portion of the uterine horn (15, 17, 18).

INNERVATION OF THE OVARY AND OVIDUCT

Ovaries and oviducts are innervated by fibers in superior ovarian nerves (SON) and ovarian plexus nerves (OPN) and follow ovarian suspensory ligaments and ovarian arteries, respectively. Autonomic fibers originate from preaortic celiac and intermesenteric plexuses and afferent fibers have been traced from T_{13} and L_1 DRG in the rat (14, 15, 18). Ovarian nerves are coded for NA, ACH, NPY, VIP, SP, CGRP, and other peptides and innervate ovarian vasculature, stroma, and interstitial tissue but do not appear to directly innervate follicles or corpora lutea (3, 4). Some examples of coexistence of peptides and/or classical transmitters in ovarian nerves have been revealed (18, 19). Afferent nerves supply collaterals to autonomic ganglia projecting to the ovary providing the basis for reflex regulation of blood flow and other ovarian functions (18).

Nerves to the oviduct generally follow SON and OPN, providing rich intrinsic plexuses of terminals coded for NA, ACH (1, 3), VIP (3, 20–22), NPY (3, 20–22), SP (3, 4, 15, 20, 23), CGRP, and other peptides (4, 24, 25) that innervate smooth-muscle fascicles, vasculature, and mucosa in the rat and the human (21). Prominent subepithelial plexuses of SP- and CGRP-coded nerves suggest sensory and/or reflex functions (3, 4, 15, 18). NA-, ACH-, NPY- (21), VIP- (20) and SP-coded (23) fibers are concentrated at the oviduct-uterine junction and probably participate in oviductal sphincter mechanisms. NPY and VIP may relax oviductal smooth muscle by prejunctional inhibition of cholinergic-mediated smooth-muscle contraction (22). In addition to their afferent functions, nerves coded for CGRP or SP may release these peptides in the periphery following stimulation and thereby participate in local effector responses (9) in the oviduct. For example, CGRP relaxes oviductal smooth muscle and influences blood flow (26), whereas SP induces oviductal smooth-muscle contraction and inhibits VIP-dependent relaxation (23). Taken together, available evidence demonstrates that several classes of nerves interact to mediate oviductal sensation, contraction, and blood flow in support of gamete and blastocyst transport.

INNERVATION OF THE UTERUS AND UTERINE CERVIX

Uterine innervation by NA-coded nerves has been extensively studied and is generally similar in all species examined, but innervation densities vary (1). Uterine horn (corpus) innervation density is less than that of cervix or oviduct. NA fibers form plexuses in association with the vasculature (see Fig. 1) and among myometrial smooth-muscle fascicles (see Figs. 2 and 3) (3, 21, 27, 28). Preterminal and terminal branches are characterized by varicosities (see Figs. 2 and 3) that contain NA (27, 28). At the ultrastructural level, these varicose terminals contain synaptic vesicles and are often observed in close proximity to vascular and myometrial smooth-muscle cells (see Figs. 1–3) (27, 28). Physiological and pharmacological data demonstrate direct NA-mediated vasoconstrictor responses in uterine vasculature (29) and that NA exerts mainly a concentration-dependent, postjunctional inhibitory effect on rat myometrial contraction (10, 12, 22). In addition, a number of studies demonstrate that NA nerves influence myometrial contractions through sex steroid-sensitive αNA stimulatory as well as βNA inhibitory receptor mechanisms (13, 22).

Uterine innervation by ACH-coded nerves has been described in many species (1, 30) and is extensive in rat (3, 27) and human (28). Uterine ACH nerves originate from principal neurons in PG (5, 14). In most species, ACH innervation densities are greater than those of NA: Cervix (Fig. 5), vagina, and oviduct are more richly innervated than uterine body or horns (3, 27, 28). Prominent ACH fiber plexuses are associated with the vasculature, myometrium, endocervix, vaginal lamina propria, and endometrium; ACH terminals ramify just under the epithelium and some appear to penetrate the epithelium (3).

It is well established that ACH nerves provide a major motor innervation to myometrium (1, 22). This correlates well with the numerous ACH-coded PG principal neurons, projecting a rich ACH-coded innervation (see Fig. 5) to the uterus and cervix (3, 5). Physiological and pharmacological studies (10, 13, 22) have elucidated the roles and interactions of some subclasses of neurons innervating rat uterus and cervix. In neurally intact rats, stimulation of hypogastric or pelvic nerves is followed by voltage- and frequency-dependent cervical and uterine horn mechanical responses that are nerve-mediated since they are blocked by tetrodotoxin. Both uterine horns and cervix contract in response to hypogastric or pelvic nerve stimulation; however, uterine horns respond best following hypogastric nerve stimulation while the cervical response is greater following pelvic nerve stimulation. Furthermore, these mechanical responses are markedly reduced by treatment with the ganglionic blocker hexamethonium and completely blocked by atropine (10). In like manner, electrical field stimulation of isolated rat cervical myometrium evoked atropine- or tetrodotoxin-sensitive contractions that are not affected by NA antagonists. In addition, contractions induced by ACH are also blocked by atropine or scopolamine, whereas neostigmine, a cholinergic agonist, enhances contractions. Taken together, these data demonstrate that the motor innervation of the cervix is cholinergic in nature and probably involves muscarinic receptor mechanisms. The NA innervation appears to be largely inhibitory since NA inhibits spontaneous contractions or contractions induced by electrical stimulation; the NA-induced inhibition is blocked by the βNA antagonist propranolol suggesting a role for βNA receptor mechanisms in inhibition of cholinergic-dependent cervical contractions (13, 22). Since the effect of NA on spontaneous contractions is potentiated by the αNA antagonist phenoxybenzamine, αNA receptors may also influence cervical contractions. Subsequent studies led to the conclusion that, while there is evidence that NA may inhibit ACH-dependent cervical contractions by a prejunctional mechanism, the postjunctional actions of NA directly on myometrial smooth muscle play a more prominent role in myometrial contraction (22). ACH fibers are also distributed to the endometrium and glands (3, 30) and guinea pig uterine mucus secretion is activated by cholinergic nerve action (30).

Uterine horns, and especially the cervix, are innervated by NPY- (3, 6, 20–22, 31) and VIP-coded (3, 5, 11, 20, 22) nerves, which distribute to myometrium and vasculature and also provide a few fibers to the mucosa. The innervation density of NPY-coded nerves is greater than that of VIP (3, 8, 20, 32). NA-, ACH-, NPY-, and VIP-coded uterine nerves originate from PG neurons coded for these same molecules (5, 6, 8, 20, 32). In rat, about 90% of PG neurons are coded for ACH, 60% NPY, 42% VIP, and 6% NA suggesting that most PG neurons contain—and probably release—combinations of classical transmitters and peptides (Papka, unpublished). For example, subclasses of PG neurons innervating cervix can be differentiated by their coding for NA and/or NPY and sensitivity to 6-hydroxydopamine treatment (6OHDA, a NA neurotoxin that abolishes nerves coded for NA) (6, 8). Target-specific coding is revealed in that nerves coded for NA + NPY (6OHDA sensitive) innervate predominantly vascular smooth muscle, while those coded for NPY but not NA (6OHDA insensitive), innervate vasculature and myometrium. Myometrium is also innervated by nerves coded for NA but not NPY (6OHDA sensitive). Further, destruction of NA- and NA + NPY-coded nerves by 6OHDA resulted in increased NPY- and VIP-coded innervation densities in the cervix. This suggests that NPY and VIP axons in the cervix sprouted terminals that invaded sites formally occupied by 6OHDA sensitive, NA-, and NA + NPY-coded terminals, possibly in response to a target-dependent trophic factor such as nerve growth factor (6, 8, 22, 33).

Neurally evoked myometrial contractions in rat cervix are potentiated by ACH but inhibited by atropine, tetrodotoxin, VIP, or NPY in a concentration-dependent manner suggesting a nerve-mediated cholinergic mechanism (22). Further, neither VIP nor NPY altered cervical myometrial contractile responses to ACH or to the cholinergic agonist carbacholine. Taken together, these results support the conclusion that NPY and VIP inhibit cholinergic-dependent myometrial contractions through a prejunctional mechanism and that VIP and NPY exert little inhibitory effect directly on myometrial smooth muscle (11, 22). Many studies demonstrated direct vasoconstrictor effects for NPY in uterus and cervix of several species (29, 31) in accordance with NPY-mediated vasoconstrictor actions observed in other tissues (2). In contrast, VIP induces uterine vasodilation through a direct action in a concentration-dependent manner and is more potent in this respect than SP or ENK (34). Recent studies report that NPY augments vasoconstriction evoked by other agents and inhibits vasodilation evoked by SP or ACH but not that evoked by VIP or CGRP (29).

SP-coded nerves are present in many tissues (2, 35), including the uterus in rat (see Fig. 4) (3, 4, 7, 8, 15, 20, 36), human (37, 38), and other species (20, 34, 37). SP-coded afferent nerves distribute to blood vessels, myometrium, and form prominent subepithelial plexuses in endometrium, endocervix, vaginal, and portio vaginalis mucosa; some intraepithelial terminals are also present. SP-coded inner-vation density is less than that for nerves coded for NPY, VIP, or CGRP and similar to NKA or CCK. Afferent peptidergic innervation densities are more extensive in cervix and vagina than in uterine horns in rat (3, 4, 6–8, 24, 25) and human (26). A large body of evidence demonstrates that SP is a transmitter in certain primary afferent nerves in many tissues (2, 35). SP-, CGRP-, NKA-, and CCK-coded nerves in most tissues are permanently destroyed in adult rats treated in neonatal life with capsaicin (CAP, a neurotoxin that destroys C-type, primary afferent nerves) (2, 35), including rat reproductive organs and PG (4, 7, 8, 36). Nerves coded for SP and CGRP have been traced to lumbosacral DRG neurons (15, 36), whereas autonomic neurons innervating uterus are not coded for these peptides and neither CGRP- nor SP-coded fibers are 6OHDA-sensitive (4–6, 8, 24, 26, 38). Taken together, these observations demonstrate that uterine and vaginal nerves coded for SP, CGRP, NKA, or CCK are C-type primary afferent nerves. However, since some CGRP- and CCK-coded nerves are insensitive to CAP treatment, they may belong to classes of primary afferents other than C-type fibers (4, 7, 8, 24, 38). Whether these two classes of CCK- and CGRP-coded primary afferent nerves also have distinct functions remains to be elucidated.

Most SP-coded nerves are also coded for CGRP (see Fig. 4), NKA, CCK (2, 8) or other putative peptide transmitters (2); but not all CGRP-coded uterine nerves also contain SP (4, 7, 8). SP and CGRP do not coexist in NA uterine nerves since SP- and CGRP-coded uterine nerves are insensitive to 6OHDA (6, 24). However, it is possible that SP or CGRP may coexist in ACH-coded uterine nerves as observed in some other tissues (2, 9). The functional significance of co-localization of multiple transmitters in nerve terminals has not been fully elucidated, but there is good evidence that the co-release of CGRP with SP augments and prolongs the effects of SP. For example, CGRP may inhibit SP endopeptidase activity, thus prolonging SP effects (2, 9).

SP dose-dependently contracts smooth muscle and evokes vasodilation in most tissues (2, 9) including the female reproductive tract (26, 34). The augmentation of mechanical and electrical myometrial activity by SP is not diminished by adrenergic or cholinergic blockers, suggesting a direct stimulatory effect by SP on myometrium (26, 34). As a vasodilator in myometrium, SP is less potent than VIP and similar to ENK (34). Recent evidence demonstrates that SP-mediated vasodilation is inhibited by NPY suggesting that interactions between SP and NPY may regulate uterine blood flow (29). Finally, SP reportedly promotes smooth muscle growth (2). On the other hand, CGRP inhibits human myometrial spontaneous contractions in a dose-dependent manner and inhibits the contractile effect of SP on the myometrium. This inhibition is not affected by βNA or muscarinic blockade (26). Similar direct inhibition of spontaneous myometrial contractions by CGRP have been reported in rat uterus (39). CGRP, as well as SP, VIP, and ACH, has been shown to promote uterine vasodilation (29).

The prominent mucosal distributions of afferent terminals coded for SP, CGRP, NKA, CCK, or other peptides provide ideal anatomical arrangements for sensory functions in the uterus, cervix, and vagina. These subsets of afferent nerves probably serve distinct functions in addition to conduction of sensory modalities to the spinal cord. Stimulation of their peripheral terminals might release these peptides in uterus and cervix via axon response or local effector mechanisms (9, 26). In this manner, these peptides, which are known to have direct effects on myometrial and vascular smooth muscle, probably participate in local regulation of myometrial contractions, vascular perfusion, and permeability in response to sensory stimulation. Also, since collaterals of primary afferent nerves coded for CGRP, NKA, SP, CCK, and GAL have been observed in close association with autonomic neurons in the PG (4–6, 8), the release of these peptides in the PG, following stimulation of their endometrial or endocervical terminals, might influence autonomic transmission to myometrial and/or vascular smooth muscle, providing an anatomical basis for local regulation of reflex actions.

GAL is widely distributed in the nervous system including rat primary afferent nerves (8, 40) but not in autonomic neurons innervating the uterus (8). Sparse to modest distributions of GAL-coded nerves, mostly in myometrium and a few with the vasculature, have been reported in the female reproductive tract (8, 40). Evidence suggests that GAL exerts a direct stimulatory effect on myometrial contraction (40). Numerous GAL-coded terminals are arranged in close association with PG neurons that provide autonomic innervation to uterine vasculature and myometrium (8, 40). Since GAL inhibits myenteric plexus cholinergic transmission (41), GAL may also inhibit PG cholinergic transmission. GAL-coded L_6 DRG neurons provide afferent innervation to rat uterus and some, but not all, DRG GAL-coded neurons are also coded for CGRP. Further, GAL-coded DRG neurons and terminals in IMG, PG, or cervix are resistant to CAP and 6OHDA treatment, which destroyed SP-, NKA- and CGRP-coded, and NA-coded nerves, respectively. Thus, GAL-coded uterine nerves belong to a type of primary afferent nerve other than C-type afferents and consist of at least two subclasses—GAL and GAL + CGRP—which may have distinct functions (8).

Nerves coded for gastrin releasing peptide (GRP) in rat oviductal, uterine, and vaginal smooth muscle (42) and ENK- and ANP-coded terminals in PG (5, 43) have been reported. Pharmacological studies demonstrated that GRP exerted a direct, estrogen-sensitive effect on uterine and cervical myometrial contraction. Bombesin, a peptide structurally similar to GRP but of nonmammalian origin, had similar effects (42). A moderate distribution of ENK-coded terminals have been observed in close association with PG autonomic neurons suggesting that ganglionic release of ENK, or ANP, may influence autonomic transmission to myometrium (5, 43). Ultrastructural immunohistochemical studies localized both peptides in large, dense-core vesicles in PG terminals. Since these terminals also contain small, clear "cholinergic type" synaptic vesicles, ENK and/or ANP is probably co-stored and co-released with ACH in PG (43). No PG autonomic neurons were coded for ENK or ANP, and it was concluded that cell bodies of origin for ENK- and ANP-coded nerves and terminals are probably in spinal cord (5, 43). ENK exerts a prejunctional inhibition on cholinergic transmission in ganglia (44); therefore, ENK, released from terminals in the PG, might exert a similar effect on cholinergic transmission to the female reproductive tract. ANP exerts a dose-dependent inhibitory effect on rat spontaneous myometrial activity (39); but how the ANP-coded terminals might influence PG autonomic transmission remains to be clarified.

UTERINE INNERVATION, HORMONAL MILIEU, AND REPRODUCTION

Various classes of uterine nerves and myometrial contractile responses are sensitive to sex steroids. Nerves innervating uterine horns (body) are more sensitive than those innervating cervix, while those innervating bladder are not affected (10, 11, 13, 27), NA and ACH nerve distributions and actions are enhanced during estrus or following estrogen treatment, diminished during pregnancy, and reappear in the postpartum period in rat (10, 27) and human (28), thereby adapting myometrial sensitivity and blood flow to gestational requirements (29, 31). αNA excitatory receptors dominate in circular myometrium, while βNA inhibitory receptors dominate longitudinal myometrium (13); as pregnancy advances, there is a shift to βNA domination facilitating fetal spacing and retention. In the last hours of pregnancy, the estrogen/progesterone ratio reverses—favoring estrogen—resulting in αNA receptor dominance in myometrium facilitating parturition (12, 13).

NPY- and VIP-coded uterine nerves show similar sex steroid sensitivities, but VIP-coded cervical nerves are only slightly affected (11, 22). Thus, near the end of gestation, the waning VIP inhibition over uterine myometrial contractions would facilitate myometrial contractions initiating parturition. But, retention of VIP-mediated inhibitory action in cervical myometrium may be required to inhibit cholineric motor innervation of sphincter mechanisms thereby facilitating passage of fetuses through the cervical canal. Whether these specific influences of sex steroids on certain classes of nerves innervating the uterus are due to direct effects of hormones on neurons or to target-specific trophic factors, such as nerve growth factor, remains to be elucidated (33).

Uterine and cervical afferent nerves are predominantly C-type primary afferents (4, 7) conveying nociceptive, pain, and probably non-nociceptive sensations and are more sensitive in an estrogen-dominated milieu (16, 17, 45). Stimuli from uterine horns are conveyed by hypogastric nerves but not pelvic nerves, whereas passage of fetuses through the cervical canal or vaginal stimulation activates only the pelvic nerves (17). Other examples of reproductive responses and behaviors dependent on afferent innervation of proximal vagina and cervix include facilitation of female rat mating posture, myometrial contractions facilitating passage of sperm through the cervix and uterus to the oviduct (1, 16, 17, 46), and activation of a neuroendocrine reflex essential to augment the corpus luteal progesterone secretion required to maintain pregnancy (7, 36, 45). Stimulation of the vaginal-cervical region increases the threshold for detection and tolerance of pain, but not tactile, stimuli in rats (16, 36, 46) and women (47). This analgesic effect is dependent on peptidergic, C-type primary afferent nerves since it is markedly reduced following vaginal-cervical stimulation in adult rats treated with capsaicin as neonates (46) and in women who ingest diets rich in capsaicin-containing chili peppers (47). The vaginal-cervical stimulation-dependent analgesic response may be important in modulation of pain during parturition.

Thus, a complex, sex steroid-sensitive, neural substrate integrates uterine sensation, myometrial contraction, and blood flow. Several subclasses of primary afferent nerves and terminals in uterus arise from lumbosacral DRG neurons and are coded for combinations of the putative peptide transmitters SP, NKA, CCK, CGRP, GAL, and others. They provide the afferent components for visceral reflexes and neuroendocrine responses important for reproductive processes and behavior. Specific targets in uterus and cervix are innervated by autonomic nerve terminals originating predominantly from PG and IMG neurons coded for combinations of NA or ACH and NPY or VIP, and probably other peptides. Available evidence also suggests that the mechanisms underlying functional interactions between uterine afferent and efferent nerves include release of transmitters from afferent peripheral terminals or ganglionic collaterals, direct actions on myometrial smooth muscle and vasculature, and prejunctional inhibition of myometrial efferent nerve action.

REFERENCES

1. Bell C. Autonomic nervous control of reproduction: circulatory and other factors. Pharmacol Rev 1972;24:657-713.
2. Hökfelt T, Millhorn D, Seroogy K, et al. Coexistence of peptides with classical neurotransmitters. Experientia 1987;43:768-80.
3. Papka RE, Cotton JP, Traurig HH. The comparative distribution of neuropeptide tyrosine, vasoactive intestinal polypeptide-, substance P-immunoreactive, acetylcholinesterase-positive and noradrenergic nerves in the reproductive tract of the female rat. Cell Tissue Res 1985;242:475-90.
4. Papka RE, Traurig HH. Substance K-, substance P-, and calcitonin gene-related peptide-immunoreactive nerves in female reproductive organs. In: Henry JL, et al., eds. Substance-P and neurokinins. New York: Springer-Verlag, 1987:229-31.
5. Papka RE, Traurig HH, Klenn P. The paracervical ganglia of the female rat: histochemistry and immunohistochemistry of neurons, SIF cells and nerve terminals. Am J Anat 1987;179:243-57.
6. Papka RE, Traurig HH. Distribution of subgroups of neuropeptide Y-immunoreactive and noradrenergic nerves in the female rat uterine cervix. Cell Tissue Res 1988; 252:533-41.
7. Traurig HH, Papka RE, Rush ME. Effects of capsaicin on reproductive function in the female rat: role of peptide-containing primary afferent nerves innervating the uterine cervix in the neuroendocrine copulatory response. Cell Tissue Res 1988;253:573-81.
8. Papka RE, Traurig HH. Galanin-immunoreactive nerves in the female rat paracervical ganglion and uterine cervix: distribution and reaction to capsaicin. Cell Tissue Res 1989;257:41-51.
9. Holzer P. Local effector functions of capsaicin-sensitive sensory nerve endings: involvement of tachykinins, calcitonin gene-related peptide and other neuropeptides. Neuroscience 1988;24:739-68.
10. Sato S, Hayashi RH, Garfield RE. Mechanical responses of the rat uterus, cervix, and

bladder to stimulation of hypogastric and pelvic nerves in vivo. Biol Reprod 1989;40:209-19.

11. Stjernquist M, Alm P, Ekman R, Owman C, Sjöberg NO, Sundler F. Levels of neural vasoactive intestinal polypeptide in rat uterus are markedly changed in association with pregnancy as shown by immunocytochemistry and radioimmunoassay. Biol Reprod 1985;33:157-63.

12. Legrand C, Maltier JP, Benghan-Eyene Y. Rat myometrial adrenergic receptors in late pregnancy. Biol Reprod 1987;37:641-50.

13. Maltier JP, Benghan-Eyene Y, Legrand C. Regulation of myometrial β2 adrenergic receptors by progesterone and estradiol-17β in late pregnant rats. Biol Reprod 1989;40:531-40.

14. Baljet B, Drukker J. The extrinsic innervation of the pelvic organs in the female rat. Acta Anat 1980;170:241-67.

15. Nance DM, Burns J, Klein, CM, Burden HW. Afferent fibers in the reproductive system and pelvic viscera of female rats: anterograde tracing and immunocyto-chemical studies. Brain Res Bull 1988;21:701-9.

16. Komisaruk BR. Nature of the neural substrate of female sexual behavior in mammals and its hormonal sensitivity. In: Hutchinson JB, ed. Biological determinants of sexual behavior. New York: John Wiley & Sons, 1978:349-93.

17. Peters LC, Kristal MB, Komisaruk BR. Sensory innervation of the external and internal genitalia of the female rat. Brain Res 1987;408:199-204.

18. Klein CM, Burden HW. Substance P- and vasoactive intestinal polypeptide (VIP)-immunoreactive nerve fibers in relation to ovarian postganglionic perikarya in para- and prevertebral ganglia: evidence from combined retrograde tracing and immunocytochemistry. Cell Tissue Res 1988;252:403-10.

19. McNeill DL, Burden HW. Peripheral pathways for neuropeptide Y- and cholecystokinin-8-immunoreactive nerves innervating the rat ovary. Neurosci Lett 1987;80:27-32.

20. Huang WM, Gu J, Blank MA, Allen JM, Bloom SR, Polak JM. Peptide-immunoreactive nerves in the mammalian female genital tract. Histochem 1984;16:1297-1310.

21. Owman C, Stjernquist M, Helm G, Kannisto P, Sjöberg NO, Sundler F. Comparative histochemical distribution of nerve fibers storing noradrenaline and neuropeptide Y (NPY) in human ovary, fallopian tube and uterus. Med Biol 1986;64:57-65.

22. Stjernquist M, Owman C. Interaction of noradrenaline, NPY and VIP with the neurogenic cholinergic response of the rat uterine cervix in vitro. Acta Physiol Scand 1987;131:553-62.

23. Forman A, Andersson KE, Maigaard S, Ulmsten U. Concentrations and contractile effects of substance P in the human ampullary-isthmic junction. Acta Physiol Scand 1985;124:17-23.

24. Ghatei MA, Gu J, Mulderry PK, et al. Calcitonin gene-related peptide (CGRP) in the female rat urogenital tract. Peptides 1985;6:809-15.

25. Inyama CO, Wharton J, Su HC, Polak JM. CGRP-immunoreactive nerves in the genitalia of the female rat originate from dorsal root ganglia $T_{11}-L_3$ and L_6-S_1: a combined immunocytochemical and retrograde tracing study. Neurosci Lett 1986;69:13-8.

26. Samuelson UE, Dalsgaard CJ, Lundberg JM, Hökfelt T. Calcitonin gene-related

peptide inhibits spontaneous contractions in human uterus and fallopian tube. Neurosci Lett 1985;62:225-30.

27. Garfield RE. Structural studies of innervation on nonpregnant rat uterus. Am J Physiol 1986;251:C41-54.

28. Morizaki N, Morizaki J, Hayashi RH, Garfield RE. A functional and structural study of the innervation of the human uterus. Am J Obstet Gynecol 1989;160:218-28.

29. Fallgren B, Edvinsson L, Ekblad E, Ekman R. Involvement of perivascular neuropeptide Y nerve fibers in uterine arterial vasoconstriction in conjunction with pregnancy. Regul Pept 1989;24:119-30.

30. Hammarstrom M. Autonomic nervous control of cervical secretion in the guinea-pig. Acta Physiol Scand 1989;135:367-71.

31. Jorgensen JC, Sheikh SP, Forman A, Norgard M, Schwartz TW, Ottesen B. Neuropeptide Y in the human female genital tract: localization and biological action. Am J Physiol 1989;257:E220-7.

32. Gu J, Polak JM, Su HC, Blank MA, Morrison JFB, Bloom SR. Demonstration of paracervical ganglion origin for the vasoactive intestinal peptide-containing nerves of the rat uterus using retrograde tracing techniques combined with immunocytochemistry and denervation procedures. Neurosci Lett 1984;51:377-82.

33. Lara HE, McDonald JK, Ojeda SR. Involvement of nerve growth factor in female sexual development. Endocrinology 1989;126:364-75.

34. Ottesen B, Gram BR, Fahrenkrug J. Neuropeptides in the female genital tract: effect on vascular and non-vascular smooth muscle. Peptides 1983;4:387-92.

35. Fitzgerald M. Capsaicin and sensory neurons—a review. Pain 1983;15:109-30.

36. Nance DM, King TR, Nance PW. Neuroendocrine and behavioral effects of intrathecal capsaicin in adult female rats. Brain Res Bull 1987;18:109-14.

37. Heinrich D, Reinecke M, Forssmann WG. Peptidergic innervation of the human and guinea pig uterus. Arch Gynecol 1986;237:213-9.

38. Franco-Cereceda A, Henke H, Lundberg JM, Petermann JB, Hökfelt T, Fischer JA. Calcitonin gene-related peptide (CGRP) in capsaicin-sensitive substance P-immunoreactive sensory neurons in animals and man: distribution and release by capsaicin. Peptides 1987;8:399-410.

39. Bek T, Ottesen B, Fahrenkrug J. The effect of galanin, CGRP and ANP on spontaneous smooth muscle activity of rat uterus. Peptides 1988;9:497-500.

40. Stjernquist M, Ekblad E, Owman C, Sundler F. Immunocytochemical localization of galanin in the rat male and female genital tracts and motor effects in vitro. Regul Pept 1988;20:335-43.

41. Tamura K, Palmer JM, Wood JD. Galanin suppresses nicotinic synaptic transmission in the myenteric plexus of guinea-pig small intestine. Eur J Pharmacol 1987;136:445-6.

42. Stjernquist M, Ekblad E, Owman C, Sundler F. Neuronal localization and motor effects of gastrin-releasing peptide (GRP) in rat uterus. Regul Pept 1986;13:197-205.

43. Papka RE, Traurig HH, Wekstein M. Localization of peptides in nerve terminals in the paracervical ganglion of the rat by light and electron microscopic immunohistochemistry: enkephalin an atrial natriuretic factor. Neurosci Lett 1985;61:285-90.

44. Konishi S, Tsunoo A, Otsuka M. Enkephalins presynaptically inhibit cholinergic transmission in sympathetic ganglia. Nature 1979;282:515-6.

45. Toner JP, Adler NT. Influence of mating and vaginocervical stimulation on rat uterine activity. J Reprod Fertil 1986;78:239-49.

46. Rodriguez-Sierra JF, Skofitsch G, Komisaruk BR, Jacobowitz, DM. Abolition of vagino-cervical stimulation-induced analgesia by capsaicin administered to neonatal, but not adult rats. Physiol Behav 1988;44:267-72.

47. Whipple B, Martinez-Gomez M, Oliva-Zarate L, Pacheco P, Komisaruk BR. Inverse relationship between intensity of vaginal self-stimulation-produced analgesia and level of chronic intake of a dietary source of capsaicin. Physiol Behav 1989;46(2): 247-52.

48. Gulbenkain S, Wharton J, Polak JM. The visualization of cardiovascular innervation in the guinea pig using an antiserum to protein gene product 9.5 (PGP9.5). J Auton Nerv Syst 1987;18: 235-47.

49. DeCamilli P, Cameron R, Greengard P. Synapsin I (protein I), a nerve terminal-specific phosphoprotein, I. Its general distribution in synapses of the central and peripheral nervous system demonstrated by immunofluorescence in frozen and plastic sections. J Cell Biol 1983;96:1337-54.

19

Cytokine Signaling Between the Immune and Reproductive Systems

Thomas G. Wegmann,[1] Larry Guilbert,[1] Radslav Kinsky,[2] and Gerard Chaouat[2]

[1]Department of Immunology, University of Alberta, Edmonton, Canada, and [2]U. 262 INSERM, Clinique Universitaire Baudelocque, Paris

T here appears to be no necessity for an intact maternal immune system in order to achieve successful reproduction under germ-free conditions. Croy and her colleagues have shown that mice that are doubly recessive for the scid and beige mutations, thereby displaying neither B- nor T-cell function and very little NK activity, can nevertheless reproduce in a pathogen-free environment (1). Therefore, it is apparent that whatever influence the maternal immune system has on reproductive outcome is adjunctive rather than essential. Nevertheless, there is a body of literature which indicates that manipulating the maternal immune response can influence reproductive outcome both positively and negatively (2). There have been a number of reports that immunizing chronically aborting human females with either paternal or pooled third-party lymphocytes can bias pregnancy toward the production of live offspring (3). However, only one double-blind clinical trial has been reported to date (4), and thus judgment must be reserved about the human clinical situation. The mouse presents a clearer picture. Clark et al. described how CBA females, when pregnant by DBA/2 males, undergo increased spontaneous abortion (5), especially as a function of maternal age (6). Thereafter, we determined that this increased fetal resorption could be reversed upon immunization with BALB/c cells bearing the paternal haplotype, but not by the paternal DBA/2 cells themselves (7). Subsequent work revealed that the CBA female was unable to immunologically respond to DBA/2 cells, but if immunized by BALB/c cells, would generate a response that would cross-react with cells of the H-2^d haplotype, including DBA/2 cells themselves (8). The responses included both B- and T-cell immunity, as well as the ability to make nonspecific NK and CTL suppressor factors at the maternal:fetal interface (9). A seminal observation from these experiments was that successful immunization to prevent fetal resorption led to an increase in both placental as well as fetal weights (9), recalling earlier observations made by others of a similar nature without the effect on fetal survival.

This led to the postulate that cells of the immune system could influence reproductive outcome by the secretion of cytokines, which would in turn lead to improved growth and functioning of reproductive tissues (10).

This working hypothesis led us to explore the consequences for the fetoplacental unit of deleting maternal T-cells during pregnancy. In all strain combinations examined to date, treating pregnant females with polyclonal and monoclonal antibodies directed against various T-cell subsets leads to decreased placental uptake of tritiated thymidine in vivo, as well as decreased placental phagocytosis of latex particles (11). This is sometimes, but not always, reflected in placental weight, fetal weight, or fetal survival (12). In abortion-prone mice, the rate of fetal resorption is increased by such treatment. In other strain combinations, a dramatic effect is seen in terms of reduction of fetal viability, as well as reduction of placental and fetal weights in the remaining viable fetuses. In other strain combinations, no such effects are seen (13). A particularly striking example is that of the MRL/lpr/lpr mouse, which has a recessive disorder that is similar to human lupus erythematosis in that it has a general T-cell-mediated autoimmunity. These mice have abnormally large placentas and strikingly high rates of phagocytosis within their placentas, when compared to sister-strain mice without the disease. Both parameters can be brought down to normal by treatment with anti-T-cell monoclonal antibodies during pregnancy. In addition, spleen cells from these animals, but not normal sister-strain spleen cells, can prevent the fetal loss observed in haplotype-compatible CBA females when mated to DBA/2 males (13).

The above experiments indicate a positive influence of T-cells on reproductive outcome. Emphasizing this further is the observation that an intact maternal T-cell system is necessary to achieve prevention of abortion in CBA females mated to DBA/2 males and immunized by BALB/c spleen cells. Thus, midgestational removal of T-cells by anti-T-cell antibodies after active paternal cell immunization leads to a high rate of fetal loss, even though antipaternal antibody is present in the serum of the CBA female (13).

Not all immune influences are positive with respect to reproductive outcome. There is a growing awareness that natural killer cells play a role in facilitating abortion in mice. Baines and his colleagues first observed that there is an influx of NK cells in the early stages of fetal resorption associated with CBA by DBA/2 matings (14). They also showed that treatment of these mice with anti-asialo-GM-1 antibody could prevent the abortion (15). These observations have recently been confirmed and generalized, in that double-stranded RNA molecules such as poly(I):poly(C), which are known to be activators of natural killer cells, can induce abortion in mice. More to the point, spleen cells from mice treated in this manner can adoptively transfer abortion but not if the spleen cells are treated with anti-asialo-GM-1 antibody to eliminate NK activity. These results make it unlikely that the adoptive transfer effect is due to nonspecific toxicity of poly(I):poly(C), and, therefore, more directly implicate NK cells in fetal resorption. Furthermore, this effect pertains to a number of strain combinations, BALB/c, CBA, and C57Bl/6. One intriguing observation is that inbred pregnancies are more susceptible to this treatment than outbred ones, suggesting that, as in the CBA × DBA/2J case, active antipaternal cell immunization may lead to resistance of NK cell-associated fetal demise. Experiments to test this are in progress (16).

One plausible way to explain these results is that the increased fetal resorption seen in the CBA × DBA/2 mating combination is a consequence of microbial infection. There is evidence that CBA × DBA/2 matings in germ-free facilities do not show increased fetal resorption, whereas siblings reared under ordinary animal-room circumstances have high resorption rates (17). It is possible that microbial infection at the maternal:fetal interface leads to the observed increased natural killer-cell activation and subsequent fetal loss. The above results indicate that regardless of the cause of spontaneous fetal resorption, it certainly can be induced by injecting activated natural killer cells. Thus there can be both positive and negative influences of immune cells on reproductive outcome. This points to cell-signaling between local immune cells and the cells of the fetal placenta, or in other words, "crosstalk" at the maternal:fetal interface.

DECIDUAL: TROPHOBLAST INTERACTIONS

A number of cells present in the maternal immune system appear among the decidual reaction during murine pregnancy. These include T-cells, macrophages, large granular lymphocytes, and natural killer cells. T-cells have been reported to migrate into the decidua shortly after the appearance of class I antigens in ontogeny and more so in allogeneic as compared to syngeneic pregnancy (18). This is also reflected in the draining lymph nodes, which are also larger in the former versus the latter type of pregnancy (reviewed in reference 19). Thus, some sort of maternal immune recognition appears to be taking place as a result of the allogeneic fetoplacental unit's presence (19). However, there is no evidence for the generation of cytotoxic lymphocytes (CTLs) in this area, and indeed, substances have been described that block the generation of such cells by apparently interfering with the effects of IL-2. The nature of these substances is currently under investigation (20). Recent experiments of Head and her colleagues call into question the relevance of cytotoxic lymphocytes as being of potential harm to the fetoplacental unit. It appears that ordinary CTLs cannot kill trophoblastic target cells even though the trophoblast has the appropriate MHC class I gene product. The antigen can be recognized by T-cells because the trophoblast target cells can serve as antigen-specific cold target inhibitors, preventing the CTLs from killing susceptible targets in the same culture (21). IL-2 activated NK cells, on the other hand, are effective at killing trophoblastic target cells (22). Thus, perhaps the most relevant cells in the placenta with respect to potential damage to the fetoplacental unit are NK cells, both from this evidence and from the in vivo work cited above. Also of importance here are two other types of cells that will be mentioned briefly. The first is the uterine gland cell, because it has been implicated by in situ hybridization studies as the principal uterine source of the cytokine, termed CSF-1 (23), the production of which is primarily under the control of estrogen and progesterone (24). A second cell of emerging importance is the as yet relatively poorly characterized metrial gland cell. Although it is bone marrow derived, it is apparently not affected by the presence of mutations that otherwise eliminate B, T, and NK functions. Recent evidence indicates that the metrial gland cell can also produce CSF-1, as well as possibly other growth factors such as LIF (25). There are also reports that metrial gland cells can kill trophoblastic target cells, although the evidence is as yet meager in this regard (26). Clearly, we need to understand a lot more about de-cidua:trophoblast interactions than we do currently.

THE ROLE OF CYTOKINES IN FERTILITY REGULATION

Because we had observed growth effects on the fetoplacental unit following immu-nization to prevent fetal resorption, we instituted a search to see whether immune system cytokines might influence the growth of placental cells. We found that members of the CSF family, including GM-CSF, IL-3, and CSF-1, were particularly effective at stimulating proliferation and phagocytosis in placental cells (27). A proportion of the cells so stimulated were found to be cytokeratin-positive and vimentin-negative, indicating that they might be trophoblastic in nature (28, 29). That GM-CSF can influence trophoblast development has recently been confirmed in a number of different systems. For example, it is clear that GM-CSF is most effective at stimulating a pure 7.5-day ectoplacental cone trophoblast (30). It is less effective on day 12 trophoblast, which was the stage we initially studied, and does not work at all on day 14 trophoblast. Drake and Head have also confirmed that purified murine midgestational trophoblast cells are responsive to GM-CSF (31). In addition, Robertson and her colleagues have found that GM-CSF promotes more rapid and efficient murine embryonic implantation into uterine epithelial mono-layers in culture (32). All of these experiments indicate that the CSF cytokines have a paracrine role to play in trophoblast growth and may influence their function as well.

An autocrine role is also apparent from recent experiments. The results indicate that the human choriocarcinomas BEWO, JEG, and JAR show reduced proliferation in the presence of anti-GM-CSF antibody. These trophoblastoid tumor cells also show reduced proliferation in the pressence of antibody reacting with the receptor for CSF-1 (anti-c-fms antibody). When added to human term trophoblast cell cultures, CSF-1 approximately doubles the rate of excretion of human chorionic gonadotropin and human placental lactogen from these cells. GM-CSF affects HCG secretion and, in addition, increases the rate of syncytium formation within these cultures. Anti-GM-CSF antibody, on the other hand, prevents these cells from spontaneously syncytializing (33). Thus, there is emerging evidence that the CSF family of cytokines and lymphokines have paracrine and autocrine roles to play in the functioning of trophoblast.

The postulated paracrinological role is reinforced by observations in ro-dents that indicate that both CSF-1 and GM-CSF are released at the maternal-fetal interface. CSF-1 is increased a thousandfold in uterine fluids as a result of its excretion by uterine gland cells and possibly other cells as a result of stimulation by estrogen and progesterone (34). In addition, a role for local uterine, decidual, and DLN T-cells in producing CSF-1 cannot be ruled out at this time. GM-CSF is released at the maternal:fetal interface in mice (35), and in rats as well (36), and more so in allogeneic than in syngeneic pregnancy (37). This release is reduced by in vivo depletion of maternal T-cells with monoclonal antibody, indicating that it is at least under T-cell control, if not made by local T-cells in the mother (35). Thus, there is evidence that CSF-1 and GM-CSF are released at the maternal:fetal interface and that they have an influence on cells of the placental trophoblast, both in terms of inducing proliferation and in terms of promoting such vital functions as endocrine release. Moreover, our recent studies indicate an autocrine role for these cytokines in placental cells and choriocarcinomas (33). Recent studies indicate that there is a pronounced in vivo effect of some of these cytokines on fertility as well (38). We have found that injection of GM-CSF, as well as IL-3, can prevent abortion in the CBA × DBA/2 mating combination. GM-CSF also leads to increased fetal and placental weight. TNFα and γ-interferon, on the other hand, as well as IL-2, have a negative effect on pregnancy, causing abortion in strains where it does not ordinarily occur (38). Thus, there is not only evidence for the presence of these various cytokines in the placenta, but also evidence that they have either positive or negative effects on pregnancy outcome.

CONCLUSION

It is necessary to continue to examine the influence of maternal immunity and immune system cytokines on reproductive success and failure. The mouse model offers an economical, efficient, and relevant way of achieving that goal. Recent developments allow a generalization of pregnancy failure to all murine strains that have been tested to date. It is now imperative to use this model to examine the various means of preventing pregnancy failure and to study in the context of this model the nature of the maternal immune response, both at the cellular and at the molecular level on both the maternal and the fetal side of the maternal:fetal interface. In addition, analogous experiments to those reviewed above are required to rule out or in an immune system influence on uterine contractility.

REFERENCES

1. Croy AA, Chapeau C. Evaluation of the pregnancy immunotrophism hypothesis by assessment of the reproductive performance of young, adult mice of genotype scid/scid.bg/bg. J Reprod Fertil 1990.
2. Gill TJ III, Wegmann TG, eds. Immunoregulation and fetal survival. New York: Oxford University Press, 1987.
3. Beard RW, Sharp F, eds. Early pregnancy loss: mechanisms and treatment. Ashton-under-Lyne, Lancs, UK: Peacock Press, 1988.
4. Mowbray JF, Liddell H, Underwood JL, Gibbings C, Reginald PW, Beard RW. Controlled trial of treatment of recurrent spontaneous abortion by immunization with paternal cells. Lancet 1985;I:941.
5. Clark DA, McDermott M, Szewzuk MR. Cell impairment of host versus graft reaction in pregnant mice, II. Selective suppression of cytotoxic cell generation correlates with soluble suppressor activity and successful allogeneic pregnancy. Cell Immunol 1980;52:106.

6. Clark DA, Chaput A, Tutton D. Active suppression of host versus graft reaction in pregnant mice, VII. Spontaneous abortion of CBA × DBA/2 fetuses in the uterus of CBA/J mice correlates with deficient non-T suppressor cell activity. J Immunol 1986;136:1668.

7. Chaouat G, Kiger N, Wegmann TG. Vaccination against spontaneous abortion in mice. J Reprod Immunol 1983;5:389.

8. Chaouat G, Kolb J-P, Kiger N, Stanislawski M, Wegmann TG. Immunological concomitants of vaccination against abortion in mice. J Immunol 1985;134:1594.

9. Chaouat G, Kolb J-P, Chaffaux M, et al. The placenta and the survival of the fetal allograft. In: Gill TJ III, Wegmann TG, eds. Immunoregulation and fetal survival. New York: Oxford University Press, 1987:239-51.

10. Wegmann TG. Fetal protection against abortion: is it immunosuppression or immunostimulation? Ann Immunol Inst Pasteur 1984;135D:309.

11. Athanassakis I, Bleackley RC, Paetkau V, Guilbert L, Barr PJ, Wegmann TG. The immunostimulatory effects of T-cells and T-cell lymphokines on murine fetally derived placental cells. J Immunol 1987;138:37.

12. Athanassakis I, Chaouat G, Wegmann TG. The effects of anti-CD4 and anti-CD8 antibody treatment on placental growth and function in allogeneic and syngeneic murine pregnancy. Cell Immunol 1990.

13. Chaouat G, Menu E, Athanassakis I, Wegmann TG. Maternal T cells regulate placental size and fetal survival. Regional Immunol 1988;1:143-8.

14. Gendron R, Baines MG. Infiltrating decidual natural killer cells are associated with spontaneous abortion in mice. Cell Immunol 1988;113:261-7.

15. De Fougerolles R, Baines MG. Modulation of the natural killer cell activity in pregnant mice alters the spontaneous abortion rate. J Reprod Immunol 1987;11:147-53.

16. Kinsky R, Delage G, Rosin N, Ming NT, Hoffman M, Chaouat G. A murine model of NK mediated resorption. Biol Reprod 1990.

17. Hamilton MS, Hamilton BL. Environmental influences in immunologically associated recurrent spontaneous abortion in CBA/J mice. Am J Reprod Immunol 1987;11:237.

18. Lala PK, Parhar RS, Kearns M, Johnson S, Scodras JM. Immunological aspects of the decidual response. In: Clark DA, Croy, BA, eds. Reproductive immunology. New York: Elsevier, 1986:190.

19. Hunziker RD, Wegmann TG. Placental immunoregulation. CRC Critical Rev Immunol 1986;6:245-85.

20. Clark DA, Falbo M, Rowley RB, Banwatt D, Stendronska-Clark J. Active suppression of host-versus-graft reaction in pregnant mice, IX. Soluble suppressor activity obtained from allopregnant mouse decidua that blocks the cytolytic effect response to IL-2 is related to transforming growth factor-beta. J Immunol 1988;141:3833.

21. Zuckermann FA, Head JR. Murine trophoblast resists cell mediated lysis, II. Resistance to natural cell-mediated cytotoxicity. Cell Immunol 1988;116:274.

22. Head JR, Drake BL, Zuckerman FA. Immunobiological features of human trophoblast. In: Wegmann TG, Nisbett-Brown E, Gill TJ III, eds. Molecular and cellular immunobiology of the maternal-fetal interface. New York: Oxford University Press, 1990:ch 10.

23. Pollard JW, Arceci RJ, Bartocci A, Stanley ER. Colony stimulating factor 1: a growth factor for trophoblasts? In: Wegmann TG, Nisbett-Brown E, Gill TJ III, eds. Molecular

and cellular immunobiology of the maternal-fetal interface. New York: Oxford University Press, 1990: ch 17.

24. Pollard JW, Bartocci A, Arceci R, Orlofsky A, Ladner MB, Stanley ER. Apparent role of the macrophage growth factor, CSF-1, in placental development. Nature 1987;330:484.

25. Croy A, Guilbert L, Brown MA, et al. Characterization of cytokine production by the metrial gland and granulated metrial gland cells (submitted).

26. Stewart I, Mukhtar DDY. The killing of mouse trophoblast cells by granulated metrial gland cells in vitro. Placenta 1988;9:417.

27. Athanassakis I, Bleackley RC, Paetkau V, Guilbert L, Barr PJ, Wegmann TG. The immunostimulatory effect of T cells and T cell lymphokines on murine fetally-derived placental cells. J Immunol 1987;138:37.

28. Guilbert L, Athanassakis I, Branch DR, et al. The placenta as an immune:endocrine interface. In: Wegmann TG, Nisbett-Brown E, Gill TJ III, eds. Molecular and cellular immunobiology of the maternal-fetal interface. New York: Oxford University Press, 1990:ch 18.

29. Athanassakis I, Vassiliadis S, Wegmann TG, Guilbert L. Fetally-derived murine placental cells simultaneously display trophoblast and macrophage characteristics (submitted).

30. Armstrong D, Chaouat G. Effects of lymphokines and immune complexes on murine placental cell growth in vitro. Biol Reprod 1989;38:400-6.

31. Head J, Drake B. 1989. Personal communication.

32. Robertson S, Lavranos T, Seamark RF. In vitro models of the maternal-fetal interface. In: Wegmann TG, Nisbett-Brown E, Gill TJ III, eds. Molecular and cellular immunobiology of the maternal-fetal interface. New York: Oxford University Press, 1990:ch 13.

33. Guilbert L, et al. 1990. (in preparation).

34. Bartocci A, Pollard JW, Stanley ER. Regulation of colony-stimulating factor 1 during pregnancy. J Exp Med 1986;164:956.

35. Wegmann TG, Athanassakis I, Guilbert L, et al. The role M-CSF and GM-CSF in fostering placental growth, fetal growth, and fetal survival. Transplant Proc 1989;21:566. And: Crainie M, Guilbert L, Wegmann TG. 1989. Unpublished observations.

36. Shiverick K. 1989. Personal communication.

37. Athanassakis I. 1988. Ph.D. Thesis, University of Alberta. And: Hui L, Guilbert L, Wegmann TG. 1988. Unpublished observations.

38. Chaouat G, Menu E, Clark DA, Dy M, Minkowski M, Wegmann TG. Control of fetal survival in CBA × DBA/2 mice by lymphokine therapy. J Reprod Fertil 1990.

PART

V

CLINICAL AND THERAPEUTIC CONSIDERATIONS

20

Overview of Studies on Labor

Alexander Turnbull

*Nuffield Department of Obstetrics and Gynaecology, University of
Oxford, and Maternity Department, John Radcliffe Hospital,
Headington, Oxford, England*

My first papers (1, 2) were concerned with difficult labor, especially due to uterine dysfunction. I found less difference than I expected between the contraction patterns in normal labor and so-called hypertonic dysfunction. This type of dystocia was almost unknown in multiparae with previous vaginal delivery, and when I found that, compared with primigravidae, such multiparae had quicker labors despite weaker contractions, I argued that to some extent "hypertonic dysfunction" must be associated with a deficiency in the factors that promote cervical softening and dilatability.

In Aberdeen in 1961, A. Anderson and I began to investigate the onset of labor, both spontaneous and induced. We published several papers on the mechanism by which hypertonic saline induced abortion and showed that the process was *not* associated with any reduction in urinary pregnanediol secretion (3). In another study (4), we obtained evidence for a potential fetal role in the control of human labor from finding that the higher the estriol level at 34 weeks (dependent on fetal mechanisms), the earlier would be the onset of labor; whereas the higher the estrone level at 34 weeks (dependent on maternal mechanisms), the later the onset of subsequent labor.

In clinical studies on induction labor, we investigated the role of amniotomy and showed that oxytocin had to be "titrated" in gradually increasing dosages following amniotomy to get the best results. We published these studies (5, 6) together with an account of the results of this approach in the population we served (7, 8) and were initially pleased when they became regarded as the standard U.K. work on the induction of labor. Subsequently, automatic equipment was developed to provide oxytocin titration (10). Our original aim was simply to achieve more efficient induction when indicated, as before, but after our work, the induction rate in the United Kingdom began to rise, and we became concerned about the possible ill effects. We helped draw attention to the increased risk of neonatal jaundice associated with induction (15) and, in a later retrospective study, showed how much more efficient was spontaneous than induced labor (21). Induction rates in the

United Kingdom gradually fell in the late 1970s, the peak being reached about 1975.

Interested in the spontaneous initiation of labor, we published a variety of studies on uterine contractility, cervical dilatation, and other factors on the subsequent length of gestation (9). I was still interested enough in induction of labor that as soon as a supply of prostaglandin F_2 (PGF_α) became available, I promoted a study showing that PGs did not have the antidiuretic effects of oxytocin (11). This work was done in Cardiff, where I was fortunate enough to be awarded a long-term MRC grant in 1972 to investigate the endocrine control of labor, and it became possible to build up a sizable research team.

After moving to Oxford in 1973, we investigated sheep and human pregnancy, including corticosteroids in the human mother and fetus and maternal estradiol and progesterone levels in relation to the onset of human labor (13, 14). Ultimately, we found that these investigations failed to clarify the control system for human labor. We clarified the role of the fetal cortisol surge in ovine parturition, showing that it induced 17α-hydroxylase and 17,20-lyase enzymes within the fetal placenta, which enabled progesterone to be metabolized to 17α-hydroxyprogesterone, then to androstenedione, and ultimately to estrone, as the fetal placenta was already rich in aromatase enzyme. With low progesterone and high estrogen levels, the maternal placenta began to synthesize $PHG_{2\alpha}$ and initiated parturition (16). In human pregnancy, we also turned to PGs and were among the first to measure their levels in amniotic fluid in pregnancy and labor and to show that the fetal membranes were their likely source (12, 18). Later, we found that vaginal or cervical distension in the pregnant and puerperal ewe caused release of PGs into the maternal circulation and that this was initiated by a surge of oxytocin occurring immediately after the manipulation. Thus, the "Ferguson" reflex in the ewe led not only to oxytocin release but also to increased PG production. In the human, we found that vaginal stimulation and amniotomy (but not amniocentesis) caused a sharp increase in maternal PG levels, but not oxytocin, and we began to stress that the control system for human parturition must be localized within the uterus (17, 20). Later we found that the surge of PGs following amniotomy was not responsible for the onset of labor; when labor began after amniotomy this was associated with a later surge of PGFm (25). Subsequently, we showed that the process of cervical softening and dilatation in labor was associated with local production of PGs (PGE especially) by cervical tissues of both the ewe and the human (22, 23). We also found that the highest levels of PGs in maternal peripheral blood occurred immediately following the delivery of the placenta in the third stage (26).

Many of our studies were directed at the problem of preterm labor. We first published a review in which "preterm" was defined as earlier than 37 weeks' gestation rather than below 2.5 kg, which had previously been used. We found that by excluding "small" for date-mature infants, preterm labor was seen as carrying greater risks of neonatal death than stillbirth. We were also able to simplify causation into (*a*) those in whom preterm delivery was "unexplained" and associated with apparently normal pregnancy, (*b*) those in whom preterm delivery was associated with a pregnancy complication such as antepartum hemorrhage, and (*c*) those in whom predelivery was elective to avoid jeopardy to the mother or fetus (19). We later found that PG levels were lower in preterm than in term labor (24), but subsequently showed that this was mainly in "unexplained" cases. Where preterm labor was associated with a complication such as chorio amnionitis, levels of PGs produced by amnion and chorion were much increased (29, 30).

Throughout all these studies we were dependent on having excellent, sensitive, and specific radioimmunoassays for steroids, prostaglandins and oxytocin. These were, in the main, established by T. Flint and M. Mitchell and run by dedicated technicians. Our main problem was to develop an assay for a stable PGE metabolite. This was finally achieved by L. Dermers during a sabbatical visit to the department. Subsequently, S. Brennecke et al. (28), utilized this assay in a review of the levels of the metabolite during human pregnancy and parturition. A. L. Bernal established the methods for culture of cells of the amnion, chorion, decidua, and placenta, which we have used in recent years (29, 30). All these techniques served us well after the ending of the long-term MRC grant in 1982.

We were among the first to realize that there was difficulty in differentiating patients, apparently in established preterm labor who would go on to delivery, from those in whom labor would stop spontaneously and the pregnancy continue. A. Anderson, who died in 1983, showed that at least 50% of preterm "labors" settled spontaneously and that in those with intact membranes, the percentage settling was even higher. We tried to differentiate these women unsuccessfully by various methods such as measuring uterine contractions, checking on cervical dilation, or measuring prostaglandin metabolite levels in peripheral blood, but none proved effective.

It was not until B. Castle and I recorded fetal breathing movements (FBM) that we found a means of predicting the likely outcome of preterm labor (27). If FBM were present, labor was likely to settle; if FBM were absent, labor was likely to progress to delivery. These findings have now been confirmed in workers in several countries, including the United States, and I recently reviewed the findings up to 1988 (31).

REFERENCES

1. Turnbull AC. Uterine action in normal and abnormal labor. J Obstet Gynaecol Br Emp 1957;64:321-33.
2. Turnbull AC. Amniotic pressure, cervical dilatation and the cervix in labour. In: A symposium on physical methods of measurement in obstetrics and gynaecology. J Obstet Gynaecol Br Cwlth 1962;69:1047-8.
3. Klopper AI, Turnbull AC, Anderson ABM. Changes in steroid hormone excretion during abortion in mid pregnancy following the intra amniotic injection of hypertonic saline. J Obstet Gynaecol Br Cwlth 1966;73:390-8.
4. Turnbull AC, Anderson ABM, Wilson GR. Maternal urinary oestrogen excretion as evidence of a fetal role in determining gestation at labour. Lancet 1967;II:627-9.
5. Turnbull AC, Anderson ABM. Induction of labour, I. Amniotomy. J Obstet Gynaecol Br Cwlth 1967;74:849-54.

6. Turnbull AC, Anderson ABM. Induction of labour, II. Intravenous oxytocin "titration." J Obstet Gynaecol Br Cwlth 1968;75:24-31.

7. Turnbull AC, Anderson ABM. Induction of labour, III. Results with amniotomy and oxytocin "titration." J Obstet Gynaceol Br Cwlth 1968;75:32-41.

8. Anderson ABM, Turnbull AC, Baird Sir Dugald. The influence of induction of labour on caesarean section rate, duration labour and perinatal mortality between 1938 and 1966. J Obstet Gynaecol Br Cwlth 1968;75:800-11.

9. Anderson ABM, Turnbull AC. Relationship between length of gestation and cervical dilatation, uterine contractility and other factors during pregnancy. Am J Obstet Gynecol 1969;105:1207-14.

10. Francis JG, Turnbull AC, Thomas FF. Automatic equipment for the induction of labour. J Obstet Gynaecol Br Cwlth 1970;77:594-602.

11. Roberts G, Anderson ABM, McGarry J, Turnbull AC. Absence of antidiuresis during administration of prostaglandin F2α. Brit Med J 1970;2:152-4.

12. Keirse MJNC, Turnbull AC. Prostaglandins in amniotic fluid during late pregnancy and labour. J Obstet Gynaecol Br Cwlth 1973;80:970-3.

13. Cawson JM, Anderson ABM, Turnbull AC, Lampe L. Cortisol, cortisone and 11-deoxycortisol levels in human umbilical and maternal plasma in relation to the onset of labour. J Obstet Gynaecol Br Cwlth 1974;81:737-45.

14. Turnbull AC, Patten PT, Flint APF, Keirse MJNC, Jeremy JY, Anderson ABM. Significant fall in progesterone and rise in oestradiol levels in human peripheral plasma before the onset of labour. Lancet 1974;I:101-4.

15. Calder AA, Moar VA, Ounsted MK, Turnbull AC. Increased bilirubin levels in neonates after induction of labour by intravenous PGE_2 or oxytocin. Lancet 1974;II:1339-42.

16. Anderson ABM, Flint APF, Turnbull AC. Mechanism of action of glucocorticoids in the induction of ovine parturition; effect on placental steroid metabolism. J Endocrinol 1975;66:61-70.

17. Flint APF, Forsling ML, Mitchell MD, Turnbull AC. Temporal relationship between changes in oxytocin and prostaglandin F levels in response to vaginal stimulation in the pregnant and puerperal ewe. J Reprod Fertil 1975;43:551-4.

18. Keirse MJNC, Hicks BR, Turnbull AC. The fetal membranes as a possible source of amniotic fluid prostaglandins. Br J Obstet Gynaecol 1976;83:146-51.

19. Rush RW, Keirse MJNC, Howat P, Baum JD, Anderson ABM, Turnbull AC. Contribution of preterm delivery to perinatal mortality. Br Med J 1976;2:965-6.

20. Mitchell MD, Flint APF, Bibby J, Brant J, Arnold JM, Anderson ABM, Turnbull AC. Rapid increases in plasma prostaglandin concentrations after vaginal examination and amniotomy. Br Med J 1977;2:1183-5.

21. Yudkin P, Frumar AM, Anderson ABM, Turnbull AC. A retrospective study of induction of labour. Br J Obstet Gynaecol 1979;86:257-65.

22. Ellwood DA, Mitchell MD, Anderson ABM, Turnbull AC. Specific changes in the in vitro production of prostanoids by the ovine cervix at parturition. Prostaglandins 1980;19:479-88.

23. Ellwood DA, Mitchell MD, Anderson ABM, Turnbull AC. In vitro production of prostanoids by the human cervix during pregnancy: preliminary observations. Br J Obstet Gynaecol 1980;87:210-4.

24. Sellers SM, Mitchell MD, Bibby JG, Anderson ABM, Turnbull AC. A comparison of prostaglandin levels in term and preterm labour. Br J Obstet Gynaecol 1981;88:362-6.

25. Sellers SM, Mitchell MD, Anderson ABM, Turnbull AC. The relationship between the release of prostaglandins at amniotomy and the subsequent onset of labour. Br J Obstet Gynaecol 1981;88:1211-6.

26. Sellers SM, Hodgson HT, Mitchell MD, Anderson ABM, Turnbull AC. Raised prostaglandin levels in the third stage of labour. Am J Obstet Gynecol 1982;144:209-12.

27. Castle BM, Turnbull AC. The presence or absence of fetal breathing movements predicts the outcome of preterm labour. Lancet 1983;II:471-3.

28. Brenecke SP, Castle BM, Demers LM, Turbull AC. Maternal plasma prostaglandin E_2 metabolite levels. Br J Obstet Gynaecol 1985;92:345-9.

29. Lopez Bernal A, Hansell DJ, Alexander S, Turnbull AC. Steroid conversation and prostaglandin production by chorionic and decidual cells in relation to term and preterm labour. Br J Obstet Gynaecol 1987;94:1052-8.

30. Lopez Bernal A, Hansell DJ, Canete Soler R, Keeling JW, Turnbull AC. Prostaglandins, chorioamnionitis and preterm labour. Br J Obstet Gynaecol 1987;94:1156-8.

31. Turnbull AC. The early diagnosis of impending premature labour. Eur J Obstet Gynecol and Reprod Biol 1989;33:11-24.

21

Control of Parturition: Scientific and Clinical Aspects

Andrew A. Calder

Department of Obstetrics and Gynaecology, University of Edinburgh,
Centre for Reproductive Biology, Edinburgh, Scotland

Myometrial contractility represents the essence of parturition. In the presence of concerted and established uterine contractility, the pregnancy cannot be sustained; in its absence, parturition cannot take place. Thus, it is entirely apt that investigators whose subject is parturition have focused on the nature and control of myometrial contractility. While this remains a subject of endless fascination that will continue to preoccupy investigators for many years to come, we must not lose sight of the central purpose of uterine contractility, which is to bring about expulsion of the uterine contents via the birth canal.

Parturition varies widely in its complexity from species to species. In the human, the maternal bony pelvis presents an obstacle course through which the fetus must pass with little room to spare, by engaging in a series of contortions in the form of rotations, flexions, and extensions of the fetal head as it descends and passes through the maternal pelvis. These maneuvers, which medical students and midwives must learn as the *mechanisms of labor,* add to the complexity of an already complex process, and in some clinical instances, abnormalities in the shape and size of these bony passages or in the shape, size, or situation of their passenger may lead to greatly increased difficulty.

These mechanical aspects of parturition might be considered to concern the "hard tissues" of the birth canal and fetus. Of greater interest to the physiologist, however, are the soft tissues of the birth canal, notably the uterine cervix. Every working obstetrician knows that labors differ from the agonizingly protracted to the ridiculously straightforward. Easy labors are much less the result of unusually efficient myometrial contractility than of an enhanced facility of the soft tissues of the birth canal to yield. Nulliparous women have longer and more difficult labors than their multiparous sisters, less because their uterus has not learned the art of contractility, but rather because their cervix has learned to dilate more readily.

Until comparatively recently the uterine cervix was seen as fulfilling a passive role in the process of parturition, simply being stretched open in response to the muscular activity of the uterine corpus. It has become increasingly clear, however, that the cervix engages in active and dramatic changes without which parturition would be infinitely more difficult, if not impossible. The central theme of this presentation is the importance of recognizing the intimate relationship between corpus and cervix and of the need for those separate components of the uterus to act in concert during both pregnancy and parturition. The maintenance of pregnancy requires myometrial quiescence and cervical rigidity. The accomplishment of delivery requires myometrial contractility and cervical compliance. Parturition therefore requires not only the activation of the myometrium, but also complex and integrated change within the tissue of the cervix that will facilitate dilatation. Both corpus and cervix, therefore, are required to undergo a dramatic role reversal between pregnancy and parturition, and for optimal performance, each must do so in harmony with the other. However dramatic these changes might be, it is important to recognize that the transition from the state of pregnancy maintenance to the process of expulsion does not occur rapidly, but rather gradually through that part of late pregnancy which is best described as "prelabor."

PRELABOR

The descriptive term *prelabor* has been employed for at least 60 years to highlight that phase lasting 5 or 6 weeks preceding the onset of clinical labor, when important physiological changes take place in both corpus and cervix. It is during this prelude to parturition that the myometrium demonstrates the build-up in spontaneous contractility that culminates in established labor. It is more than 100 years since John Braxton Hicks of Guy's Hospital, London, described the phenomenon of uterine contractions occurring before labor (1) and more than 30 years since

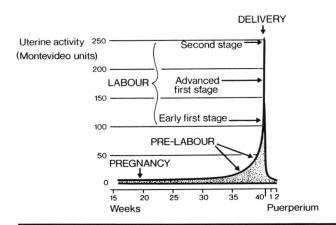

Fig. 1. The pattern of development of uterine contractility during pregnancy, prelabor, and delivery (after Caldeyro-Barcia and colleagues; see reference 2).

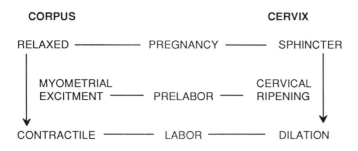

Fig. 2. The relationship between corpus and cervix during the transition from pregnancy to labor.

Roberto Caldeyro-Barcia and his colleagues (2) demonstrated the gradual increase in both the frequency and intensity of myometrial contractions during the last 5 or 6 weeks of pregnancy (see Fig. 1).

Equally important, however, are the changes taking place in the cervix that are embraced by the term *cervical ripening*. The long, closed, and relatively rigid structure of midpregnancy changes in both shape and consistency to become softer, shorter, and already beginning to dilate, even before the onset of labor. This shape change has been documented by Anderson and Turnbull (3) and by Hendricks et al. (4).

The critical importance of prelabor lies in the fact that it is characterized by those two fundamental changes—myometrial sensitization and cervical ripening—and that normal physiology demands that they should take place in concert, in a clearly synchronized fashion (Fig 2).

CERVICAL RIPENING

Although the cervix and corpus both belong to the same organ, the uterus, they differ so considerably in structure and composition as almost to deserve separate organ status. Whereas the corpus is predominantly composed of smooth muscle, the muscle content of the cervix is much less abundant. The predominant element in the cervix is collagen, fibrils of which are bound together into dense bundles that confer on the tissue the rigidity that characterizes its nonpregnant state. The collagen is embedded in a ground substance of large-molecular-weight proteoglycan complexes that consist of a core protein to which are attached glycosaminoglycan branches (GAGs). These are long chains of highly negatively charged repeating disaccharides containing one hexosamine (glucosamine or galactosamine) and one uronic acid (glucuronic or iduronic). The cervix contains a variety of GAGs, such as heparin and heparan sulfate and chondroitin and dermatan sulfate, the latter being the most abundant GAG in the cervix of women. The relationship between the ground substance and the collagen appears to be important in orientating the collagen fibers and determining the mechanical strength of the tissue. The binding affinity of GAGs to collagen increases with greater chain length and charge density. GAGs that contain iduronic as opposed to glucuronic acid, such as dermatan sulfate, bind strongly and promote tissue stability (5), while hyaluronic acid binds least strongly and acts to destabilize the collagen fibrils.

Cervical ripening appears to be associated with a qualitative change in the GAG content of the ground substance with a move to replace those with a strong binding affinity to collagen by those with a lower affinity and also with more hydrophilic properties so that the water content of the tissue increases. The net effect of these changes is to bring about a scattering of the collagen fibrils and thereby reduction in the tensile strength of the tissue.

Cervical ripening is, however, also associated with a reduced collagen concentration. This can be seen when collagen concentration is measured biochemically (6, 7), but is more obvious when the tissue is studied histologically, which may reflect the fact that a lower proportion of the collagen in the ripened cervix exists as intact fibers 8.

In addition to the influence on collagen binding of changes in the ground substance, there is probably also an activation of lytic enzymes, including collagenase and leukocyte elastase. The involvement of leukocytes, which may be seen to infiltrate cervical tissue during the ripening process, highlights the similarities between cervical ripening and tissue inflammation.

The tissue changes of cervical ripening are subject to endocrine control, which bears many similarities to the control of myometrial contractility. Thus, it appears that many of the endocrine and paracrine substances that have been highlighted in this volume are also intimately concerned in the control of cervical function. This seems hardly surprising in view of the need for myometrial and cervical function to be coordinated.

The influence of the placental steroids on the cervix appears to mirror their influence on the myometrium. Thus, progesterone would appear to favor maintenance of the pregnancy by inhibiting collagenase activity and the synthesis of prostaglandins, notably prostaglandin E_2 within cervical tissue. Estrogens appear to have the opposite effect in that they promote cervical softening and perhaps stimulate prostaglandin activity within the tissue. The prostaglandins themselves appear to exert a crucial regulating function within the tissue. Prostaglandin E_2 is known to be activated during cervical ripening and has been employed with great effect in clinical practice to ripen the unripe cervix. The one substance that does not appear to obey the rules and that seems to have contradictory roles in relation to uterine contractility and cervical ripening is relaxin, which has long been supposed to inhibit uterine contractility while favoring cervical softening.

BIOLOGICAL CONTROL OF PARTURITION

We may therefore view parturition as the antithesis of pregnancy, the latter being containment of the fetus, the former expulsion. The myometrium in the uterine corpus moves from a state of quiescence to one of powerful contractility, while the connective tissue of the cervix moves from a state of rigidity to one of distensibility.

It is now widely accepted that the control of these changes is generated from within the uterus itself rather than by maternal systemic mechanisms. The evidence for this comes from many sources, but among the most dramatic and significant observations are the reports of the outcome in the wholly exceptional circumstance in which twins are conceived in adjacent uteri, which results from failure of fusion of the mullerian ducts. This most unusual biological occurrence has been reported twice in the literature (9, 10), and in both instances the parturition of each twin was clearly separated by a significant time interval.

The control of parturition resides within the fetus, placenta, and membranes. Much of the evidence for this is detailed and discussed elsewhere in this book. Suffice it here to suggest that there are probably two separate routes whereby fetal, endocrine, and other changes bring to bear their influence on the myometrium and the cervix—namely, a bloodborne system via the umbilical cord to the placenta and a second route principally influencing the fetal membranes as a result of the fetus modifying the composition of its amniotic fluid. The result is activation of the myometrial cell and modification of the cervical collagen. Where the latter is concerned, changes may be brought about within the cervical stroma as a result of alterations in the level of circulating hormones, and it is clearly recognized as a result of the work of Ellwood et al. (11, 12) that prostaglandins, notably PGE_2 are synthesized and released within the cervical stroma during the processes of cervical ripening and parturition. The purpose of prostaglandins derived from the amnion, however, is less clearly established, although the demonstration by Nakla et al. (13) that amniotic derived PGE_2 can cross the fetal membranes escaping the metabolic activity of the chorion increases the likelihood that PGE_2 from this source has an important biological role.

It may be worth emphasizing that the first area of cervical tissue that would come under the influence of such prostaglandin is the part closest to the internal cervical os. This is the portion of cervical tissue most in need of softening to allow effacement of the cervix to proceed, and one might postulate that in the process of cervical effacement that area of tissue is softened prior to being "taken up" toward the corpus, thereby exposing the next area of tissue to the influence of prostaglandins of amniotic origin. This region of internal cervical os and adjacent fetal membranes might therefore be seen to represent the critical focus in terms of parturition to which highly specific biological changes must be directed. Support for such a view comes from the clinical observations that infection in that area of critical focus may well be responsible for preterm delivery and also from experience with attempts at induction of labor. If the "forewaters" are ruptured by amniotomy in an attempt to induce labor when the cervix remains unripe, the outcome of induction is generally unsatisfactory (14). This may be because the ability of the fetal membranes to transmit prostaglandin E_2 to the adjacent cervical tissue has been removed. In contrast, if in such cases prostaglandin E_2 is delivered to that very point by means of an extra-amniotic catheter, cervical ripening may be accelerated and an altogether more successful outcome attained (15).

CLINICAL CONTROL OF PARTURITION

The clinical imperative for control of parturition stems from the need to prevent preterm delivery in some cases and to induce labor in others. In attempting to meet these needs safely and reliably, many different techniques and pharmacological agents have been explored. Most have borne little resemblance to physiological control mechanisms, but not surprisingly, the most successful techniques have been those with a sound physiological basis.

Inhibition and Suppression of Preterm Labor

The delivery of the fetus while yet immature now represents the biggest single problem in modern obstetrics. The cost in terms of perinatal death and long-term handicap is colossal, and consequently a more perfect understanding of the mechanisms responsible and better therapeutic intervention must be energetically pursued. Betamimetic therapy, while theoretically appropriate, has in practice proved extremely disappointing. Although prostaglandin inhibitors carry theoretical risks of adverse effects on the fetal ductus arteriosus (16), the benefits of such therapy may yet be seen to outweigh these dangers, especially when applied prior to 30 weeks' gestation. More work is required to clarify this contentious issue.

Induction and Acceleration of Labor

Obstetric history shows a bizarre catalog of techniques directed toward interruption of pregnancy. In medieval times, various exotic concoctions were prescribed, but most of these had little or no effect. In more recent times, the emphasis moved toward mechanical interference in the form of balloons and bougies inserted through the cervix, and it is now recognized that such benefit as these interventions brought was probably the result of stimulation of the release of prostaglandins within the tissues. Amniotomy was introduced by Thomas Denman of the Middlesex Hospital around 1760, and became known as the "English method" of labor induction. Amniotomy has stood the test of time and, despite serious attendant hazards, remains the cornerstone of labor induction today.

In an effort to provoke cervical ripening, agents such as estradiol (17) and relaxin (18) have been employed with apparent success, but these have never become established in clinical practice. Likewise, oxytocin, which in the past was often given in the form of prolonged intravenous infusion, has been shown to be of little value for this purpose (19). The preeminent agent for cervical ripening is prostaglandin E_2, and this is best given by local routes of administration, either vaginally or pericervically. Prostaglandin $F_{2\alpha}$ may also be effective, but is generally considered to be less satisfactory.

Likewise, as an agent for labor induction, prostaglandin $F_{2\alpha}$ is the poor relation of prostaglandin E_2. It loses out heavily on grounds of potency, specificity, and toxicity, and its use can only be supported if PGE_2 is not available. For this reason, it will not be considered futher here and the remainder of this discourse will center on the use of PGE_2. Local routes of administration hold the key to success. The delivery of prostaglandins locally within the genital tract has greatly enhanced their value. Extra-amniotic administration of PGE_2 in a gel or solution is the most effective method of cervical ripening requiring very low doses and consequently minimizing side effects (20). Some might consider it unacceptably invasive and consequently hazardous. Theoretically, infection may be introduced, although in practice this has not been a significant complication and although hemorrhage may be provoked and inadvertent rupture of the membranes may occur, these have proved to be extremely rare in practice. The vaginal route (21) has the beauty of simplicity, although much of the prostaglandin may be absorbed systemically, so larger doses are required. The compromise between those two routes lies in the endocervical technique (22), which is less invasive and consequently potentially less hazardous than the extra-amniotic route and may allow more specific delivery of the active agent to the target tissue. The dose required is also much smaller than that required with vaginal therapy. This technique is, however, only appropriate for cervical ripening. If the cervix is already effaced and partially dilated, there is no endocervical target to attack. Using gels, the fate of therapy placed in the endocervical canal is by no means certain, so that the possibility of the prostaglandins ending in the vagina or the extra-amniotic space cannot be ruled out. Much interest has therefore surrounded the search for suitable vehicles for prostaglandin delivery, and a variety of pessaries and gels have been developed for this purpose with varying release and absorption profiles. The objectives must be maximum efficiency, economy of dosage, minimal side effects, and greatest possible safety margins. To this, we may now add the view of the consumer, namely, the expectant mother. In modern obstetrics, no method, however effective and safe, will be widely acceptable if mothers find it highly disagreeable.

A RATIONAL APPROACH TO PHARMACOLOGICAL CONTROL OF LABOR

Modern obstetrics offers three principal methods in induction or augmentation of labor: (*a*) prostaglandins, especially PGE_2, which is best administered by local routes within the genital tract (oral or intravenous administration may have a limited place); (*b*) amniotomy, and (*c*) oxytocin, namely, the synthetic oxytocin "syntocinon," which is administered by intravenous infusion, with the dose rate being titrated against the myometrial response. These three weapons should be employed either separately or in combination. The modern art of labor induction and augmentation depends on a rational approach whereby these different interventions are tailored to the individual clinical situation. The essence of success lies first in establishing the distance the individual has already traveled along the course of pregnancy, prelabor, and parturition.

Let us consider two diametrically opposite clinical situations. Mother A left to her own devices will be in established labor of spontaneous onset tomorrow. Mother B left alone will still not be in labor 3 weeks hence. Both are at term, and both have indications for delivery by induction of labor, but because of the vastly different proximity of spontaneous labor their responses to intervention are likely to be very different. The closer the individual mother has reached to the spontaneous onset of labor, the easier and more successful will labor induction be. Conversely, the more distant the prospect of spontaneous labor, the more complicated and unsatisfactory is intervention likely to be. How can we distinguish between these mothers? The best guide is obtained by pelvic assessment and calculation of the Bishop score (23), especially if she is a primigravida. A high score presages the spontaneous onset of labor in the near future. A low score indicates that this is a much more distant prospect. Mother B (who will almost certainly show a low Bishop score) will respond poorly if induction is attempted by amniotomy and intravenous oxytocin titration. The response will be disappointing, with a high probability of prolonged labor, fetal distress, cesarean section, and birth asphyxia (24). In contrast, mother A, on the threshold of spontaneous labor, may require nothing more than amniotomy for a successful and satisfactory outcome.

Of central importance is the correct timing of amniotomy. If we consider the developing arc of prelabor, latent labor, active labor, and delivery (Fig. 3), amniotomy may be carried out at any point in that spectrum. It will certainly be more difficult if the cervix is unripe, but it can be accomplished. This, however, is misguided clinical practice. Amniotomy should not be performed until the cervix is ripe. To do so is to increase dramatically the risk of fetal and maternal complications. Ideally, the cervix should be fully effaced and beginning to dilate and the fetal presenting part should not be high. These conditions are even more favorable if the uterus has already begun to show contractility. Thus, if these conditions do not prevail, local administration of prostaglandin E_2 should be performed to bring them about. Even if the cervix is ripe, it may still be appropriate to initiate labor with a single application of vaginal PGE_2 (for example 1-mg PGE_2 in gel) and then to add in the influence of amniotomy once contractions are becoming established. Such a policy was found to be highly effective by Kennedy et al. (25). This study compared the obstetric outcome of two groups, each of 50 mothers with a ripe cervix, who required induction of labor. These mothers were randomly allocated to a group receiving a single vaginal tablet of PGE_2 (3 mg) whose membranes were ruptured 3–6 h later at the point when uterine contractility was becoming established, or to a group in whom amniotomy was performed at the outset and followed immediately by intravenous infusion of syntocinon.

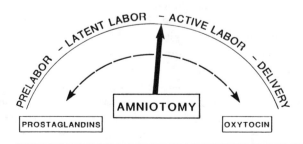

Fig. 3. Schematic representation to show the optimal application of prostaglandins, oxytocin, and amniotomy in the control of human labor.

The obstetric results in terms of length of labor, mode of delivery, and neonatal condition were very similar in the two groups, but the former method (local prostaglandins) proved superior in respect of a lower incidence of postpartum hemorrhage and of neonatal jaundice. The clearest area of advantage, however, was seen in respect of the mothers' assessment of the techniques, as shown in Table 1. The clear statement of maternal preference for the prostaglandin technique is one of the most compelling arguments in favor of this approach.

What then is the place of oxytocin in current obstetrics? It remains a potent and useful drug, but it is of little or no value prior to amniotomy. The increased activity of endogenous prostaglandins that amniotomy induces (26) seems essential to sensitize the myometrium to oxytocin, and therefore, oxytocin should not be used before amniotomy has been performed.

We have, therefore, three weapons at our disposal: amniotomy, oxytocin, and prostaglandins. The secret of successful labor induction or augmentation of nonprogressive labor lies in using each to its maximum potential, as illustrated in Figure 3 and summarized below.

Prostaglandins, especially PGE_2, are highly effective for ripening the cervix and inducing labor. If the cervix is already ripe, a small dose of PGE_2 may be all that is required to initiate labor that resembles spontaneous labor as closely as possible.

Amniotomy is of central importance. Although it is possible for an infant "in the caul" of intact membranes, it is the general rule for the membranes to rupture or be ruptured during labor. Such rupture is associated with heightened activity of endogenous prostaglandins. The timing of amniotomy is crucial. Performed too early, before the cervix is ripe, the influence of the membranes in the process of cervical ripening is lost, and this may lead to increased complications. In contrast, if we delay it too long, we may lose the advantage of its uterine sensitizing influence. The optimal timing for amniotomy therefore lies at the transition between latent labor and active labor.

Oxytocin is a potent myometrial stimulant if the uterus is primed to respond to it by prostaglandins, either endogenous or exogenous. It must be given intravenously, and many mothers find this disagreeable. In most instances of labor induction, a proper combination of prostaglandin therapy and amniotomy may allow the use of oxytocin to be avoided, but it remains the therapy of final resort to carry labor through to delivery if this is required.

Table 1. Mother's assessment of labor induction techniques.

Mother's Response	Amniotomy, Plus Oxytocin	Vaginal PGE_2 Tablet
Favorable	8	43
Noncommittal	16	7
Unfavorable	26	0
Total	50	50

CONCLUSIONS

Clinical intervention in pregnancy, as in any other aspect of medicine, is by nature an interference with normal physiology. In most instances, however, the motivation behind such intervention will be the pathological departure of the individual pregnancy from normal biological controls. Hitherto, attempts to suppress parturition or to induce it have been far from physiological in their nature. However, as knowledge increases, it may become increasingly possible to apply therapeutic interventions that come closest to reproducing or restoring normal physiology. In the interests of optimal clinical outcome for every pregnancy, this is an objective devoutly to be pursued.

REFERENCES

1. Braxton Hicks J. On the contractions of the uterus throughout pregnancy: their physiological effects and their value in the diagnosis of pregnancy. Obstet Soc 1872;13:216-27.
2. Caldeyro-Barcia R. Uterine contractility in obstetrics. Proc 2nd Int Cong Gynecol Obstet, vol 1. Montreal, 1959:65-78.
3. Anderson ABM, Turnbull AC. Relationship between length of gestation and cervical dilatation uterine contractility and other factors during pregnancy. Am J Obstet Gynecol 1969;105:1207-14.
4. Hendricks CH, Bremner WR, Kraus G. Normal cervical dilatation pattern in late pregnancy and labor. Am J Obstet Gynecol 1970;106:1065.
5. Obrink B. A study of the interactions between monomeric tropocollagen and glycosaminoglycans. Eur J Biochem 1973:387-400.
6. Kleissl HP, van der Rest M, Naftolin F, Glorieux FH, de Leon A. Collagen changes in the human cervix at parturition. Am J Obstet Gynecol 1978;130:748-53.
7. Granstrom L, Ekman G, Ulmsten U, Malmstrom A. Changes in the connective tissue of corpus and cervix uteri during ripening and labour in term pregnancy. Br J Obstet Gynaecol 1989;96:1198-202.
8. Junqueira LCU, Zugaib M, Montes GS, Toledo DMS, Kirsztian RM, Shigihara KM. Morphologic and histochemical evidence for the occurrence of collagenolysis and for the role of neutrophilic polymorphnuclear leukocytes during cervical dilatation. Am J Obstet Gynecol 1980;138:273-81.
9. Williams B, Cummings G. An unusual case of twins: case report. J Obstet Gynaecol Br Emp 1953;319-21.
10. Mingeot RA, Keirse MJ. Twin pregnancy in a pseudodidelphys. Am J Obstet Gynecol 1971;111:1121-2
11. Ellwood DA, Anderson ABM, Mitchell MD, Turnbull AC. A significant increase in the in-vitro production of prostaglandin E_2 by ovine cervical tissues at term. J Endocrinol 1979;81;133P-4.
12. Ellwood DA, Mitchell MD, Anderson ABM, Turnbull AC. The in-vitro production of prostanoids by the human cervix during pregnancy: preliminary observations. Br J Obstet Gynaecol 1980;87:210-4.
13. Nakla S, Skinner K, Mitchell BF, Challis JRG. Changes in prostaglandin transfer across human fetal membranes obtained after spontaneous labor. Am J Obstet Gynecol, 1986;155:1337-41.

14. Calder AA. Management of the unripe cervix. In: Keirse MJNC, Anderson ABM, Bennebrock Gravenhorst J, eds. Human parturition. The Hague: Leiden University Press, 1979:201-17.

15. Calder AA, Embrey MP, Tait T. Ripening of the cervix with extra-amniotic prostaglandin E_2 in viscous gel before induction of labour. Br J Obstet Gynaecol 1977;84:264.

16. Moise KJ, Huhta JC, Sharif DS, Ou C-N, Kirshon B, Wasserstrum N, Cano L. Indomethacin in the treatment of premature labor: effects on the fetal ductus arteriosus. N Eng J Med 1988;319(6):327-31.

17. Gordon AJ, Calder AA. Oestradiol applied locally to ripen the unfavourable cervix. Lancet 1977;II:1319.

18. MacLennan AH, Green RC, Bryant-Greenwood GD, Greenwood FC, Seamark RF. Ripening of the human cervix and induction of labour with purified porcine relaxin. Lancet 1980;I:220.

19. Forman A, Ulmsten U, Banyai J, Wingerup L, Uldbjerg N. Evidence for a local effect of intracervical prostaglandin E_2-gel. Am J Obstet Gynecol 1982;143:756.

20. Calder AA. The human cervix in pregnancy—a clinical perspective. The cervix in pregnancy and labour. Edinburgh: Churchill Livingstone, 1981:103.

21. MacKenzie IZ, Embrey MP. Cervical ripening with intravaginal PGE_2 gel. Br Med J 1977;2:1381.

22. Ulmsten U, Kirstein-Pedersen A, Stenberg P, Wingerup L. A new gel for intracervical application of prostaglandin E_2. Acta Obstet Gynaecol Scand 1979;84(suppl):19.

23. Bishop EH. Pelvic scoring for elective induction. Obstet Gynecol 1964;24:266.

24. Calder AA. Methods of induction of labour. In: Studd J, ed. Progress in obstetrics and gynaecology, vol 3. Edinburgh: Churchill Livingstone,1983:86-100.

25. Kennedy JH, Stewart P, Barlow DH, Hillan E, Calder AA. Induction of labour: a comparison of a single prostaglandin E_2 vaginal tablet with amniotomy and intravenous oxytocin. Br J Obstet Gynaecol 1982;89:704-7.

26. Keirse MJNC. Endogenous prostaglandins in human parturition. In: Keirse MJNC, Anderson ABM, Bennebroek Grovenhorse J, eds. Human parturition. The Hague: Leiden University Press, 1979:101-41.

22

Analysis of Uterine Contractility

Martti Pulkkinen

*Department of Obstetrics and Gynecology, University of Turku,
Turku, Finland*

C linical findings about uterine contractility usually derive from measurements of intrauterine pressure (IUP) made with a fluid-filled, open-ended catheter during labor, after rupture of membranes, or with an abdominal pressure sensor. The basis of contractility studies is physiological parameters like membrane potential, contraction threshold in the electrical field, contractile force of an excised piece of uterine smooth muscle, and generation and propagation of electrical activity in situ.

When comparing the environments in which in situ examination of the female reproductive duct (i.e., the upper part [oviduct] and the lower part [uterus]), must be made, it is the uterine physiologist who has the most direct approach to the organs under study. The human oviduct is only 0.2–2 mm in diameter, but the uterus, usually no more than a slit with no real cavity, widens during pregnancy to form a hydrodynamically sound basis for pressure studies. Surface electrical potentials, measured at several locations along the oviduct, give the best overall picture of its function (1). The electrical potential that precedes the mechanical activity reflects its force, and excitation-contraction coupling usually functions without disturbance (2). The intestinal tract is a good subject for transport studies generally, and the findings are often applicable also to the uterus (3). In this chapter, we shall look at the clinical data base and the events that should be analyzed in connection with uterine contractility.

THE NATURE OF CONTRACTILITY
Electrical Activity

Propagation of Activity.   To express direction of propagation unambiguously, the terms *procervical* and *profundal* are useful and would parallel the terms *prouterine* and *pro-ovarian* used for ovum transport. These terms are also valuable because they express direction without reference to position (compare with "upward" and "downward") (4), and they are not associated with gastroenterology (compare with "peristaltic" and "antiperistaltic") (5), urology ("antegrade" and "retrograde") (6), or infectious diseases ("ascending" and "descending") (7), all of which are used in literature to describe direction of propagation.

For the analysis of velocity of propagation (cm or mm/sec), the concept "velocity vector" is valuable, because in an oval organ with considerable wall thickness the assumption that activity is propagated linearly seldom holds good. When observations of either direct electrical or mechanical activity are made simultaneously at two or more places in the uterus, what is usually measured is in fact a vector of the real velocity of propagation (8). Single smooth-muscle cells are covered by collagen types I and V, but cell bundles are covered by collagen type III and fibronectin, perhaps forming insulating layers that direct the velocity vector (9).

Synchronic/Asynchronic Activity. Synchronic activity is seen electrophysiologically as a propagation front reaching the billions of cells in the uterus in a short time and synchronizing their function. It is characteristic of synchronic activity that the contraction cycle is symmetrical in form (Fig. 1). There is rapid rise in pressure, high amplitude, but low cycle frequency.

Train Discharge and Spike Activity. Several spikes following each other with high frequency, a train discharge, are associated with high force of labor (5, 8). Sine-form activity (or plateau-type action potentials) in the smooth muscle of both the intestinal tract (3) and the oviduct (1) is connected with nonpropulsion.

Conduction Distance. Conduction distance is best determined clinically by ultrasound (Fig. 2). At the time of sampling of chorionic villi (pregnancy weeks 9–14), an artificial "fibroid" is often observed (i.e., a local uterine contracture, bulging into the cavity, even at the placental site). In a series of 1581 patients, the incidence of such a contracture was 38.3 percent, its average diameter at 16–20 weeks being 27.7 mm with the radius naturally corresponding to the conduction distance (10). When, later in pregnancy, the radius lengthens and the event becomes phasic, through the mechanisms described by Garfield (see Chapter 3), the full evolution of uterine activity leads either to abortion or delivery.

Mechanical Activity

Contraction and Contracture. It is important to distinguish between contraction, a physiological pressure cycle, and contracture, an unphysiological state of sustained contraction. The endocrine background for phasic contraction during pregnancy is the cessation of progesterone action (Fig. 3) and the effects of this on conduction: junctional resistance and gap junctions. The cellular events are different in the phasic (contraction) and tonic (contracture) states (2).

Response, Reaction, Sensitivity. The dose-response curves for a given agent (e.g., oxytocin) show the responsiveness as maximum response (hyperresponsive) and reactivity (hyperreactivity) as the slope of the curve (11). The term *sensitivity* should be used only to describe the possible shift in a dose-response curve or –log ED.

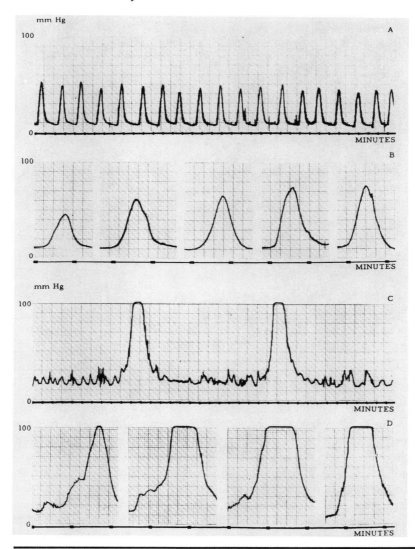

Fig. 1. In the symmetric pressure cycles at term (*A*) only active pressure and rate of rise increase as clinical labor progresses (*B*). Another patient, also at term, has a completely different pattern (*C*), which shows low active pressure and high-frequency activity of irregular shape. High-amplitude pressure cycles are infrequent, and there is "climbing" rise in pressure (Braxton-Hicks contractions). As labor progresses, the climbing character disappears (*D*). (From Csapo A, Sauvage J, The evolution of uterine activity during human pregnancy, Acta Obstet Gynecol Scand 1969;47:193, with permission of The Scandinavian Society.)

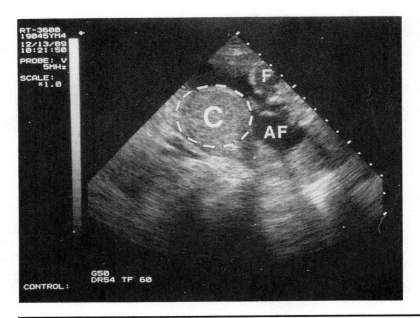

Fig. 2.   A local contracture (C), 25 mm in diameter, bulges into the amniotic fluid (AF) close to the fetus (F). Maintenance of pregnancy clearly depends on propagation block. (Courtesy O. Piiroinen, M.D.)

Pressure Cycle.   IUP includes the following: active pressure (AP), or amplitude of cycle; resting pressure (RP), a better term than *tonus* and already employed by classic smooth-muscle physiologists (12); active pressure area (APA = area above RP) or total APA (TAPA = area above zero mmHg); time of rise in pressure (T_r), describing propagation of activity; frequency (F) of pressure cycles, calculated in periods of between 10 and 30 min; symmetry in shape. A synchronic, well-propagating contraction is a symmetric pressure cycle that varies only in height. The climbing character of IUP, known as Braxton-Hicks contractions, disappears when clinical labor begins (see Fig. 1).

Deviation from symmetry, most variable during the relaxation period, reflects difficulties of propagation (uncoordination). During the menstrual cycle, uterine activity undergoes well-known changes: At day 16, low AP, high F, low AP/T_r, and irregular rise in pressure reflect a local, nonpropagating asynchronic activity; at day 2, high AP, low F, and high AP/T_r indicate a propagating synchronic activity. The oxytocin-induced change occurs in the ascending phase of the pressure cycle, expressed as an increase in AP/T_r (12, 13).

Measuring the Force

The force of the uterus in both menstruation and labor is basically the wall tension (wT), but the inactive and elastic uterine area controls IUP. Amniotic pressure

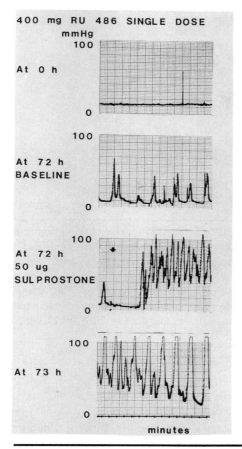

Fig. 3. Physiological uterine activity (increased active pressure, low frequency, and no change in low resting pressure) induced within 72 h by antiprogesterone (400-mg mifepristone). After low-dose prostaglandin, this became unphysiological (high resting pressure, high frequency) for a short time. Thereafter, effective physiological activity caused abortion. (From Pulkkinen MO, Piiroinen O, Vainikka J, A study of the effect of mifepristone (antiprogesterone) followed by prostaglandin on uterine activity and fetal heart rate in patients having a termination of pregnancy, Arch Gynecol Obstet 1989;244:78, with permission of Springer-Verlag, Berlin.)

results from muscle activity and elasticity. A uterine pressure of 70–80 mmHg can be achieved by as little as 10–4 cm shortening of the uterine circumference, provided there is no elasticity. Uterine pressure increases linearly in time at a rate determined by the ratio of the active/inactive portion (14).

According to Pascal, pressure P = force F/area A. In the closed spheroid uterus, P = (2w/R)T, where w = wall thickness and R = radius. In practice this

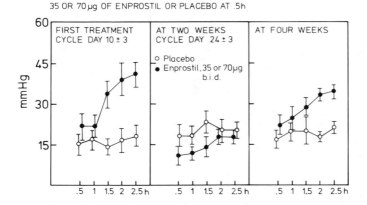

Fig. 4. Oral dose of enprostil (PGE$_2$-derivate) increases the resting pressure for many hours during day 1of treatment. After 2 weeks of daily intake of the drug, the uterus is more relaxed than after placebo treatment and does not react significantly to prostaglandin; 4 weeks later in the early cycle, response to enprostil is attenuated. (From Pulkkinen MO, Acute and chronic effects of oral enprostil, a synthetic dehydroprostaglandin E$_2$ on uterine contractility. In: Prostaglandins, leukotriens, and essential fatty acids, 1989;36:17, with permission of Churchill Livingstone Publishers.)

means that a small, nonpregnant uterus generates, with the same T, much higher IUP than a large, pregnant uterus. The nonpregnant uterus can generate pressures as high as 300 mmHg, but the term uterus, less than 100 mmHg. The increase in elasticity limits RP, except when the muscle is excessively stretched, as in polyhydramnions (15).

The importance of uterine elasticity for the contractility measured is demonstrated by patients receiving oral PGE-derivate over a long period of time. At first, oral intake of enprostil increases RP for many hours. After daily intake of the drug for 2 weeks, there is a marked change in the character of IUP. RP is lower than with placebo treatment (late cycle), and oral intake of prostaglandin does not change it. After 4 weeks, there is still a response, but it is attenuated (Fig. 4). This is more readily explained by an increase in uterine wall elasticity through the effect of prostaglandin on the collagens that mediate the force than by changes in smooth-muscle function (16).

CLINICAL ANALYSES

Data for clinical analysis are based on either electrical or mechanical activity. The electrophysiological signals are mediated either by intrauterine electrodes (8) or through abdominal surface potentials, ASPs (17). IUP signals are at present observed through open-ended catheters or through microtransducers at the tip of the catheter.

Electrical Activity

Electromyogram. In an electromyogram (EMG), the electrical activity picked up by extracellular electrodes is analyzed after appropriate amplification. By obtaining the EMG with a bipolar electrode and by combining the EMG data with IUP data (open-ended catheter), Wolfs and van Leeuwen have described normal human labor in detail (8). The gradual synchronization of uterine activity is reflected in the increasing regularity of pressure wave form, amplitude, and dp/dt. Low-voltage, irregular EMG comes gradually in a series of bursts, while the amplitude increases. The bursts are subsequently restricted to the rising phase of the pressure cycle. Even a low dose of oxytocin may bring about this change, but if it does not, the change cannot be induced by an increased dose. If forced, the mechanical activity is unphysiological (high F, high RP), like the electrical activity (continuous, high-frequency, low-voltage EMG). The force of the contraction is dependent on refractory time, reflecting the "negative staircase" of the parturient uterus (8).

Abdominal Surface Potentials. Many attempts to catch skin potentials have been impaired either by low signal-to-noise ratios or short recording times. Computer-processed abdominal surface potentials (ASP), graphically and two-dimensionally displayed as topograms, may prove to be of clinical value in assessing the progress of labor (17). These data give support to the theory of Caldeyro-Barcia that uterine activity in the active phase of labor starts often, but not always, from the high fundal lateral areas and progresses procervically. The front of relaxation moves in the opposite direction to the contraction (Fig. 5).

Mechanical Activity

Fluid-Filled Catheters. The open-ended catheter measures IUP until the fluid batch is absorbed or the catheter is blocked by debris. Easy to use and low in price, such catheters have been widely employed clinically, but for research purposes the information they give is not sufficiently precise. The time lag between pressure change and measured change is 80 msec (18). The frequency response under optimal conditions is sufficient for recording IUP.

In the nonpregnant uterus, which has no real cavity, but only a slit, a microballoon tip, a sponge tip, or just an open-ended catheter records the resultant of all contractile activity from those parts of the uterine wall surrounding the tip. In the pregnant uterus, following the laws of hydrodynamics, IUP (isometric contraction) can only be measured reliably before rupture of membranes (4, 12). IUP measured after membrane rupture will vary according to the degree of pressure "leakage." At the postpartum stage, pressure recording makes sense for a short period only, when the internal os of the cervix is accidentally blocked by a clot. The microballoon technique, widely used earlier (4, 7, 12), gives reliable results, but requires special skill and is laborious.

Microtransducer Catheters. The sensor is a silicon semiconducting unbonded strain gauge with the sensor surface on the side of the catheter tip. The reaction

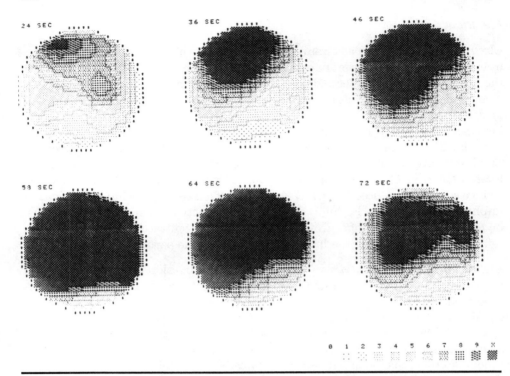

Fig. 5. Abdominal surface potentials: a topogram of synchronous uterine activity pattern during active clinical labor. Note that the pacemaker area is fundal/lateral and relaxation is opposite to contraction. (From Takagi K et al., A topographic investigation of the site of the origin and subsequent propagation of uterine contractions in spontaneous labor and their clinical significance, Asia-Oceania J Obstet Gynecol 1986;12:377, with permission of the University of Tokyo Press.)

time is <1 msec. In the test chamber, both fluid-filled and microtransducer catheters give identical pressure recordings (12, 18). Microtransducer catheters are easy to use but uneconomical in an obstetric ward.

IUP recorded with a microtransducer at the tip of the catheter depends on the form and position of the catheter (Fig. 6). If not "baked" to fit the axis of the uterine cavity, artificial RPs of 100 mmHg and more can be recorded. Measured RP depends on the discrepancy between the flexion of the uterus and the flexion of the catheter. In practice, it is usually possible to obviate artificial change in RP (or AP) through skillful introduction of the device. IUP is higher if recorded fundally than if recorded at a lower level (Table 1). Depending on whether the sensor is dorsal, ventral, or lateral, the AP may change (18). In a dysmenorrheic patient, the pressure-velocity can be as high as 120 mmHg/sec (19). When recording IUP with the fixed microballoon technique, again in a dysmenorrheic patient, the "high" rate

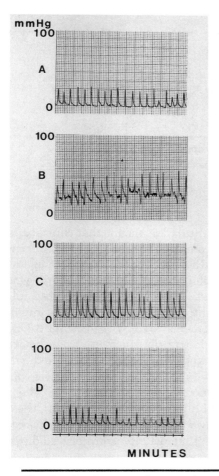

Fig. 6. A microtransducer catheter (Millar) gives the same intrauterine pressure at the beginning (A) and at the end (D) of this experiment, the position of the pressure sensor being ventral/fundal. When the position of the sensor is dorsal/fundal, there is an artificial rise in resting pressure (B), and when lateral/fundal, resting pressure is normal, but active pressure (C) is slightly higher.

of rise in pressure decreased from 12 to the normal 6 mmHg/sec when an antiprostaglandin was administered (20); in other words, there was a 10-fold difference in the pressure-velocity recorded with different techniques. It is important to note that the resultant force measured by the fluid-filled catheter derives from a larger area of the uterine wall than that measured by the microtransducer.

Direction of Propagation

The clinical practice of measuring IUP at a single location fails to reveal the direction of the activity and thus the direction of the transport itself (menstrual

Table 1. Uterine activity at two locations.

	Fundal		Middle-Low	
	E	D	E	D
Active pressure	41	99	10	52
Resting pressure (mmHg average)	16	51	15	23

Note: Pressure microsensors were 30 mm apart.

E = eumenorrheic patients, and D = dysmenorrheic patients.

For E, n = 5; for D, n = 10.

blood, fertilized egg, "passenger" fetus, placenta). This means that clinical analyses of uterine contractility are descriptively incomplete, in spite of all the information obtained through IUP or EMG. When all the activity in the oviduct propagates, and transports the ovum in the uterine direction, it is designated 1.0, but when all activity is pro-ovarian, it is designated 0.0 (1). In uterine physiology this would be a good way of describing the transport of the intrauterine passenger. The importance of a mathematical model for transport is demonstrated by the theoretical calculation that pro-uterine activity only (1.0) would transfer the ovum from the ovary to the uterus in 1 min instead of 3 days. If we apply the same principle to the uterus, the probability that the menstrual blood will move procervically on cycle day 1 is approximately 0.6, a familiar figure in oviduct physiology (Table 2) (1). The propagation of uterine activity at ovulation could affect, among other things, the site of implantation. During pregnancy, when delivery is approaching, a change occurs in the direction of propagation (5, 8, 17). In ewes, all activity is procervical during the late postpartum period (P = 1.0) (5).

Contractility in the Nonpregnant State

Analysis of uterine contractility in the nonpregnant state has provided precise information about physiological changes during the menstrual cycle (12). In the late luteal phase, nonpropagating, asynchronic, high-frequency activity becomes

Table 2. Direction of propagation in 15 patients at cycle day 1.

	Number of observations
Procervical	33
Profundal	18
Uncoordinated	10

Note: IUP was at two locations 30 mm apart; probability of procervical transfer of menstrual blood = 0.65 (33 of 51).

propagating, synchronic, low-frequency activity during bleeding. In dysmenorrhea, a disease with high endometrial and menstrual blood prostaglandins associated with a high progesterone level at the time of onset of bleeding, high RP decreases the blood flow and causes anoxic pain. Relief of pain after administration of antiprostaglandins is associated with decrease of RP, F, and rate of rise in pressure, but not AP. Antiprostaglandins do not affect conduction velocity, even when pressure-velocity is decreased by low AP (20).

Uterine contractility has been analyzed in connection with several diseases, but the procedure has not gained acceptance in gynecological practice (21).

Contractility During Human Pregnancy

Early Pregnancy. Analyses of uterine activity induced by luteectomy (22) or antiprogesterones (23) have given content to the term *physiological uterine activity*. Physiological activity includes high AP, low F, low RP, high rate of rise in pressure, as well as the symmetrical shape of the pressure cycle, all of which indicate good propagation and synchrony (see Figs. 1 and 3). If the same process is induced by prostaglandins, a totally different picture emerges: initially low AP, high F, and high RP, lasting for several hours if a long-acting derivate is used. During the physiological evolution of the activity, the fetus is usually living and the mother without pain, but after administration of prostaglandins the fetus dies and the mother is in pain (23). When progesterone action is at first blocked by an antiprogesterone, the prostaglandin-created unphysiological response is of short duration and the uterus is hyperresponsive and hyperreactive. The end result of blocking progesterone action and increasing prostaglandin action (Csapo's see-saw [7]) is a perfect physiological activity that very quickly leads to clinical abortion (see Fig. 3). To achieve the same result simply by withdrawal of progesterone, it is necessary to reach a very low serum progesterone level (4 ng/ml) before there is full evolution of IUP and the oxytocin response (OR) (22). With antiprogesterones, a progesterone action is achieved that corresponds to a serum progesterone level of 4–10 ng/ml, this estimate being based on a comparison of IUP findings in luteectomy and antiprogesterone studies.

Term Pregnancy. The classic descriptions by Caldeyro-Barcia (24), Reynolds (25), and Csapo (4) of the gradual evolution of IUP and OR as pregnancy progresses do not call for comment. Clinicians have to face two main problems: induction of labor and progress of labor. Analyses of uterine activity are important for determination of fetal well-being. It is particularly important in practice to determine the relationship between the pressure cycle and fetal heart rate.

Induction of Labor: In a series of 821 patients, the 50-mU single-shot oxytocin test, combined with analyses of baseline IUP, was the best way of predicting the success of an induction, mirrored in the cervix (26). It is possible to make some prediction about the duration of induced labor through APA and F.

The clinical value of measuring IUP during labor has been much discussed (27, 28). Monitoring IUP to determine the appropriate oxytocin regimen for induction of labor has reduced the frequency of neonatal jaundice and blood exchange. This is not due to the reduction of the total dose of oxytocin, but to better control of IUP (26).

   Progress of Labor: This field of obstetrics has suffered as a result of the poor correlation and overlapping of IUP-values obtained at the stages of no clinical labor, early labor, normal labor, and dysfunctional labor ever since the time of the basic studies by the pioneers (4, 24, 25, 29, 30). Computerized processing of data on-line in digital print-out, as torrs/min (UAU-units), utilizing either voltage-controlled oscillator systems (31) or uterine activity integrals (UAIs), as kilo Pascal seconds (32), has resulted in some progress, but in obstetric practice no general agreement has been reached and IUP analyses have not been widely accepted (27, 28). Probably the lack of information about direction of propagation has led to confusion in this field. The Montevideo and Alexandria units describe uterine activity superficially, and greater precision is required in order to describe properly the physiological progress of labor. The form of the pressure cycle (Fig. 1) and the direction of the force generated should be included in analyses of contractility, before full clinical benefit is to be gained. Although dysfunctional labor is one of the commonest conditions dealt with in obstetrics, its diagnosis is still based on cervical dilatation curves and not on measured uterine dysfunction, which has already been well described in Reynolds' textbook on uterine physiology (25).

   Uterine Activity and Fetal CTG: When uterine pressure (UP) signals are sampled at the 1-Hz rate in connection with CTG, the patterns recognized are RP and the pressure cycle. Four basic methods have been developed for identifying a contraction: (*a*) fixed absolute RP threshold, (*b*) smoothed and differentiated UP signal, using the first, second, or third derivate, (*c*) UP signal smoothed by an exponential function with a given time constant using 10 sec average fast part and 100 sec average slow part of contraction, and (*d*) relation of threshold to RP, calculated as the mode or modified mode of frequency distribution over a given epoch. The duration of a contraction is calculated by simple subtraction. Frequency is expressed either as the interval between contractions (seconds) or as the number of contractions within a certain period. Manual measurement of area is time consuming, but the algorithm for a computer program is simple. Converting the electrical voltage of the UP signal into pulses gives the same result as the algorithm (31). When equal, the maximal slopes of the contraction and relaxation indicate the symmetry of the contraction. For references in this area, see Stigsby (33).

CONCLUSION

Analysis of uterine contractility in clinical research should include several parameters. The force of labor, or wall tension, cannot at present be measured directly. Only indirect methods are possible. Intrauterine pressure measurements should be performed, if possible, in a closed system. By electrophysiological means, using advanced technology, it should be easier to determine the direction of the forces of transporation, expressed as the mathematical probability of propulsion. If the mechanical and electrophysiological data, properly observed and analyzed, were computerized, this could solve a number of clinical problems. It could determine, for instance, the likelihood of abortion or premature labor, distinguish false from true labor, and make the correct on-line diagnosis of dysfunctional labor. After more than 100 years of work in this area, we are still reaping imperfect clinical benefits (34, 45). Theorists of initiation/onset of labor, which is really a will o' the wisp, should pay careful attention to analyses of uterine contractility, which show that physiological contractility can only occur when, after unbalancing of the pregnancy-maintaining and labor-inducing factors, the propagation of activity allows it to proceed.

REFERENCES

1. Pulkkinen MO, Talo A. Tubal physiologic consideration in ectopic pregnancy. Clin Obstet Gynecol 1987;30:164-72.
2. Garfield RE, Blennerhassett MG, Miller SM. Control of myometrial contractility: role and regulation of gap junctions. Oxf Rev Reprod Biol 1988;10:436-90.
3. Karaus M, Wienbeck M. Motor patterns in the colon. In: Kumar D, Gustavsson S, eds. Gastrointestinal motility. Chichester: John Wiley & Sons.
4. Csapo A, Sauvage J. The evolution of uterine activity during human labor. Acta Obstet Gynecol Scand 1968;47:181-212.
5. Naaktgeboren C, Pool C, Weijden GC, Taverne MAM, Schoof AG, Kroon CH. Electrophysiological investigations on uterine motility in ewes during pregnancy and birth. Z Tierzuchtg Zuchtungsbiol 1975;92:220-43.
6. Ulmsten U. Uterine activity and blood flow in normal and dysmenorrheic women. In: Dawood MY, McGuire JL, Demers LM, eds. Premenstrual syndrome and dysmenorrhea. Baltimore: Urban & Schwarzenberg, 1985:103-24.
7. Csapo A. Force of labor. In: Iffy L, Kaminetzky HA, eds. Principles and practice of obstetrics and perinatology. New York: Wiley Medical, 1981:761-99.
8. Wolfs GMJA, Leeuwen M. Electromyographic observations on the human uterus during labor. Acta Obstet Gynecol Scand 1979;90(suppl):1-61.
9. Pulkkinen MO, Lehto M, Jalkanen M, Näntö-Salonen K. Collagen types and fibronectin in the uterine muscle of normal and hypertensive pregnant patients. Am J Obstet Gynecol 1984;149:711-7.
10. Saari-Kemppainen A, Karjalainen O, Ylöstalo P. A randomized study of ultrasound screening during pregnancy [Abstract]. XII World Congress Gynecology and Obstetrics. Rio de Janeiro, 1988.
11. Garfield RE, Beier S. Increased myometrial responsiveness to oxytocin during term and preterm labor. Am J Obstet Gynecol 1989;161:454-61.
12. Csapo A. The diagnostic significance of the intrauterine pressure. Obstet Gynecol Survey 1970;25:403-35, 515-43.
13. Seitchik J, Chatkoff ML. Oxytocin-induced uterine hypercontractility wave forms. Obstet Gynecol 1976;48:436-41.
14. Coren RL, Csapo AI. The intra-amniotic pressure. Am J Obstet Gynecol 1963;85:470-83.
15. Wood C. Myometrial contractility in pregnancy and labor. In: Kellar RJ, ed. Modern trends in obstetrics. Glasgow: Butterworths, 1969:56-109.
16. Pulkkinen MO. Acute and chronic effects of oral enprostil, a synthetic dehydro-

prostaglandin E_2, on uterine contractility. In: Prostaglandins, leukotriens, and essential fatty acids, 1989;36:15-9.

17. Takagi K, Matsuura M, Sakata H, Takagi S. A topographic investigation on the site of origin and subsequent propagation of uterine contractions in spontaneous labor and their clinical significance. Asia-Oceania J Obstet Gynecol 1986;12:371-83.

18. Åkerlund M, Bengtson LPh, Ulmsten U. Recording of myometrial activity in the non-pregnant human uterus by a microtransducer catheter. Acta Obstet Gynecol Scand 1978;57:429-33.

19. Smith RP. Pressure-velocity analyses of uterine muscle during spontaneous dysmenorrheic contractions in vivo. Am J Obstet Gynecol 1989;160:1400-5.

20. Pulkkinen MO. The pathophysiology of primary dysmenorrhea. Acta Obstet Gynecol Scand 1983;113(suppl):63-7.

21. Bengtson LPh. Hormonal effect on human myometrial activity. Vitamine and Hormones 1973;31:257-303.

22. Csapo A, Pulkkinen M. Indispensability of the human corpus luteum in the maintenance of early pregnancy luteectomy evidence. Obstet Gynecol Survey 1978;33:69-81.

23. Pulkkinen MO, Piiroinen O, Vainikka J. A study of the effect of mifepristone (antiprogesterone) followed by prostaglandin on uterine activity and fetal heart rate in patients having a termination of pregnancy. Arch Gynecol Obstet 1989;244:75-8.

24. Caldeyro-Barcia R, Poseiro JJ. Physiology of the uterine contraction. Clin Obstet Gynecol 1960;3:386-408.

25. Reynolds SRM. Physiology of the uterus. New York: Hoeber, 1949.

26. Enkola K, Pulkkinen MO. Induction of human labor at term: uterine activity, inducibility, duration and neonatal jaundice. Acta Physiol Hungarica 1985;65:281-8.

27. Gordon AJ. Measurement of uterine activity—a useful clinical tool? Br J Obstet Gynaecol 1984;91:209-10.

28. Rodriguez MH, Masahi DI, Phelan JP, Diaz GD. Uterine rupture: are intrauterine pressure catheters useful in the diagnosis? Am J Obstet Gynecol 1989;161:666-9.

29. Csapo A. The theoretic, diagnostic and prognostic value of the intrauterine pressure. Bibl Gynaecol 1966;42:93-124.

30. Csapo A. Extraovular pressure—its diagnostic value. Am J Obstet Gynecol 1964;90:493-504.

31. Hon EH, Paul RH. Quantitation of uterine activity. Obstet Gynecol 1973;42:368-70.

32. Steer PJ, Beard RW. Normal levels of active contraction area in spontaneous labour. Br J Obstet Gynaecol 1984;91:211-9.

33. Stigsby B, Nielsen PV, Doeller M. Computer description and evaluation of cardiotocograms. Eur J Obstet Gynecol Reprod Biol 1986;21:61-86.

34. Schatz F. Beitrage zur physiologischen Geburtskunde. Arch Gynaek 1872;3:58-144.

35. Heinricius G. En metod att grafiskt atergiva kontraktiones hor en icke gravid livmoder. Finsk Lakaresallsk Handl 1889;31:349-53.

23

Clinical Management of Dysmenorrhea and Labor

Robert H. Hayashi

The University of Michigan Medical Center, Ann Arbor

$\boxed{C}$ urrent etiologic, diagnostic, and therapeutic principles and theories regarding the clinical entities of dysmenorrhea and dystocia are presented in this chapter. These two clinical entities have uterine contractility as their basic pathophysiologic abnormality. *Dysmenorrhea* (difficult monthly flow), sometimes referred to as painful menstruation, has an excessive amount of uterine contractility. *Dystocia* (difficult labor) is associated with inefficient or not enough uterine contractility. From a therapeutic standpoint, dysmenorrhea would require an ablation of uterine contractility, and dystocia, an enhancement of uterine contractility.

DYSMENORRHEA

It has been estimated that over 50% of women have dysmenorrhea and that in about 10%, the severity of the discomfort renders an individual incapacitated 1–3 days each month. It is certainly one of the more frequent reasons for a gynecologic office visit and accounts for significant absenteeism of the work/school force.

Dysmenorrhea is classified as primary or secondary. *Primary dysmenorrhea* is the occurrence of painful cramps during menstruation in the absence of macroscopically identifiable pelvic pathology. *Secondary dysmenorrhea* is the occurrence of painful cramps or pelvic pain during menstruation in the presence of macroscopically identifiable pelvic pathology such as endometriosis, adenomyosis, chronic pelvic inflammatory disease, leiomyomata, pelvic adhesions, intrauterine polyps, or an intrauterine device (1).

Primary dysmenorrhea only occurs with ovulatory cycles and usually appears within 6–12 months after menarche (1). The discomfort begins several hours before or just after the onset of the menses. The discomfort is most severe and may be incapacitating on the first or second day of menstruation. In over half of the patients with dysmenorrhea, systemic symptoms occur including nausea and vomiting, fatigue, diarrhea, low backache, and headache. Primary dysmenorrhea is a symptom complex of young women. If the onset of the symptoms of dysmenorrhea begin more than 2 years after menarche, one should be suspicious of secondary dysmenorrhea.

Although the exact etiology of primary dysmenorrhea is not known, it has been attributed to several factors, including behavioral and psychological ones, uterine ischemia, increased vasopressin release, and increased uterine prostaglandin production and release. Psychological factors have not been demonstrated convincingly to play a primary role in dysmenorrhea, but may certainly modulate symptoms or should be evaluated in patients who have not responded to medical therapy. Preliminary studies have suggested that there may be increased circulating vasopressin levels in women with primary dysmenorrhea during menstruation (2). Exogenously infused vasopressin has also been shown to induce symptoms in women on the first day of menstruation (3). In 1965 Pickles et al. first reported increased concentrations of prostaglandin $F_{2\alpha}$ in menstrual fluid and the endometrium of dysmenorrheic women (4). Since then, many studies have found increased production of both prostaglandin E_2 and $F_{2\alpha}$ by the endometrium of women with primary dysmenorrhea, and this production appears to peak during the first 48 h of menstrual flow. These studies have been detailed and cited in an excellent review by Dawood (1).

Of the increased uterine contractility seen in primary dysmenorrhea, no single, consistent abnormality has been observed; however, the following four abnormalities in various combinations have been shown to occur in most dysmenorrheic women: increase in resting tonus, active intrauterine pressure, frequency of contractions, and incoordinate or dysrhythmic uterine activity (5). Objective evaluation of uterine activity can be accomplished by use of a balloon-tipped catheter attached to a micropressure transducer. Interpretation of the data from assessment of uterine activity has taken various forms, but all have demonstrated increased uterine activity in primary dysmenorrhea and have been useful in demonstrating therapeutic effects of drugs. The Scandinavian investigators have used "total pressure area" under the curve as an end point (6). Schulman et al. utilized the following calculations to establish a concept of a contractility index; the total time of active pressure divided by the total time of resting pressure per 10-min period (7). Smith, utilizing a microprocessor distribution analysis system, digitized analog data with an X-Y digitizer to develop a 2-dimensional plot of uterine pressure versus frequency and a 3-dimensional plot of the above plus time (8). Using an intrauterine thermistor probe to reflect local uterine blood flow, Akerlund et al. demonstrated that when uterine activity is abnormal and increased, uterine blood flow decreases (9). This observation has suggested a theory that the excessive uterine activity of dysmenorrhea results in uterine ischemia, which is responsible for the pain and discomfort of this entity.

For successful therapy of primary dysmenorrhea, the clinician should have ruled out all of the usual conditions associated with secondary dysmenorrhea mentioned earlier. Psychological support for the patient is also an important component of therapy. The basic principle of therapy for primary dysmenorrhea is to decrease the excessive uterine contractility associated with the onset of menstruation. Since primary dysmenorrhea occurs only in ovulatory cycles, one therapeutic approach is to use combination-type oral contraceptives to cause anovulation. If the patient desires birth control, this is the agent of choice. It is the main method of therapy since its introduction with a therapeutic efficacy for primary dysmenorrhea of 90% or over (1). Anovulatory cycles are associated with a significant decrease of prostaglandin production at menstruation (10). The secretory phase of the cycle is necessary for the increased production of prostaglandins at menstruation. Decreased uterine contractility associated with pain relief in dysmenorrheic women treated with oral contraceptives has been documented (6). In another study, Ekstrom et al. measured uterine contractility in dysmenorrheic and nondysmenorrheic subjects before and after therapy with oral contraceptives (11). They also administered two agonists, prostaglandin $F_{2\alpha}$ and vasopressin, before and after therapy, to attempt to elicit the same symptoms of dysmenorrhea in response to elicited uterine contractility. They found that fewer symptoms were elicited by the two agonists after oral contraceptive therapy with the same relative uterine contractility elicited before therapy. This suggested other possible mechanisms of the therapeutic effect of oral contraceptive besides a reduced uterine reactivity to the agonists.

In patients with primary dysmenorrhea who do not require contraception, inhibitors of prostaglandin synthetase are very effective (60%–90%) (1). Also, these drugs are taken only during the period of symptomatology—that is, the first few days of the menstrual period. Of the five classes of prostaglandin synthetase inhibitors, three of the classes—indole-acetic acid derivates, fenemates, and arylproprionic acids—have been shown to have efficacy in primary dysmenorrhea, whereas two—benzoic acid derivatives and buterophenones—have not (1). Suppression of endometrial production of prostaglandins resulting in significant reduction of uterine contractility with accompanying relief of the symptoms of primary dysmenorrhea has been shown with naproxin (12), mefenamic acid (13), indomethacin (14), and ibuprofen (15). Another class of tocolytic drugs, the β-sympathomimetic drugs have also been shown to be efficacious in the treatment of primary dysmenorrhea. Isoxsuprine (16), salbutamol (17), and terbutaline (9) have been more effective than placebo, but because of a higher incidence of side effects, they have been relegated to a second line of therapeutics for primary dysmenorrhea. Because of their effect on uterine contractility, calcium channel blockers have also been evaluated to treat primary dysmenorrhea. Nifedipine has been shown to provide rapid relief of symptoms in primary dysmenorrhea, but with bothersome side effects of facial flushing or headache (18). Forman et al. demonstrated that nifedipine has additive uterine relaxant effects after initial treatment of primary dysmenorrhea with prostaglandin synthetase inhibitor (19). The therapeutic advantages of calcium channel blockers are yet to be elucidated, and their use is only after other doses of drugs have failed. For patients on combination oral contraceptives and still symptomatic, the addition of prostaglandin synthetase inhibitor has been successful (1).

In summary, primary dysmenorrhea is a symptom complex of unknown etiology associated with ovulatory cycles. Excessive uterine activity beginning several hours before the menstrual flow and lasting up to 48 h is associated with this symptom complex. Excessive prostaglandin production by the endometrium and increased uterine response to vasopressin have been documented. Principal modes of therapy include inducing anovulation with combination oral contraceptives and use of prostaglandin synthetase inhibitors singly or in combination depending on the patient's needs and response. Other therapeutic approaches include the use of tocolytic drugs such as β-sympathomimetics and calcium channel blockers.

LABOR

In order for labor to be successful, the physiologic alterations must occur to change the cervix from a firm sphincter consisting of interwoven bundles of collagen fibrils to a ripe, soft, easily dilated structure that will allow passage of the products of conception. Studies utilizing cervical biopsies in pregnant women obtained in early and late pregnancy have demonstrated progressive decrease of collagen content, increasing collagenolytic and elastase activity, and a parallel increase of polymorphonuclear leukocytic infiltration of the cervical tissues as pregnancy approached term (20). This study tied the infiltration of leukocytes to the enzyme degradation of the collagen organization of the cervical tissue in the process of cervical ripening. Another more recent study provides evidence of a close correlation between the biochemical composition of the cervix and the clinical course of delivery in terms of cervical dilatation (21). It also demonstrated the role of prostaglandin E_2 in the process of cervical ripeness. Cervical biopsy specimens were obtained from three groups of patients: 10 women with a favorable cervix and spontaneous labor, group A; 12 women with an unfavorable cervix, given prostaglandin E_2 intracervically and induced labor, group B; and 5 women with an unripe cervix and spontaneous labor, group C. The total amount of collagen and nonextractable collagen content were significantly higher in group C. The collagenolytic activity was most elevated in group B. The results of this study support the concept that collagen is an important regulator of the cervical function in late pregnancy and term labor and that prostaglandin E_2 mimics the spontaneous cervical-ripening process.

The other element necessary for successful labor is coordinated uterine contractility. The physiologic process by which this comes about is discussed elsewhere in this book.

Labor is defined in its broadest sense as the succession of painful uterine contractions resulting in progressive changes in the cervix and the eventual expulsion of the uterine contents. When this progression of changes slows or ceases, the labor process is abnormal and is called *dystocia*. The clinical management of dystocia requires definitions of normal limits of the progressive changes. These progressive changes are cervical dilatation and descent of the presenting part. Once labor begins, the clinician can monitor the progress of labor by vaginal digital examination to estimate these changes over time. In order to make the diagnosis of dystocia, the clinician will need to know the normal limits of labor progress.

Friedman and coworkers have popularized a simple concept of graphic analysis by plotting estimated measurements of cervical dilatation and station of the presenting part versus time in hours (23). They submitted data for computer analysis from a large number of patients whose cervical dilatation and station of the presenting part were followed closely in labor in a number of hospitals and derived mean rates of cervical change and descent of the presenting part for nulligravids and multiparous patients. Patients whose rate of progress fell below these limits were liable to have a surgical or instrumental delivery. Their labors were considered abnormal.

Classically, labor is divided into four phases. The first is the latent phase, when the uterine activity causes very subtle changes of the cervix. Usually the cervix reaches a dilation of 3 cm over 21 h in a nulligravida and 4 cm over 14 h in a multipara. At these respective cervical dilatations, the rate of dilation increases to over 1 cm/h in response to increasing uterine contractility (24). The active phase or first stage of labor begins when the cervix is dilating progressively from the latent phase to full dilatation. The mean rate of cervical dilation of the first stage of labor according to Friedman is 1.2/h in the nulligravida and 1.5/h in the multipara (24). It is in the late part of the first stage of labor (about 7 cm dilation) that the fetal presenting part begins to progressively descend.

Dystocia in the first stage of labor can be depicted as follows: Slow-slope active phase is when the rate of cervical dilatation is less than normal. Arrest of cervical dilation is when the cervix fails to change over a 2-h period after the patient has entered the active phase of labor. Descent disorders are usually manifest in the second stage of labor. Failure of descent by the time of full cervical dilation is almost always due to absolute cephalopelvic disproportion and contraindicates the use of oxytocin augmentation. Protracted descent can be diagnosed when descent is proceeding at <1 cm/h in nulliparous labor and at <2 cm/h in the multiparous labor. This is difficult to diagnose due to fetal head molding. A useful adjunct to assess descent is by abdominal palpation of fetal head remaining above the symphysis pubis. Arrest of descent is diagnosed when descent is stopped for >1 h in the nullipara and >30 min in the multipara.

Clinical management of dystocia in the first stage of labor should include evaluation of the four "P's": pelvis, passenger, position, and power. A most important cause of dystocia is cephalopelvic disproportion (CPD). Clinical pelvimetry is done on all patients who are in labor to assess the pelvic architectural type as described by Caldwell and Molloy to determine adequacy for a vaginal delivery. X-ray pelvimetry has not been used for many years not only due to the theoretical risks to the fetus of gamma radiation, but moreover to the fact that the information provided by pelvic measurements is not completely predictive of CPD because the fetal head may mold to fit through relatively small pelvic dimensions. Recently, Morgan and Thurnau developed a fetal-pelvic index (FPI) that compared ultrasound measurements of the fetal head and abdominal circumferences to X-ray measurement of the pelvic inlet and midpelvic planes. Initial studies of FPI claim 85% sensitivity and 92% specificity in predicting difficult midpelvic deliveries or shoulder dystocia (26). This approach deserves further clinical trial. A practical maneuver to assess the potential for the unengaged fetal head to enter the pelvic inlet is the Muller-Hillis maneuver. The fetal brow and suboccipital region of the head are grasped through the maternal abdomen and downward pressure is applied in the axis of the pelvic inlet at the height of a uterine contraction (25). Gentle fundal pressure is also applied at this time while another person evaluates the descent of the head vaginally. When the cervix is 5-cm dilated, this maneuver can also be done (fundal pressure) to determine descent, flexion, and rotation of the presenting part.

Clinical estimation of fetal weight by palpation is important in evaluating the "passenger" and making a decision regarding prophylactic cesarean delivery to prevent shoulder dystocia or CPD. Studies evaluating the accuracy of clinical estimation of fetal weight have consistently reported a tendency to estimate toward the mean birthweight, meaning that the small babies are overestimated and the large babies are underestimated. Many investigators have published different techniques and formulations of mensuration for sonographically estimating fetal weight; however, because of technical limitations of ultrasound in clinical practice, a 10%-15% error of estimated fetal weight may be inevitable. Recently Watson et al. demonstrated in a prospective study of 100 patients where clinical estimation of fetal weight was as accurate as ultrasound (about 8% error) even at both extremes of weight (27).

Determining the position of the fetal head in relation to the maternal pelvis may help to understand a delay in the progress of labor. An occiput posterior sometimes results in a prolonged deceleration phase of late active phase of labor as the occiput slowly rotates to an anterior position. The deflexed fetal head may not negotiate the pelvic canal since large fetal head dimensions are presented to the pelvic canal compared to a well-flexed fetal head.

Evaluation of the "powers" or uterine contractility by the clinician is discussed in another chapter, but is a cornerstone in the management of dystocia. If uterine contractility is found to be insufficient to keep the progress of labor within normal limits, then an ecbolic agent should be used. Dilute oxytocin infusion is the method of choice and is also discussed elsewhere in this volume.

Management of a prolonged latent phase of labor includes either uterotonic stimulation or heavy maternal sedation. Oxytocin induction is effective 85% of the time, but an equal proportion of patients will respond likewise to therapeutic rest and not have to be exposed to the potential risks of oxytocin. The advantage of sedation is rest and respite from painful uterine contractions for the mother. About 10% will not respond to sedation and may require oxytocin.

Management of the active phase after evaluation of the "P's" will usually involve the use of oxytocin to augment labor. Other issues of management that are controversial at present include the issue of the role of artificial rupture of membranes in the management of labor. The suggestion that artificial rupture of membranes is often effective in ameliorating arrest disorders has not been verified by objective data (28). However, the timing of the rupture of membranes may have some influence as to its enhancement of labor. The later in labor, the better are its benefit whereas early amniotomy apparently has little benefit (29). Another controversy in labor management is the role that epidural anesthesia may play in the etiology of dystocia. Friedman observed a significant prolongation of both the deceleration phase and the second stage following epidural anesthesia (24). In a recent, large retrospective study in Israel using a historic control group, Niv et al. found that despite an increased use of labor epidural anesthesia of over 50% compared with 0.17% in the control group, and with no significant change in obstetric practice at one hospital over the study period, the rate of instrumental delivery was unchanged (30). With careful attention to dosage and the application of a segmental block to minimize effect on the muscular tone of the pelvic diaphragm, labor epidural appears to have minimal cause for dystocia.

Maternal upright posture may provide benefit. The hormones of pregnancy, especially relaxin, loosen the pelvic joint ligaments such that the interspinous diameter of the midpelvis may widen by as much as 1.5 cm when a woman moves from a supine to squatting position (31). The upright position will also maximize the effect of gravity in dilating the cervix and vagina. Also, the axis of the fetus and the birth canal are aligned. Despite these theoretical advantages, the fact that no study has controlled for confounding variables, there exists a persistent uncertainty concerning the influence of maternal posture on labor progress.

Management of the second-stage abnormalities deal primarily with descent disorders. Use of oxytocin in protracted descent is generally not of benefit unless a demonstrable cause of decreased uterine contractility has been demonstrated. Arrest of descent, on the other hand, often responds to oxytocin. The adage that "tincture of time" can be used in the management of the second stage is reasonable provided that fetal well-being is being closely monitored. Molding of the fetal head to the birth canal takes time as does internal rotation of an occiput posterior or transverse position to anterior position. Maternal exhaustion or inappropriate expulsive efforts may also prolong the second stage. Pelvic operative delivery is an appropriate approach, provided the clinician has thorough knowledge of the instrument use, position of fetal head, knowledge of the pelvic architecture, and experience or experienced help. The issue of the use of midforceps is controversial and outside the scope of this chapter. Suffice it to say that this author is confident that thoughtful use of this modality is proper in carefully selected situations.

In summary, the clinical management of dysmenorrhea and dystocia for the most part requires good medical skills to make a proper diagnosis so that use of appropriate medication to diminish excessive uterine contractility in primary dysmenorrhea or enhance uterine contractility in active-phase dystocia will be therapeutic. Dystocia, however, requires a clear understanding of confounding variables and many mitigating factors for proper complete management.

REFERENCES

1. Dawood MY. Dysmenorrhea. J Reprod Med 1985;30:154-67.
2. Akerlund M, Stromberg P, Forsling ML. Primary dysmenorrhea and vasopressin. Br J Obstet Gynaecol 1979;86:484-7
3. Akerlund M, Stromberg P, Forsling ML, et al. Inhibition of vasopressin effects on the

uterus by a synthetic analogue. Obstet Gynecol 1983:62:309-12.

4. Pickles VR, Hall WJ, Best FA, et al. Prostaglandins in endometrium and menstrual fluid from normal dysmenorrheic subjects. Br J Obstet Gynaecol 1965;72:185.

5. Woodbury RA, Torpin R, Child GP, et al. Myometrial physiology and its relation to pelvic pain. JAMA 1947;134:1081-5.

6. Hauksson A, Ekstrom P, Juchnicka E, et al. The influence of a combined oral contraceptive on uterine activity and reactivity to agonists in primary dysmenorrhea. Acta Obstet Gynecol Scand 1989;68:31-4.

7. Schulman H, Duvivier R, Blattner P. The uterine contractility index: a research and diagnostic tool in dysmenorrhea. Am J Obstet Gynecol 1983;145:1049-58.

8. Smith RP: Distribution analysis of intrauterine pressure in non-pregnant dysmenorrheic women. Am J Obstet Gynecol 1984;149:271-3.

9. Akerlund M, Anderson KE, Ingemarsson J. Effects of terbutaline of myometrial activity, uterine blood flow, and lower abdominal pain in women with primary dysmenorrhea. Br J Obstet Gynaecol 1976;83:673-8.

10. Chan WY, Dawood MY. Prostaglandin levels in menstrual fluid of non-dysmenorrheic and of dysmenorrheic subjects with and without oral contraceptive or ibuprofen therapy. Adv Prostaglandin Thromboxane Res 1980;8:1445-7.

11. Ekstrom P, Juchnicka E, Laudanski T, Ekerlund M. Effect of an oral contraceptive in primary dysmenorrhea-changes in uterine activity and reactivity to agonists. Contraception 1989;40:39-47.

12. Lundstrom V, Green K, Suanborg K. Endogenous prostaglandins in dysmenorrhea and the effect of prostaglandin synthetase inhibitors (PGSI) on uterine contractility. Acta Obstet Gynecol 1979;87:51-6.

13. Smith RP, Powell JR. Intrauterine pressure changes during dysmenorrhea therapy. Am J Obstet Gynecol 1982;143:286-92.

14. Lundstrom V, Green V, Wigvist N. Prostaglandins, indomethacin and dysmenorrhea. Prostaglandins 1976;11:893-907.

15. Dawood MY. Ibuprofen and dysmenorrhea. Am J Med 1984;77:87-94.

16. Nesheim BI, Walloe L. The use of isoxuprine in essential dysmenorrhea: a controlled clinical study. Acta Obstet Gynecol 1976;55:315-6.

17. Lalos O, Joelsson J. Effects of salbutamol on the nonpregnant human uterus in viva: a hysterometric study in dysmenorrheic women. Acta Obstet Gynecol 1981;60:549-52.

18. Sandahl B, Ulmsten U, Andersson KE. The trial of the calcium antagonist nefedipidine in the treatment of primary dysmenorrhea. Arch Gynecol 1979;227:147-51.

19. Forman A, Andersson KE, Ulmsten U. Combined effects of diflunisal and nifedipine on uterine contractility in dysmenorrheic patients. Prostaglandins 1982;23:237-46.

20. Junqueira LCU, Zuqaib M, Montes GS, et al. Morphologic and histochemical evidence for the occurrence of collagenalysis and for the role of neutrophilic polymorphonuclear leukocytes during cervical dilatation. Am J Obstet Gynecol 1980;138:273-81.

21. Ekman G, Malmstrom A, Uldbjerg N, et al. Cervical collagen: an important regulator of cervical function in term labor. Obstet Gynecol 1986;67:633-6.

22. Rajabi MR, Dean DD, Baydoun SN, et al. Elevated tissue levels of collagenase during dilation of uterine cervix in human parturition. Am J Obstet Gynecol 1988;159:971-6.

23. Friedman EA. Graphic analysis of labor. Am J Obstet Gynecol 1954;68:1568-75.

24. Friedman EM. Labor: clinical evaluation and management, 2nd ed. New York:

Appleton-Century-Croft, 1978.

25. Caldwell WE, Moloy HC. Anatomical variations in the female pelvis and their effect in labor with a suggested classification. Am J Obstet Gynecol 1933;26:479-505.

26. Morgan MA, Thurnau GR, Fishburne JI Jr. The fetopelvic index as an indicator of fetal-pelvic disproportion: a preliminary report. Am J Obstet Gynecol 1986;155: 608-13.

27. Watson WJ, Soisson AP, Harlass FE. Estimated weight of the term fetus: accuracy of ultrasound vs clinical examination. J Reprod Med 1988;33:369-71.

28. Friedman EA, Sachtleban MR. Amniotomy and the course of labor. Obstet Gynecol 1963;22:755-70.

29. Seitchik J, Holden A, Castillo M. Amniotomy and the use of oxytocin in labor in nulliparous women. Am J Obstet Gynecol 1985;153:848-54.

30. Niv D, Ber A, Rudick V, Leylein Y, David MP, Geller E. Mode of vaginal delivery and epidural analgesia. Isr J Med Sci 1988;24:80-3.

31. Russell JGB. Moulding of the pelvic outlet. Br J Obstet Gynaecol 1969;76:817-20.

24

The Role of Systemic and Intrauterine Infection in Preterm Parturition

Roberto Romero, Cecilia Avila, Carol Ann Brekus, and Moshe Mazor

Department of Obstetrics and Gynecology, Yale University School of Medicine, New Haven, Connecticut

T he mechanisms responsible for the initiation of human parturition have long been a subject of study for reproductive biologists. In addition to the intrinsic scientific interest of this subject, the understanding of the physio-pathology of human labor has significant clinical relevance. The single most important risk factor for adverse pregnancy outcome is untimely birth (1–3). While prolonged pregnancy increases the risk of intrauterine death, premature birth is the leading cause of perinatal morbidity and mortality worldwide. In addition, premature infants have an increased risk of long-term handicaps such as mental retardation, blindness, and bronchopulmonary dysplasia. The cost to society in terms of acute and chronic medical care and long-term handicaps makes prematurity the most serious complication of pregnancy.

A growing body of evidence suggests that intrauterine infection plays a key role in the pathogenesis of preterm labor and delivery (4–6). This chapter reviews the evidence supporting a role for infection in the onset of preterm labor. The cellular and biochemical mechanisms by which infection may lead to preterm labor and delivery are also discussed.

Three lines of evidence support a role for infection in the onset of labor: (*a*) The administration of bacteria or bacterial products to animals results in either abortion or labor (7–14); (*b*) systemic maternal infections such as pyelonephritis, pneumonia, and typhoid fever are associated with the onset of labor; and (*c*) localized intrauterine infection is associated with preterm labor and delivery (15–28).

Animal Evidence. Those in the field of veterinarian medicine have long recognized the importance of naturally occurring infection in spontaneous abortion. Bang in 1897 described abortions in cattle due to gram-negative microorganisms (7). Experimental evidence has also indicated that the administration of bacteria or bacterial products such as endotoxin induces abortion. In 1944 Zahal and Bjerknes demonstrated that the injection of Shigella and Salmonella endotoxin into mice and rabbits was capable of inducing abortion (8). Takeda and Tsuchiya confirmed this observation using *E. coli* endotoxin in pregnant mice and rabbits (9, 10). Subsequently, several investigators have replicated these findings using different animal species (11–13). The mechanisms of endotoxin-induced abortion appear to be mediated by prostaglandins (PG) as the concentration of PGF increases in serum endometrium and urine after the administration of 10 μg of Salmonella endotoxin to pregnant mice on day 16 (14). Furthermore, pretreatment of the animals with indomethacin reduced the endotoxin-induced abortion rate from 51.2% to 18% (14).

SYSTEMIC MATERNAL INFECTION

Systemic maternal febrile infections such as pneumonia, pyelonephritis, malaria, and typhoid fever have been associated with preterm labor and delivery. The rate of preterm delivery associated with maternal pneumonia ranges from 15% to 48% (15–18). Although the advent of antibiotic treatment has dramatically reduced maternal mortality from this condition, it has not affected the rate of preterm delivery. While pyelonephritis was associated with preterm delivery in the pre-antibiotic era, in the postantibiotic era, this condition is associated with preterm labor but not preterm delivery (19–23). Similarly, typhoid fever in the pre-antibiotic era carried a 60%–80% risk of abortion and preterm labor, but this risk has decreased since the introduction of antibiotic therapy (24–26). Malaria has also been associated with a 50% rate of preterm delivery (27). However, chemoprophylaxis seems to protect patients from preterm delivery (28). Collectively, these data support the concept that severe untreated systemic maternal infection is associated with preterm labor and delivery and that treatment may decrease the rate of preterm delivery in some cases (e.g., pyelonephritis, typhoid fever) but not in others (e.g., pneumonia).

The mechanisms involved in the initiation of labor in the setting of systemic infections have not been studied in the human. However, wide clinical experience indicates that maternal fever is associated with increased uterine activity. This effect has been demonstrated with parenteral administration of endotoxin to women at term. A 2- to 3-fold increase in uterine activity was noted during the chill period (15–60 min), and uterine activity gradually diminished (29). Since parenteral administration of endotoxin to animals and humans results in the production and release of cytokines, which can in turn, stimulate PG production, we have proposed that these products mediate the increase in uterine activity in the setting of febrile maternal infection (30).

INTRAUTERINE INFECTION

Despite the important role of systemic maternal infection in the etiology of preterm labor, these diseases are rare, and therefore, their attributable risk to preterm delivery is low. Recently, the association between intrauterine infection and preterm labor and delivery has become a major focus of investigation.

During pregnancy the amniotic cavity is normally sterile. Microbial invasion of the amniotic cavity can occur after rupture of membranes and even with intact membranes. To accurately assess the microbiologic state of this cavity, the method of amniotic fluid collection is critical. The two methods generally used are transabdominal amniocentesis and transcervical retrieval, either by needle puncturing of the membranes or by aspiration through an intrauterine catheter. Transcervical amniotic fluid collection is associated with an unacceptable risk of contamination with vaginal flora; therefore, when analyzing the prevalence of microbial invasion of the amniotic cavity in term and preterm labor, we will only review studies in which amniotic fluid was obtained by transabdominal amniocentesis.

There is disagreement in the literature regarding the terminology used to describe microbial invasion of the uterine cavity during pregnancy. We have previously employed the term *intra-amniotic infection* to indicate the presence of a positive amniotic fluid culture for microorganisms regardless of the presence or absence of clinical signs or symptoms of infection. The term *clinical chorioamnionitis* refers to the clinical syndrome associated with microbial invasion of the amniotic cavity. Manifestations include maternal fever, uterine tenderness, foul-smelling vaginal discharge, fetal tachycardia, and maternal leukocytosis (31). This clinical syndrome appears in only a small fraction of women with microbial invasion of the amniotic cavity. In a recent study, we found that only 12.5% of women with preterm labor (intact membranes) and a positive amniotic fluid culture had clinical chorioamnionitis (32). The presence and severity of clinical chorioamnionitis is probably related both to microbial factors and to the host response to the infection. Microbial factors include the type and virulence of the microorganism, inoculum size, and pathway of infection (hematogenous versus ascending infection). Host factors include the local and systemic cytokine response to the presence of infection and the systemic effects of these products on the host.

Microorganisms may gain access to the amniotic cavity and fetus using any of the following pathways: (*a*) by ascending from the vagina and the cervix, (*b*) by hematogenous dissemination through the placenta (transplacental infection), (*c*) by retrograde seeding from the peritoneal cavity through the fallopian tubes, and (*d*) by accidental introduction at the time of invasive procedures (e.g., amniocentesis, percutaneous blood sampling, chorionic villous sampling, or shunting) (32–38).

Indirect evidence indicates that the most common pathway of intrauterine infection is the ascending route. This evidence is as follows: (*a*) histologic chorioamnionitis is more common and severe at the site of membrane rupture than in other locations, such as the placental chorionic plate or umbilical cord; (*b*) in cases of congenital pneumonia (stillbirths or neonatal), inflammation of the chorioamniotic membranes is present in the overwhelming majority of cases; (*c*) the bacteria identified in cases of congenital infections are similar to those found in the genital tract; and (*d*) in twin gestation, histologic chorioamnionitis is more common in the first-born twin and has not been demonstrated in only the second twin. As the membranes of the first twin are generally apposed to the cervix, this is taken as evidence in favor of an ascending infection (32–38). This is consistent with our observations from the amniotic fluid microbiology in twin gestations. Indeed, in cases of microbial invasion of the amniotic cavity in twin gestation, the presenting sac was involved. When both amniotic cavities were involved, the inoculum size was larger in the presenting sac (39).

We have proposed a classification of the events leading to ascending intra-uterine microbial invasion (Fig. 1) (6). Stage I consists of an overgrowth of faculta-tive organisms or the presence of pathologic organisms (e.g., *Neisseria gonorrhea*) in the vagina and/or cervix. Bacterial vaginosis may be one of the manifestations of stage I. Once microorganisms gain access to the intrauterine cavity, they reside in the decidua (stage II). A localized inflammatory reaction leads to deciduitis and further extension, to chorionitis. The infection may invade the fetal vessels (choriovasculitis) or proceed through the amnion (amnionitis) into the amniotic cavity, leading to an intra-amniotic infection (stage III). Rupture of the membranes is not a prerequisite for intra-amniotic infection, as bacteria are capable of crossing intact membranes (40). Once in the amniotic cavity, the bacteria may gain access to the fetus by different ports of entry (stage IV). Aspiration of the infected fluid by the fetus may lead to congenital pneumonia. Otitis, conjunctivitis, and omphalitis are localized infections that occur by direct spreading of microorganisms from infected amniotic fluid. Seeding from any of these sites to the fetal circulation leads to bacteremia and sepsis. Another possible pathway for fetal sepsis is the spread of an infection located in the decidua parietalis to the decidua basalis and, from there, directly to the fetal villous circulation.

The mechanisms responsible for preterm premature rupture of mem-branes (PROM) may also be associated with ascending infection. A localized infec-

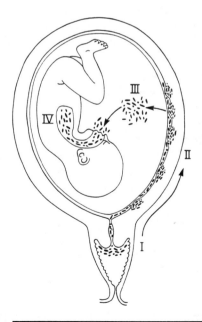

Fig. 1. The stages of ascending infection in labor.

tion in the choriodecidual junction can lead to rupture of membranes. Microbial invasion of the amniotic cavity may result from the spread of microorganisms from the localized choriodecidual nidus or by direct spread from the vagina through the site of rupture. Rupture of membranes can also result when ascending infection, as described in the previous paragraph, reaches stage III. The effect of bacterial proteases and/or host products secreted in response to bacterial infection from both sides of the membranes may lead to weakening of the membranes. This model explains why women with PROM can have either a positive or a negative amniotic fluid culture at the time of presentation. Over time, a progressive increase in the incidence of positive amniotic fluid cultures is also expected.

Table 1 illustrates the microbial isolates obtained from cases of intra-amniotic infection and preterm labor in one of our recent studies (32). The most common isolates were *Ureaplasma urealyticum*, *Fusobacterium* species, and *Mycoplasma hominis*. Fifty percent of these were polymicrobial infections. The inoculum size varied considerably, and 71% of the infections had more than 10^5 colony forming units/ml. Our observations are consistent with other studies that support a role for *Fusobacterium* (41, 42) and *Mycoplasma species* (43) in preterm labor. It is noteworthy that the most common microorganisms responsible for neonatal sepsis were not frequently isolated.

The role of *Chlamydia trachomatis* as an intrauterine pathogen has not been elucidated. This microorganism is an important cause of endocervicitis but has not been isolated from amniotic fluid (44). Recently, a case of congenital pneumonia caused by *Chlamydia trachomatis* suggests that this microorganism may be capable of causing ascending intra-amniotic infection (45).

THE ROLE OF INTRAUTERINE INFECTION IN PRETERM DELIVERY

Several lines of evidence suggest that intrauterine infection is associated with preterm labor and delivery. This evidence is derived from (*a*) microbiologic studies of the amniotic cavity, (*b*) histopathologic examination of the placenta, and (*c*) clinical and laboratory evidence of infection or inflammation in patients with preterm delivery. This section will critically review this evidence.

Studies examining the clinical circumstances surrounding preterm delivery indicate that one third of all patients presenting with preterm labor have intact membranes. A second third is associated with preterm PROM, and the remaining third results from delivery because of maternal or fetal indications (46)

To examine the role of intrauterine infection in the etiology of preterm delivery, we will review the association between microbial invasion of the amniotic cavity and spontaneous preterm labor (with or without intact membranes). However, this analysis may underestimate the real contribution of intrauterine infection to the etiology of preterm delivery, since an amniotic fluid culture only reflects the microbiologic state of the amniotic cavity. If an intrauterine infection is limited to the extra-amniotic space (e.g., deciduitis), it will not be detected with an amniotic fluid culture.

Table 1. Quantitative microbiology in 24 patients with microbial invasion of the amniotic cavity with preterm labor and intact membranes.

Patient	Organism	cfu/ml
1	*Ureaplasma urealyticum*	$>10^5$
	Fusobacterium species	5,000
2	*Ureaplasma urealyticum*	$>80,000$
3	*Ureaplasma urealyticum*	$>10^5$
	Fusobacterium species	$>10^5$
4	*Mycoplasma hominis*	1+
	Bacteroides species	$>10^5$
	Peptococcus species	$>10^5$
	Ureaplasma urealyticum	1+
5	*Mycoplasma hominis*	$>10^5$
	Ureaplasma urealyticum	
6	*Mycoplasma hominis*	$>10^5$
7	*Mycoplasma hominis*	$>10^5$
	Ureaplasma urealyticum	$>10^5$
	Gardnerella vaginalis	2+
8	*Fusobacterium* species	$>25,000$
9	*Viridans streptococci*	$>10^5$
10	*Gardnerella vaginalis*	$>10^5$
11	*Gardnerella vaginalis*	$>10^5$
12	*Fusobacterium* species	1+
13	*Bacteroides* species (4 varieties)	$>10^5$
14	*Streptococcus agalactiae*	$>10^5$
15	Mixed anaerobic flora	$>10^5$
	Mixed aerobic flora	1+
16	*Bacteroides* species	$>10^5$
	Peptococcus species	$>1,600$
17	Mixed aerobic and anaerobic flora	1+
18	Mixed anaerobic flora, gram-negative rods of three varieties	$>45,000$
19	*Staphylococcus aureus*	$>10^5$
20	*Fusobacterium* species	$>10^5$
21	*Peptostreptococcus*	$>10^5$
22	Mixed anaerobic flora	$>10^5$
23	Mixed anaerobic flora	$>5,000$
24	*Candida tropicalis*	$>8,000$

Source: From Romero R, Sirtori M, Oyarzun E, Mazor M, Avila C, Athenassiadis A, Callahan R, Sabo V, Hobbins JC, Infection and labor, V, Prevalence, microbiology and clinical significance of intraamniotic infection in women with preterm labor and intact membranes, Am J Obstet Gynecol 1989;161:817–24, with permission.

Intra-Amniotic Infection and Preterm Labor with Intact Membranes and Preterm Premature Rupture of Membranes

Table 2 displays the results of studies in which amniocentesis was performed on women with preterm labor and intact membranes (32, 41, 47–57). The mean rate of positive amniotic fluid cultures was 11.9% (90/758). Women with positive amniotic fluid cultures generally did not have clinical evidence of infection at presentation, but they were more likely to subsequently develop chorioamnionitis (42.2% [38/90] versus 4% [13/328]), to be refractory to tocolysis (62.5% [35/56] versus 13% [36/276]) and to rupture their membranes spontaneously (20% [9/46] versus 5.1% (15/292)] than were the women with negative amniotic fluid cultures (6).

Table 3 displays the results of amniotic fluid cultures from women with preterm PROM in seven published studies (56, 58–63). Positive amniotic fluid cultures occurred in 27.9% (113/404). This figure probably underestimates the true prevalence of intra-amniotic infection. Recent evidence gathered by ultrasound indicates that women with PROM and severely reduced amniotic fluid volumes have a higher incidence of intra-amniotic infection (62, 64). Since these women are less likely to have an amniocentesis, the bias in these studies is to underestimate the prevalence of infection. Another bias in these studies is that women with preterm PROM who were admitted in labor did not undergo amniocentesis. Therefore, such studies provide information about the prevalence of intra-amniotic infection in women who had preterm PROM without labor. Recently, we have documented that patients who were in preterm labor on admission had a tendency to have a higher incidence of positive amniotic fluid cultures in comparison to women admitted with PROM who were not in labor (39% versus 25%, P = 0.049). Furthermore, of patients who were not in labor on admission, 60% had a positive amniotic fluid culture when they entered active labor (65).

Placental Chorioamnionitis

Inflammation of the placenta is a host-response mechanism to a variety of stimuli such as infection and immune injury. Traditionally, acute inflammation of the chorioamniotic membranes has been considered an indicator of amniotic fluid infection (66–68, 33–38, 69, 70). This view has been based upon indirect evidence. Previous studies have demonstrated an association between acute inflammatory lesions of the placenta and the recovery of microorganisms from the subchorionic plate (71, 72) and from the chorioamniotic space (43). Bacteria have been recovered from the subchorionic plate of 72% of placentas with histologic chorioamnionitis (71). In another study, 39.1% of chorioamniotic membranes that showed diffuse inflammation had bacteria detected with Gram's and Grocott's stains in the histologic sections. Immunofluorescence studies with antibodies against Group B *Streptococcus* (GBS) and *Bacteroides fragilis* showed that 14/15 and 5/15 placentas, respectively, were positive for these organisms despite negative microbiology in most cases (73). Furthermore, we have recently found that there is an excellent correlation between positive amniotic fluid cultures and histologic chorioamnionitis (74).

Table 2. Intra-amniotic infection in women with preterm labor and intact membranes as determined by amniotic fluid studies obtained by transabdominal amniocentesis.

Author	Year	No. of Patients	Positive Cultures No. (%)	Clinical Chorioamnionitis No. (%)	PROM No. (%)	Refractory to Tocolysis No. (%)
Miller et al. (47)	1980	23	11 (47.8)	8 (72.7)	2/7 (28.5)	
Bobbitt et al. (48)	1981	31	8 (25.8)	6 (75.0)		7/8 (87.5)
Wallace and Herrich (49)	1981	25	3 (12.0)	1 (33.3)		
Hameed et al. (50)	1984	37	4 (10.8)	3 (75.0)		3/4 (75.0)
Wahbeh et al. (51)	1984	33	7 (21.2)	2 (28.5)		4/7 (57.1)
Wieble and Randall (52)	1985	35	1 (2.9)	1 (100.0)		
Leigh and Garite (41)	1986	59	7 (11.8)	4 (57.1)	4/7 (57.1)	7/7 (100.0)
Gravett et al. (53)	1986	54	13 (24.0)	5 (38.5)		5/13 (38.5)
Iams et al. (54)	1987	5	0 (0.0)			
Duff and Kopelman (55)	1987	24	1 (4.2)	0	0/1	0/1
Romero et al. (56)	1988	41	4 (9.8)			
Skoll et al. (57)	1989	127	7 (5.5)	1 (14.3)	1/7	
Romero et al. (32)	1989	264	24 (9.1)	3 (12.5)	2/24	9/16 (56.2)
Totals		758	90 (11.9)	38 (42.2)	9/46 (19.6)	35/56 (62.5)

Source: From Romero R, Mazor M, Infection and preterm labor, Clin Obstet Gynecol 1988;31:553, with permission.

Table 3. Intra-amniotic infection in women with preterm PROM as determined by amniotic fluid studies obtained by transabdominal amniocentesis.

Author	Year	No. of Patients	Positive Culture No. (%)	Success Rate (%)	Clinical Chorioamnionitis No. (%)	Neonatal Infection No. (%)
Garite et al. (58)	1979	59	9/30 (30.0)	51	6/9 (66.6)	2/9 (22.2)
Garite et al. (59)	1982	207	20/86 (23.2)	49	11/20 (55.0)	5/20 (25.0)
Cotton et al. (60)	1984	61	6/41 (14.6)	69	6/6 (100.0)	1/6 (16.6)
Broekhuizen et al. (61)	1985	79	15/53 (28.3)	66	3/15 (20.0)	8/15 (53.3)
Vintzileous et al. (62)	1985	54	12/54 (22.2)	—	2/12 (16.6)	4/12 (33.3)
Feinstein et al. (63)	1986	73	12/50 (20.0)	68	6/12 (50.0)	5/12 (41.6)
Romero et al. (64)	1988	90	39/90 (43.3)	95	—	—
Totals		623	113/404 (27.9)	59	34/74 (45.9)	25/74 (33.7)

Source: From Romero R, Mazor M, Infection and preterm labor, Clin Obstet Gynecol 1988;31:553, with permission.

Several studies have examined the prevalence of inflammation in placentas from women delivering preterm infants. The results of these studies have been reviewed in detail elsewhere (75). Russell reported that histologic chorioamnionitis was more common in women who delivered prematurely than in the entire obstetrical population (18.7% [123/659] versus 5.2% [392/7505], P < 0.01) (76). Using the data from the Collaborative Perinatal Project, Naeye and Peters found a higher incidence of histologic chorioamnionitis in the placentas of women delivering between 20 to 28 weeks than in the placentas of women delivering between 33 to 37 weeks (23% versus 11%) (68). Guzick and Winn also found that histologic chorioamnionitis was significantly more common in women with preterm delivery than in women with term deliveries (32.8% [80/244] versus 10% [253/2530], P < 0.01). If PROM was present, 48.6% (51/105) of all preterm deliveries had histologic chorioamnionitis. In the absence of PROM, 20.9% (29/139) of preterm deliveries had chorioamnionitis (77).

Clinical Evidence of Chorioamnionitis

The prevalence of endometritis is higher in women delivering preterm than in women delivering at term (PROM preterm: 18.7% [38/203] versus PROM term: 8.4% [38/454], P < 0.001; preterm intact membranes 13.1% [36/274] versus 6.4% [120/1881], P < 0.001). Furthermore, the prevalence of endometritis is the same after preterm delivery with intact membranes as after delivery with PROM. These data suggest that postpartum infection is associated with preterm delivery (78).

Maternal C-Reactive Protein

Subclinical infection is difficult to diagnose without amniocentesis. Acute-phase reactant proteins have been used as a marker of clinical infection. The most widely utilized of these proteins is C-reactive protein (CRP) (79). CRP was discovered by demonstrating that the sera from acutely ill patients could precipitate a nontype-specific somatic polysaccharide fraction from pneumococci called fraction C (80). CRP is synthesized by hepatocytes in response to interleukin-1 (IL-1), tumor necrosis factor (TNF), interleukin-6 (IL-6), and other inflammatory mediators (81–85). Peak concentrations of CRP are detected within 48 to 72 h following the onset of infection or injury. Quantitation of CRP did not become popular because it required a cumbersome technique. Recently, the availability of enzyme-linked assays and nephelometric techniques have revived clinical interest in CRP. The main limitation of CRP is that it is a nonspecific feature of the acute phase response to infection or tissue injury (83). Therefore, it is a marker of host response to injury rather than a specific indicator of infection.

Table 4 shows the prevalence of elevated CRP in women with preterm labor and PROM (86–92). The prevalence of elevated CRP is similar in women with preterm labor who are with or without PROM. An important observation is that women with preterm labor and elevated CRP are less likely to respond to tocolysis than women with normal or nondetectable serum CRP (77.7% [28/36] versus 10.4% [5/48], respectively) (90, 92). A good correlation between maternal CRP concentra-

Table 4. Prevalence of maternal C-reactive protein in women with preterm PROM and in women with preterm labor and intact membranes.

Author	Year	Definition of Positive Results	No. of Patients	Preterm Labor	
				PROM No.(%)	Intact Membranes No.(%)
Evans et al. (86)	1980	≥2 mg/dl	36	20 (55.5)	
Farb et al. (87)	1983	≥2 mg/dl	33		11 (33.0)
Hawrylyshyn et al. (88)	1983	≥1.25 mg/dl	52	23 (44.2)	
Romem and Artal (89)	1984	≥1.78–1.8 mg/dl	51	14 (27.4)	
Handwerker (90)	1984		50		15 (30.0)
Potkul et al. (91)	1985	≥0.7 mg/dl	40		16 (40.0)
Dodds and Iams (92)	1987	≥0.8 mg/dl	34		21 (61.7)
Totals			296	57/139 (41.0)	63/157 (40.1)

Source: From Romero R, Mazor M, Wu YK, Sirtori M, Oyarzun E, Mitchell MD, Hobbins JC, Infection in the pathogenesis of preterm labor, Semin Perinatol 1988;12:262–79, with permission.

tions and histologic chorioamnionitis (sensitivity 88% and specificity 96%) in a population of patients with preterm PROM has also been reported (88).

Genitourinary Infection

Colonization of the genitourinary tract with several microorganisms has been associated with prematurity, low birth weight, and PROM. We have reviewed in detail the literature concerning urinary and cervicovaginal colonization with the most common microorganisms and their relationship to preterm delivery. The interested reader is referred to this material for specific details (75).

The relationship between asymptomatic bacteriuria and preterm delivery/ low birth weight has been a controversial issue for years (93–104). We have recently employed meta-analysis to critically review the available data and have found that women with asymptomatic bacteriuria have a higher rate of prematurity/low birth weight than nonbacteriuric women. Furthermore, eradication of asymptomatic bacteriuria with antibiotic treatment results in a reduction of the rate of preterm birth/low birth weight (105).

There is convincing evidence of a relationship between gonorrhea and prematurity. Of five studies reviewed, four confirm this association (106–110). Recently, attention has been called to the relationship between bacterial vaginosis and preterm delivery (111). After reviewing the literature, we found three case-controlled studies and one cohort study that support an association between bacterial vaginosis and preterm labor. The only cohort study in which enrollment occurred in early pregnancy did not show an association between preterm labor and bacterial vaginosis (112).

Cervicovaginal colonization with GBS, *Trichomonas vaginalis,* and *Mycoplasma* species (*Mycoplasma hominis* and *Ureaplasma urealyticum*) has been implicated in the etiology of preterm birth (112–140). After a critical review of the literature, we cannot conclude that there is evidence to support an association between cervicovaginal colonization with these microorganisms and preterm birth. The relationship between *Chlamydia trachomatis* infection and preterm birth is inconclusive. In seven different studies addressing the association between cervical colonization with *Chlamydia trachomatis* and preterm birth, three supported, three negated, and one yielded inconclusive results (113, 118–122, 141).

Neonatal Sepsis

The prevalence of neonatal sepsis is 4.3/1000 live births in premature infants, in contrast to 0.8/1000 live births for term infants (143). Furthermore, the lower the birth weight, the higher the prevalence of sepsis (164/1000 for 1001 to 1500 g, 91/1000 for 1501 to 2000 g, and 23/1000 for 2001 to 2500 g) (164). The conventional interpretation of these data is that premature newborns are more susceptible to infection. The observation that at least half of the cases of sepsis are diagnosed within the first 48 h after delivery, together with the high prevalence of intra-amniotic infection in women with preterm labor and PROM, calls for a reappraisal of this traditional view. We would suggest that the higher prevalence of sepsis in the preterm newborn is partially attributable to a higher incidence of intrauterine infection in women in preterm labor. Furthermore, we propose that the onset of preterm labor in this subpopulation may be part of the repertoire of a host defense against infection.

THE ROLE OF ARACHIDONIC ACID METABOLITES AND CYTOKINES IN THE INITITION OF PRETERM LABOR

Arachidonic Acid Metabolites

A solid body of evidence supports a role for products of arachidonic acid metabolism in the onset of human parturition at term. There are fewer available data, however, to support a similar role for metabolites of arachidonic acid in preterm labor (143–150).

Prostaglandins (PG) have been measured in peripheral blood and amniotic fluid in women in preterm labor. Mitchell et al (144) found no significant difference in peripheral plasma levels of 13,14-dihydro-15-keto-PGF (PGFM) in women with preterm labor and in nonlaboring women in late pregnancy. Moreover, plasma concentrations of PGFM were significantly lower in preterm labor than in early labor at term (144). Subsequently, Sellers et al. were unable to demonstrate a significant difference in plasma PGFM concentrations between women in early preterm labor and in nonlaboring women of similar gestational ages. Furthermore, the plasma concentrations of this compound were not different in women with preterm labor who delivered within 24 h compared to those in preterm labor whose pregnancy continued and delivered at term (145). In contrast, Weitz et al. found that plasma concentrations of PGFM were significantly higher in women with preterm labor who failed tocolysis and delivered a premature infant than in women responding to this treatment (148).

Tambyraja et al (143) found that the concentration of PGFM in amniotic fluid of women in preterm labor increased as labor progressed. They could not demonstrate any predictive value of PGFM concentrations in the outcome of preterm labor treated with salbutamol. Similarly, Nieder and Augustin could not demonstrate a significant elevation in amniotic fluid PGE_2 and $PGF_{2\alpha}$ in women with premature labor when compared to women without labor of a similar gestational age (149). Recently, our group has shown that amniotic fluid concentrations of PGE_2 and its stable metabolite 11-deoxy-13,14-dihydro-15-keto-11,16-cyclo PGE_2 (PGEM-II) were significantly higher in women with preterm labor who are unresponsive to tocolysis than in those responsive to tocolysis (Figs. 2 and 3) (150). Furthermore, women with preterm labor and intra-amniotic infections had higher amniotic fluid concentrations of PGE_2, PGE-II, $PGF_{2\alpha}$ and PGFM than did women without intra-amniotic infection (151). In addition, amniotic fluid concentrations of PGE_2 and $PGF_{2\alpha}$ are increased in women with intra-amniotic infection and preterm PROM in labor (147). Therefore, there is strong evidence supporting the participation of PG in the mechanisms involved in the onset of parturition in women with intra-amniotic infection. On the other hand, it should be stressed that

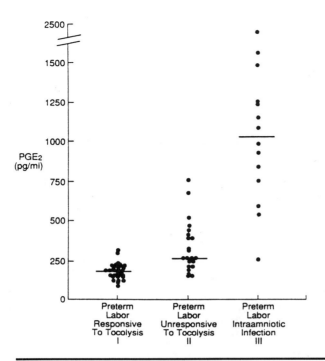

Fig. 2a. Amniotic fluid concentrations of PGE$_2$ in the three study groups. The line represents the median value for each group. Significant differences in the distribution of amniotic fluid concentration of PGE$_2$ were found among the three groups.

similar evidence supporting a role for PG in preterm labor in the absence of intra-amniotic infection is lacking.

Metabolites of arachidonic acid through the lipoxygenase pathway are also postulated to play a role in the onset and maintenance of human parturition at term (152, 153). Since some of the arachidonate lipoxygenase metabolites may act as inflammatory mediators and can stimulate uterine contractility, they may also be involved in the mechanisms responsible for preterm labor (154–156). Indeed, we have recently shown that the concentrations of 5-hydroxyeicosatetraenoic acid (5-HETE) are increased in the amniotic fluid of women in preterm labor leading to delivery, regardless of the presence or absence of infection (157). This observation is potentially important because 5-HETE can stimulate uterine contractility in a dose-dependent manner (155). Amniotic fluid concentrations of leukotriene-B$_4$ (LTB$_4$) and 15-HETE are also elevated in women with preterm labor and intra-amniotic infection (158). In contrast, we have not been able to demonstrate changes in the amniotic fluid concentrations of LTC$_4$ and 12-HETE in these patients in comparison to other women in preterm labor (158). These findings suggest that preterm labor with intra-amniotic infection is associated with selective activation of the lipoxygenase pathway of arachidonic acid.

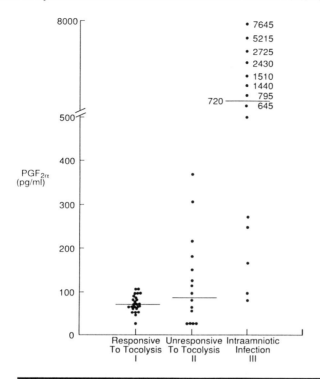

Fig. 2b.   Amniotic fluid concentrations of prostaglandin $F_{2\alpha}$ in the three study groups. The line represents the median value for each group. Significant differences in the distribution of amniotic fluid concentrations of $PGF_{2\alpha}$ were found between groups 3 and 1 and between groups 3 and 2 ($P < 0.05$). No significant difference was detected between groups 1 and 2 ($P > 0.05$).

In the setting of preterm labor, little is known about the signals controlling bioavailability of PG and lipoxygenase metabolites of arachidonic acid. Although the signals may be similar to those operating in term labor, recent work has focused on the role of bacterial products and host mediators in the generation of PG by intrauterine tissues.

Bacterial Products

PG biosynthesis in the setting of bacterial infections may be stimulated by either bacterial or host signals secreted in response to microbial presence. The traditional explanation for the onset of labor in the setting of infection has been that bacterial products directly stimulate PG biosynthesis. Indeed, several investigators have shown that bacterial products are a source of phospholipase A_2 and C and can stimulate PG production by human amnion (159–163). We have also reported that endotoxin (lipopolysaccharide or LPS) is present in the amniotic fluid of women

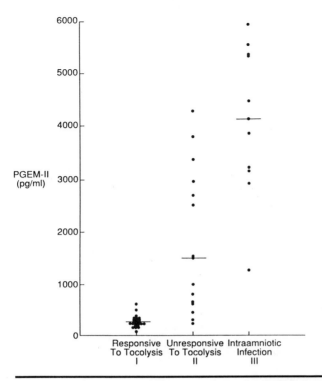

Fig. 3a. Amniotic fluid concentrations of PGEM-II in the three study groups. The line represents the median value for each group. Significant differences in the distribution of amniotic fluid concentrations of PGEM-II were found between groups 3 and 1, 3 and 2, and 1 and 2 (P < 0.05).

with gram-negative intra-amniotic infections (163) and is capable of stimulating PG production by amnion and decidua (Fig. 4) (164). Additionally, amniotic fluid concentrations of endotoxin from women with preterm labor and PROM are higher than in women with PROM and without labor (Fig. 5) (165). However, the quantities of endotoxin required to stimulate PG production by human amnion are not generally found in the amniotic fluid of women with intra-amniotic infection and preterm labor. Moreover, the overlap in endotoxin concentrations between the two groups suggests that factors other than endotoxin are involved in triggering the onset of premature labor in the setting of intra-amniotic infection. Therefore, it is possible that other bacterial products may be responsible for the stimulation of arachidonic acid metabolites by intrauterine tissues or, alternatively, that host-defense mechanisms are operative.

The observation that 28%–33% of women with preterm PROM have an intra-amniotic infection without labor suggests that the mere presence of microor-

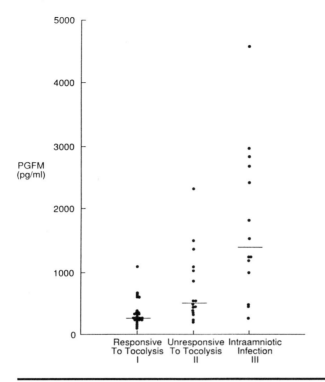

Fig. 3b. Amniotic fluid concentrations of PGFM in the three study groups. The line represents the median value for each group. Significant differences in the distribution of amniotic fluid concentrations of PGFM were found among groups 3 and 1, 3 and 2, and 1 and 2 (P < 0.05).

ganisms in the amniotic cavity is not sufficient to lead to the onset of labor (56, 58–63, 65). Furthermore, there is now evidence that effects of microbial products on PG production by intrauterine tissues are more variable than previously thought (164, 166). Recently we have examined the effect of a bacterial conditioned media on PG production by amnion and decidua and found that the effect is highly concentration dependent and that some microorganisms have an inhibitory rather than a stimulatory effect. (167).

Until recently, it was widely accepted that microorganisms alone were responsible for the ill effects and metabolic derangements associated with infection. It has now been established, however, that many of these ill effects are mediated by endogenous host products. A typical example of this is the pathophysiology of endotoxic shock. Bacterial endotoxin exerts its deleterious effects through the release of endogenous mediators such as TNF.

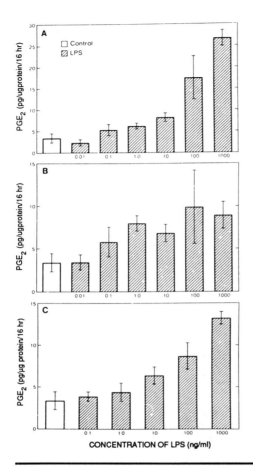

Fig. 4. The effects of bacterial endotoxin on the production of PGE_2 by human amnion cells. Panels *A, B,* and *C* show the effect of 026 *E. coli*, 055 *E. coli* and *S. typhosa*, respectively. (White bars = control; striped bars = lipopolysaccharide.)

Host Products (Cytokines)

The onset of labor in the setting of infection can be considered the pathophysiologic counterpart to endotoxin shock and, thus, a host-mediated response. In view of the pivotal role of the macrophage-monocyte system in the host response against infection and tissue injury, we have proposed that secretory products of macrophage activation may signal the onset of labor in the presence of infection (75).

Macrophages are ubiquitous cells present in the maternal (decidua), fetal, and placental compartments. These cells are activated by microbial products to secrete a wide variety of mediators including IL-1, IL-6, and TNF.

IL-1, also known as endogenous pyrogen, is produced by activated monocytes/macrophages cells in response to bacterial products such as endotoxin

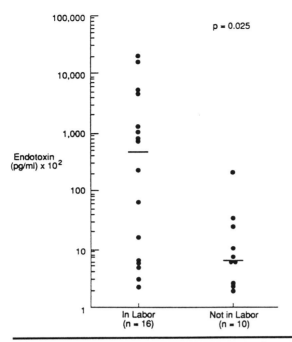

Fig. 5. Endotoxin concentration in infected amniotic fluid of women with PROM with and without labor.

(84, 171). IL-1 is pleotropic cytokine, which, along with TNF and IL-6, has been shown to mediate host responses to infection and injury. The biologic properties of IL-1 include the mediation of fever, actions of T and B lymphocytes, induction of collagenase activity, and PG biosynthesis (168).

Two biochemically related but distinct forms of IL-1 have been isolated: IL-1$_\alpha$ and IL-1$_\beta$. These two cytokines are the products of the different genes. They have the same molecular weight but a different isoelectric point (pI for IL-1 = 5; pI for IL-1$_\beta$ = 7). Despite sharing only a 25% amino acid sequence homology, IL-1$_\alpha$ and IL-1$_\beta$ bind to the same receptor. These two peptides have the same spectrum of biological activities.

In 1985 we postulated that IL-1 produced by the host (fetus or mother) could serve as a signal for the initiation of human parturition (169, 170). The evidence to support this view includes the following: (*a*) IL-1 stimulates PG production by amnion (Fig. 6), decidua, and myometrium. (*b*) Human decidua can produce IL-1 in response to bacterial products (171). (*c*) Amniotic fluid IL-1 bioactivity and concentrations are elevated in women with preterm labor and intra-amniotic infection, in contrast to amniotic fluid from patients with preterm labor but without intra-amniotic infection, which does not contain IL-1 (Fig. 7). (*d*) In women with preterm PROM and intra-amniotic infection, IL-1 bioactivity is higher in the presence of labor (172). (The data indicate that it is not the microbial presence

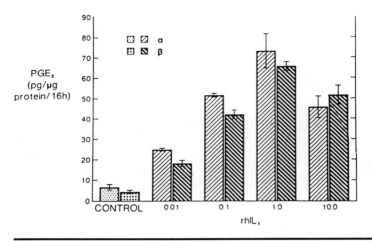

Fig. 6.   Effect of recombinant human IL-1$_\alpha$ and IL-1$_\beta$ on the production of PGE$_2$ by amnion cells in primary culture. The mean and the standard error of the mean are depicted. IL-1 concentrations are expressed in ng/ml.

in the amniotic cavity but rather the host response to bacterial presence that is associated with the onset of labor.) (*e*) In vitro perfusion of human uteri with IL-1 results in the development of regular uterine contractions.

Another potential role of IL-1 in parturition is to participate in cervical ripening. Changes in the biophysical properties of the cervix are associated with modifications in collagen and glycosaminoglycans. IL-1 stimulates collagenase activity and also has effects on the metabolism of glycosaminoglycans. Experiments conducted in rabbits have shown that the uterine cervix from term pregnancies produces more IL-1-like activity than the uterine cervix from non-pregnant animals (173).

We have also found that another monokine, TNF, may participate in the parturition associated with infection (174). TNF is secreted by activated macrophages and has similar properties to IL-1 (Table 5). Evidence suggesting a role for TNF in the onset of labor associated with infection includes the following: (*a*) TNF stimulates PG production by human amnion and decidua (175); (*b*) TNF is produced by human decidua in response to bacterial products (176); and (*c*) TNF is absent from normal amniotic fluid but is present in the amniotic fluid of women who have intra-amniotic infection and preterm labor (174).

Another cytokine that has been implicated as a major mediator of the host response to infection and tissue damage is IL-6 (177). This cytokine is produced by a wide variety of cells, such as macrophages, fibroblasts, endothelial cells, keratinocytes, and endometrial stromal cells (176-181). IL-6 elicits major changes in the biochemical, physiologic, and immunologic status of the host, including the acute-phase plasma protein response, activation of T-cells and natural killer cells,

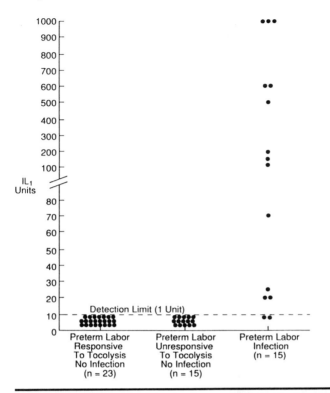

Fig. 7. IL-1-like bioactivity in the amniotic fluid of women with preterm labor. Group 1: preterm labor responsive to tocolysis with negative amniotic fluid cultures. Group 2: preterm labor unresponsive to tocolysis with negative amniotic fluid cultures. Group 3: preterm labor with positive amniotic fluid cultures. IL-1-like bioactivity is expressed in units because samples have been run in different assays. One unit of IL-1 is defined as that amount of IL-1 required to double the proliferative response of thymocytes stimulated with concanavalin A.

and stimulation and proliferation of immunoglobulin production by B-cells. IL-6 induces the production of CRP by liver cells (182). This may be important in the context of intra-amniotic infection, as clinical studies have indicated that elevated maternal serum CRP often precedes the development of clinical chorioamnionitis and the onset of preterm labor in women with preterm PROM (113). We have assayed amniotic fluid IL-6 in women in preterm labor with and without intact membranes. Low levels of IL-6 were detected in the amniotic fluid of normal women in the midtrimester and third trimester of pregnancy. Women with preterm labor with intra-amniotic infection had higher amniotic fluid levels of IL-6 than women in preterm labor without intra-amniotic infection (184).

Table 5.   Comparison of biological properties of IL-1 and TNF/cachetin.

Biological Property	IL-1	TNF/Cachetin
Endogenous pyrogen fever	+	+
Slow-wave sleep	+	+
Haemodynamic shock	+	+
Increased hepatic acute-phase protein synthesis	+	+
Decreased albumin synthesis	+	+
Activation of endothelium	+	+
Decreased lipoprotein lipase	+	+
Decreased cytochrome p450	+	+
Decreased plasma Fe/Zn	+	+
Increased fibroblast proliferation	+	+
Increased synovial cell collagenase and PGE_2	+	+
Induction of IL-1	+	+
T- or B-cell activation	+	−

Source: From Dinarello C, Clinical relevance of interleukin-1 and its multiple biological activities, Bull Inst Pasteur 1987;85:267–85, with permission.

Other bioactive agents secreted during the inflammatory process may also participate in this process. Platelet- activating factor is present in the amniotic fluid from women with preterm labor, and this lipid is capable of stimulating PGE_2 production by amnion and of stimulating myometrial contractions directly (185).

We have proposed a model (Fig. 8) in which the initiation of human parturition in the presence of infection is controlled by the host. Systemic maternal infections, such as pyelonephritis, or localized infections, such as deciduitis, could trigger parturition via the monocyte/macrophage system in peripheral blood and human decidua. Alternatively, a second host, the fetus, may signal the onset of labor when the amniotic cavity becomes infected. Preterm labor can, therefore, be viewed as an event occurring when the intrauterine or maternal environment is hostile and threatens the well-being of the fetus. From this point of view, the initiation of preterm labor may have survival value.

The evidence reviewed above indicates an association between rupture of the fetal membranes and intrauterine infection. The pathophysiology of this event may be similar to that of preterm labor. The membranes are a connective tissue organ. Bacterial infection, directly or indirectly (IL-1 and TNF) may induce the release of proteases (collagenase, elastases, etc.) from macrophages or other cell types, which then degrade the fetal membranes and lead to rupture. The reason why some infections result in preterm labor and others in PROM remains to be determined. We view them as two different expressions of the same basic phenomenon: activation of the host-defense macrophage system. Infection seems to be the main, but not the only, etiology for this chain of events.

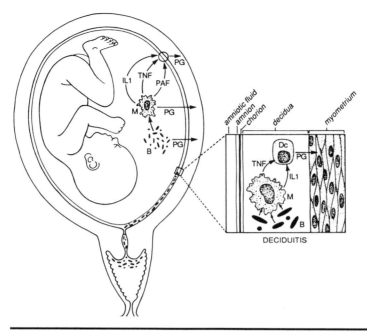

Fig. 8. Cellular and biochemical mechanisms involved in the initiation of preterm labor in cases of intrauterine infection. (B = bacteria; M = monocyte/macrophage; Dc = decidua; IL-1 = interleukin-1; TNF = tumor necrosis factor/cachectin; PG = prostaglandins; PAF = platelet-activating factor.)

MICROBIAL INVASION OF THE AMNIOTIC CAVITY: CAUSE OR CONSEQUENCE OF LABOR?

Since the amniotic cavity is normally sterile, we have considered microbial invasion of the amniotic cavity as an abnormal finding. The data presented in Tables 2 and 3 support an association between microbial invasion of the amniotic cavity and preterm labor and preterm PROM. However, these data do not provide evidence of causality. Indeed, the argument may be put forth that microbial invasion of this compartment is the consequence of labor or rupture of the membranes rather than the cause of preterm labor and preterm PROM.

Recently we completed a study to establish the prevalence of microbial invasion of the amniotic cavity in women in spontaneous labor at term. Amniotic fluid was retrieved transabdominally in a group of women undergoing primary or repeat cesarean section in active labor or who were suspected to have preterm labor but subsequently delivered a term infant by weight and pediatric examination. We found that 18.8% (17/90) of these patients had a positive amniotic fluid culture (186). Since the prevalence of microbial invasion of the amniotic cavity is similar in both women in term and preterm labor leading to preterm delivery, the argument could be made that microbial invasion is a phenomenon associated with labor per se. It is possible that microorganisms gain access to the sterile amniotic cavity when cervical dilatation exposes intact membranes to the normal vaginal flora.

Despite the similar rate of positive amniotic fluid cultures in term and preterm labor and delivery with intact membranes, there are several striking differences in these two settings. First, the inoculum size in term labor is much smaller than in preterm labor (186). Second, the concentration of IL-1, TNF, and IL-6 are several-fold higher in the setting of preterm labor than in term labor (187). Third, the prevalence and severity of histopathologic chorioamnionitis is much higher in preterm labor and delivery than in term gestation (30% versus 10%). Fourth, the prevalence of clinical chorioamnionitis is much higher in preterm than in term gestation (76). Collectively, these data indicate that there are fundamental differences between microbial invasion of the amniotic cavity in the context of a term and preterm gestation. We believe that microbial invasion of the amniotic cavity can be both a cause or a consequence of labor. Ascending microbial invasion may lead to macrophage activation and the initiation of parturition when present for an extended period of time. This may be the chain of events often associated with preterm parturition and intra-amniotic infection. However, if labor has already begun in the context of term or preterm gestation, secondary microbial invasion may occur. We believe that is the most likely sequence of events associated with microbial invasion during spontaneous term labor.

PRETERM LABOR AS A HETEROGENEOUS DISEASE

The traditional management of preterm labor has consisted of treatment with tocolytic agents and often steroid administration. This uniform approach to the problem implies that preterm labor is a unique pathologic entity for which there is a single treatment. It is now evident that tocolytic treatment has failed to prolong pregnancy beyond 48 h and to reduce perinatal morbidity and mortality (188).

We view preterm labor as a pathologic event; labor may be considered as the response of the fetomaternal pair to a variety of insults (infection, ischemia, etc). If these insults cannot be effectively handled in the context of a continuing pregnancy, then labor and delivery may occur. For example, severe maternal infections such as pyelonephritis in the pre-antibiotic era were associated with preterm labor and delivery. Today, maternal pyelonephritis can result in preterm labor, but early antibiotic treatment prevents progression toward inevitable labor and delivery in most cases. In the case of an intrauterine infection, the host can utilize the normal complement of host-defense mechanisms against infection (i.e., specific and nonspecific mechanisms) available in any other site. However, if these mechanisms fail to control the infection, labor enables the host to rid itself of the infected tissue. The presence of a second host, the fetus, adds further complexity to the solution of this problem. Nature must contend with maximizing the survival of two hosts. At term, when the fetus is mature, initiation of labor is an expedient and safe solution for both hosts. On the other hand, in the previable gestation, uterine evacuation promotes maternal survival at the expense of fetal life. For these reasons, the initiation of labor in the setting of infection can be considered to have survival value.

Up to this point, this chapter has focused on the role of infection in preterm labor. However, infection is only one of the insults that may compromise fetomaternal survival. Placental histopathologic studies would suggest that inflammation may account for probably no more than 30%–40% of cases of preterm delivery (74). This estimate correlates well with our studies of amniotic fluid microbiology (32). Therefore, other pathologic processes must be responsible for the initiation of preterm labor in the remainder of cases. We have recently established that the most common noninflammatory lesion of the placenta in the setting of preterm delivery is vascular pathology (decidual thrombosis, acute atherosis, failure of physiologic transformation of the spiral arteries, etc.) (189, 190). We propose that these vascular lesions may lead to uteroplacental ischemia and to the initiation of preterm labor and delivery. Clinical and experimental observations supporting this include (*a*) that there is an excess of intrauterine growth retardation and abruptio placenta in the setting of premature birth and (*b*) that experimental uterine ischemia in monkeys often results in the initiation of labor.

Another distinct clinical group of patients with a potentially different mechanism for preterm labor and delivery is composed of women with congenital anomalies and polyhydramnios. Uterine overdistension may activate a uterine pressor sensitive system capable of initiating uterine contractility and labor. This mechanism can be invoked to also explain the excess rate of preterm labor observed in multiple gestations.

Yet another potential mechanism for preterm labor and delivery is an immunologically mediated phenomenon induced by an allergic mechanism. Indeed, the uterus contains a large number of mast cells, and the trophoblast may constitute the antigen required for eliciting an allergic reaction. Garfield has recently reported that products of mast cell degranulation are capable of inducing myometrial contractions (191). We have also identified a group of patients in preterm labor with clinical and laboratory findings consistent with an allergy-mediated event.

The emerging picture is that preterm labor and delivery is a syndrome (Fig 9). Multiple pathological processes may lead to myometrial activation and cervical ripening. This view of preterm labor has considerable implications for the diagnosis, treatment, and understanding of the cellular and biochemical mechanisms responsible for the initiation of parturition.

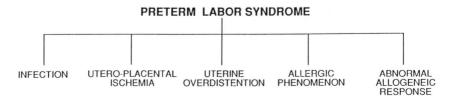

Fig. 9.   Preterm labor syndrome.

REFERENCES

1. Rush RW, Keirse MJNC, Howat P, et al. Contribution of preterm delivery to perinatal mortality. Br Med J 1976;2:965.
2. Main DM, Main EK. Management of preterm labor and delivery. In: Gabbe SG, Niebyl J, Simpson JL, eds. Obstetrics: normal and problem pregnancies. New York, Churchill Livingstone, 1986:689-737.
3. Kessel SS, Villar J, Berendes HW, et al. The changing pattern of low birth weight in the United States (1970 to 1980). J Am Med Assoc 1984;251:1978.
4. Minkoff H. Prematurity: infection as an etiologic factor. Obstet Gynecol 1983;62:137.
5. Naeye RL, Peters EC. Causes and consequences of premature rupture of fetal membranes. Lancet 1980;I:192.
6. Romero R, Mazor M. Infection and preterm labor. Clin Obstet Gynecol 1988;31:553.
7. Bang B. The etiology of epizootic abortion. J Comp Anthol Ther 1897;10:125-50.
8. Zahl PA, Bjerknes C. Induction of decidua-placental hemorrhage in mice by the endotoxins of certain gram-negative bacteria. Proc Soc Exper Biol Med 1943;54:329-32.
9. Takeda Y, Tsuchiya I. Studies on the pathological changes caused by the injection of the Shwartzman filtrate and the endotoxin into pregnant rabbits. Jpn J Exper Med 1953;21:9-16.
10. Takeda Y, Tsuchiya I. Studies on the pathological changes caused by the injection of the Shwartzman filtrate and the endotoxin into pregnant animals, II. On the relationship of the constituents of the endotoxin and the abortion-producing factor. Jpn J Exper Med 1953;23:105-10.
11. Rieder RF, Thomas L. Studies on the mechanisms involved in the production of abortion by endotoxin. J Immunol 1960;84:189-93.
12. McKay DG, Wong T-C. The effect of bacterial endotoxin on the placenta of the rat. Am J Pathol 1963;42:357-77.
13. Kullander S. Fever and parturition: an experimental study in rabbits. Acta Obstet Gynecol Scand 1977;66(suppl):77-85.
14. Skarnes RC, Harper MJK. Relationship between endotoxin-induced abortion and the synthesis of prostaglandin F. Prostaglandins 1972;1:191-201.
15. Finland M, Dublin TD. Pneumococcic pneumonias complicating pregnancy and the puerperium. JAMA 1939;112:1027-32.
16. Oxorn H. The changing aspects of pneumonia complicating pregnancy. Am J Obstet Gynecol 1955;70:1057-63.
17. Benedetti TJ, Valle R, Ledger WJ. Antepartum pneumonia in pregnancy. Am J Obstet Gynecol 1976;144:413-7.
18. Madinger NE, Greenspoon JS, Ellrodt AG. Pneumonia during pregnancy: has modern technology improved maternal and fetal outcome. Am J Obstet Gynecol 1989;161:657-62.
19. McLane CM. Pyelitis of pregnancy: a five-year study. Am J Obstet Gynecol 117-23.
20. Kass E. Maternal urinary tract infection. New York State J Med 1962;1:2822-6.
21. Hibbard L, Thrupp L, Summeril S, Smale M, Adams R. Treatment of pyelonephritis in pregnancy. Am J Obstet Gynecol 1967;98:609-15.
22. Cunningham FG, Morris GB, Mikal A. Acute pyelonephritis of pregnancy: a clinical review. Obstet Gynecol 1973;42;112-7.

23. Fan Y-D, Pastorek JG, Miller JM, Mulvey J. Acute pyelonephritis in pregnancy. Am J Perinatol 1987;4:324-6.

24. Wing ES, Troppoli DV. The intrauterine transmission of typhoid. JAMA 1930;95:405.

25. Diddle AW, Stephens RL. Typhoid fever in pregnancy: probable intrauterine transmission of the disease. Am J Obstet Gynecol 1938;38:300.

26. Stevenson CS, Glasko AJ, Gillespie EC. Treatment of typhoid in pregnancy with chloramphenicol (chloromycetin). JAMA 1951;146:1190.

27. Herd N, Jordan T. An investigation of malaria during pregnancy in Zimbabwe. C Afr J Med 1981;27:62-8.

28. Gilles HM, Lawson JB, Sibelas M, Voller A, Allan N. Malaria, anaemia and pregnancy. Ann Trop Med Pharmacol 1969;63:245.

29. Sereno JA, Poseiro JJ, Sica-Blanco Y, Pose SV. Int Cong Phys Sci.

30. Romero R, Mitchell MD, Duff GW, Durum S, Hobbins JC. A possible mechanism for premature labor in gram-negative maternal infection: a monocyte product stimulates prostaglandin release by the amnion. Presented at the 32nd Meeting of the Society for Gynecologic Investigation. Phoenix, AZ, 1985.

31. Gibbs RS, Blanco JD, St Clair PJ, Castaneda YS. Quantitative bacteriology of amniotic fluid from women with clinical intraamniotic infection at term. J Infect Dis 1982;145:1-8.

32. Romero R, Sirtori M, Oyarzun E, et al. Infection and labor, V. Prevalence, microbiology, and clinical significance of intraamniotic infection in women with preterm labor and intact membranes. Am J Obstet Gynecol 1989:817-24.

33. Blanc WA. Infection amniotique et neonatal. Gynaecologia 1953;136:101-4.

34. Blanc WA. Amniotic infection syndrome pathogenesis morphology and significance in circumnatal mortality. Clin Obstet Gynecol. 1959;2:705-12.

35. Blanc WA. Pathways of fetal and early neonatal infection: viral placentitis, bacterial and fungal chorioamnionitis. J Pediatr 1964;59:473-96.

36. Benirschke K, Clifford SH. Intrauterine bacterial infection of the newborn infant. J Pediatr 1959;54:11-8.

37. Driscoll SG. Pathology and the developing fetus. Pediatr Clin North Am 1965;12:493-514.

38. Benirschke K. Routes and types of infection in the fetus and the newborn. Am J Dis Child 1965;28:714-21.

39. Romero R, Fayek S, Avila C, et al. The prevalence and microbiology of intraamniotic infection in twin gestation with preterm labor. Am J Obstet Gynecol (submitted).

40. Galask RP, Varner MW, Petzold CR, et al. Bacterial attachment to the chorioamniotic membranes. Am J Obstet Gynecol 1984;148:915-28.

41. Leigh J, Garite TJ. Amniocentesis and the management of premature labor. Obstet Gynecol 1986;67:500-6.

42. Altshuler G, Hyde S. Clinicopathologic considerations of fusobacteria chorioamnionitis. Acta Obstet Gynecol Scand 1988;67:513-7.

43. Hillier SL, Martius J, Krohn M, Kiviat N, Holmes KK, Eschenbach DA. A case-control study of chorioamnionic infection and histologic chorioamnionitis in prematurity. N Engl J Med 1988;319:972-8.

44. Thomas G, Sbarra A, Feingold, et al. Antimicrobial activity of amniotic fluid against *Chlamydia trachomatis*, *Mycoplasma hominis*, and *Ureaplasma urealyticum*. Am J Obstet Gynecol 1988;158:16-22.

45. Thorp JM, Katz VL, Fowler LJ, Kurtzman JT, Bowes WA. Fetal death from chlamydial infection across intact amniotic membranes. Am J Obstet Gynecol 1989; 161:1245-6.

46. Arias F, Tomich P. Etiology and outcome of low birth weight and preterm infants. Obstet Gynecol 1982;60:277.

47. Miller JM, Pupkin MJ, Hill GB. Bacterial colonization of amniotic fluid from intact fetal membranes. Am J Obstet Gynecol 1980;136:796-804.

48. Bobbit JR, Hayslip CC, Damato JD. Amniotic fluid infection as determined by transabdominal amniocentesis in patients with intact membranes in premature labor. Am J Obstet Gynecol 1981;140:947-52.

49. Wallace RL, Herrick CN. Amniocentesis in the evaluation of premature labor. Obstet Gynecol 1981;57:483-6.

50. Hameed C, Tejani N, Verma UL, et al. Silent chorioamnionitis as a cause of preterm labor refractory to tocolytic therapy. Obstet Gynecol 1984;149:726-30.

51. Wahbeh CJ, Hill GB, Eden RD, et al. Intra-amniotic bacterial colonization in premature labor. Am J Obstet Gynecol 1984;148:739-43.

52. Weible DR, Randall HW. Evaluation of amniotic fluid in preterm labor with intact membranes. J Reprod Med 1985;30:777-80.

53. Gravett MG, Hummel D, Eschenbach DA, et al. Preterm labor associated with subclinical amniotic fluid infection and with bacterial vaginosis. Obstet Gynecol 1986;67:229-37.

54. Iams JD, Clapp DH, Contos DA, et al. Does extra-amniotic infection cause preterm labor? Gas-liquid chromatography studies of amniotic fluid in amnionitis, preterm labor, and normal controls. Obstet Gynecol 1987;70:365-8.

55. Duff P, Kopelman JN. Subclinical intra-amniotic infection in asymptomatic patients with refractory preterm labor. Obstet Gynecol 1987;69:L756-9.

56. Romero R, Emamian M, Quintero R, et al. The value and limitations of the gram stain examination in the diagnosis of intraamniotic infection. Am J Obstet Gynecol 1988;159:114-9.

57. Skoll MA, Moretti ML, Sibai BM. The incidence of positive amniotic fluid cultures in patients in preterm labor with intact membranes. Am J Obstet Gynecol 1989;161:813-6.

58. Garite TJ, Freeman RK, Linzey EM, et al. The use of amniocentesis in patients with premature rupture of membranes. Obstet Gynecol 1979;54:226-30.

59. Garite TJ, Freeman RK. Chorioamnionitis in the preterm gestation. Obstet Gynecol 1982;59:539-45.

60. Cotton DB, Hill LM, Strassner HT, et al. Use of amniocentesis in preterm gestation with ruptured membranes. Obstet Gynecol 1984;63:38-43.

61. Broekhuizen FF, Gilman M, Hamilton PR. Amniocentesis for gram stain and culture in preterm premature rupture of the membranes. Obstet Gynecol 1985;66:316-21.

62. Vintzileos AM, Campbell WA, Nochimson DJ, et al. Qualitative amniotic fluid volume versus amniocentesis in predicting infection in preterm rupture of the membranes. Obstet Gynecol 1986;67:579-83.

63. Feinstein ST, Vintzileos AM, Lodeiro JG, et al. Amniocentesis with premature rupture of membranes. Am J Obstet Gynecol 1986;68:147-52.

64. Gonik B, Bottoms SF, Cotton DB. Amniotic fluid volume as a risk factor in preterm premature rupture of the membranes. Obstet Gynecol 1985;65:456-9.

65. Romero R, Quintero R, Oyarzun E, et al. Intraamniotic infection and the onset of

labor in preterm premature rupture of membranes. Am J Obstet Gynecol 1988;159:661-6.

66. Gibbs RS, Blanco JD, St Clair PJ, et al. Quantitative bacteriology of amniotic fluid from women with clinical intra-amniotic infection at term. J Infect Dis 1982;145:1-8.

67. Driscoll SG. The placenta and membranes. In: Charles D, Finland M, eds. Obstetric and perinatal infections. Philadelphia: Lea & Febiger, 1973:529-39.

68. Naeye RL, Peters EC. Causes and consequences of premature rupture of fetal membranes. Lancet 1980;I:192.

69. Overbach AM, Daniel SJ, Cassady G. The value of umbilical cord histology in the management of potential perinatal infection. J Pediatr 1970;76:22-31.

70. Maudsley RF, Brix GA, Hinton NA, et al. Placental inflammation and infection: a prospective bacteriologic and histologic study. Am J Obstet Gynecol 1966;95:648-59.

71. Pankuch GA, Appelbaum PC, Lorenz RP, et al. Placental microbiology and histology and the pathogenesis of chorioamnionitis. Obstet Gynecol 1984;64:802-6.

72. Aquino TI, Zhan J, Kraus FT, Knefel R, Taff T. Subchorionic fibrin cultures for bacteriologic study of the placenta. Am J Clin Pathol 1984;81:482-6.

73. Chellam VG, Rushton DI. Chorioamnionitis and funiculitis in the placentas of 200 births weighing less than 2.5 kg. Br J Obstet Gynaecol 1985;92:808-14.

74. Romero R, Salafia CM, Athanassiadis AP, et al. The relationship between acute inflammatory lesions of the placenta and amniotic fluid microbiology. Am J Obstet Gynecol (submitted).

75. Romero R, Mazor M. Infection and preterm labor. Clin Obstet Gynecol 1988;31:553-84.

76. Russell P. Inflammatory lesions of the human placenta: clinical significance of acute chorioamnionitis. Am J Diag Gynecol Obstet 1979;2:127-37.

77. Guzick DS, Winn K. The association of chorioamnionitis with preterm delivery. Obstet Gynecol 1985;65:11-6.

78. Daikoku NH, Kaltreider DF, Khouzami VA, et al. Premature rupture of membranes and spontaneous preterm labor: maternal endometritis risks. Obstet Gynecol 1982;59:13-20.

79. Abernethy TJ, Avery OT. The occurrence during acute infections of a protein not normally present in blood. J Exp Med 1941;73:173-82.

80. Tillett WS, Francis T. Serological reactions in pneumonia with a non-protein somatic fraction of pneumococcus. J Exp Med 1930;52:561-71.

81. Hurlimann J, Thorbecke GT, Hochwald GM. The liver as the site of C-reactive protein formation. J Exp Med 1966;123:365-78.

82. Merriman CR, Pulham LA, Kampschmidt RF. Effect of leukocytic endogenous mediator on C-reactive protein in rabbits. Proc Soc Exp Biol Med 1975;149:782-6.

83. Van Lengte F. The diagnostic utility of C-reactive protein. Hum Pathol 1982;13:1061-3.

84. Dinarello CA. Clinical relevance of interleukin-1 and its multiple biological activities. Bull Inst Pasteur 1987;85:267-85.

85. Perlmutter DH, Dinarello CA, Punsal P, et al. Cachectin/tumor necrosis factor regulates hepatic acute phase gene expression. J Clin Invest 1986;78:1349-54.

86. Evans MI, Hajj SN, Devoe LD, et al. C-reactive protein as a predictor of infectious morbidity with premature rupture of membranes. Am J Obstet Gynecol 1980;138:648-52.

87. Farb HF, Arnesen M, Geistler P, et al. C-reactive protein with premature rupture of

membranes and premature labor. Obstet Gynecol 1983;62:49-51.

88. Hawrylyshyn P, Bernstein P, Milligan JE, et al. Premature rupture of membranes: the role of C-reactive protein in the prediction of chorioamnionitis. Am J Obstet Gynecol 1983;147:240-6.

89. Romem Y, Artal R. C-reactive protein as a predictor for chorioamnionitis in cases of premature rupture of the membranes. Am J Obstet Gynecol 1984;150:546-50.

90. Handwerker SM, Tejani NA, Verma UL, et al. Correlation of maternal serum C-reactive protein with outcome of tocolysis. Obstet Gynecol 1984;63:220-4.

91. Potkul RK, Moawad AH, Ponto KL. The association of subclinical infection with preterm labor: the role of C-reactive protein. Am J Obstet Gynecol 1985;153:642-5.

92. Dodds WG, Iams JD. Maternal C-reactive protein and preterm labor. J Reprod Med 1987;32:527-30.

93. Kass EH. Bacteriuria and pyelonephritis of pregnancy. Arch Intern Med 1960; 105:194-8.

94. Kincaid-Smith P, Bullen M. Bacteriuria in pregnancy. Lancet 1965;I:395-9.

95. Whalley P. Bacteriuria of pregnancy. Am J Obstet Gynecol 1967;97:723-38.

96. Kass EH. Pyelonephritis and bacteriuria: a major problem in preventive medicine. Ann Intern Med 1962;56:46-53.

97. Wilson MG, Hewitt WL, Monzon OT. Effect of bacteriuria on the fetus. N Engl J Med 1966;274:115-8.

98. Dixon HG, Brant HA. The significance of bacteriuria in pregnancy. Lancet 1967;I: 19-20.

99. Savage WE, Hajj SN, Kass EH. Demographic and prognostic characteristics of bacteriuria in pregnancy. Medicine 1967;46:385-407.

100. Robertson JG, Livingstone JRB, Isdale MH. The management and complications of asymptomatic bacteriuria in pregnancy. Br J Obstet Gynaecol 1968;75:59-65.

101. Elder HA, Santamarina BAG, Smith S, et al. The effect of tetracycline on the clinical course and the outcome of pregnancy. Am J Obstet Gynecol 1971;111:441-62.

102. Brumfitt W. The effects of bacteriuria in pregnancy on maternal and fetal health. Kidney Int 1975;8(suppl):113-9.

103. Bryant RE, Windom RE, Vineyard JP, et al. Asymptomatic bacteriuria in pregnancy and its association with prematurity. J Lab Clin Med 1964;63:224-31.

104. LeBlanc AL, McGanity WJ. The impact of bacteriuria in pregnancy—a survey of 1300 pregnant patients. Biol Med 1964;22:336-47.

105. Romero R, Oyarzun E, Mazor M, et al. Meta-analysis of the relationship between asymptomatic bacteriuria and preterm delivery/low birth weight. Obstet Gynecol 1989; 73:576-82.

106. Sarrel PM, Pruett KA. Symptomatic gonorrhea during pregnancy. Obstet Gynecol 1968;32:670-3.

107. Handsfield HH, Hodson WA, Holmes KK. Neonatal gonococcal infection: orogastric contamination with *Neisseria gonorrhea*. JAMA 1973;225:697-701.

108. Amstey MS, Steadman KT. Asymptomatic gonorrhea and pregnancy. J Am Ven Dis Assoc 1976;33:14-6.

109. Edwards LE, Barrada MI, Hamann AA, et al. Gonorrhea in pregnancy. Am J Obstet Gynecol 1978;132:637-41.

110. Stoll BJ, Kanto WP, Glass RI, et al. Treated maternal gonorrhea without adverse effect on outcome of pregnancy. South Med J 1982;75:1236-8.

111. Eschenbach DA, Gravett MG, Chen KCS, et al. Bacterial vaginosis during preg-

nancy: an association with prematurity and postpartum complications. In: Mardh PA, Taylor-Robinson D, eds. Bacterial vaginosis. Stockholm: Almqvist & Wiksell, 1984:214-22.

112. Minkoff H, Grunebaum AN, Schwarz RH, et al. Risk factors for prematurity and premature rupture of membranes: a prospective study of the vaginal flora in pregnancy. Am J Obstet Gynecol 1984;150:965-72.

113. Martius J, Krohn MA, Hillier SL, et al. Relationships of vaginal lactobacillus species, cervical *Chlamydia trachomatis*, and bacterial vaginosis to preterm birth. Obstet Gynecol 1988;71:89-95.

114. Baker CJ, Barrett FF, Yow MD. The influence of advancing gestation on group B streptococcal colonization in pregnant women. Am J Obstet Gynecol 1975;122:820-5.

115. Regan JA, Chao S, James LS. Premature rupture of membranes, preterm delivery, and group B streptococcal colonization of mothers. Am J Obstet Gynecol 1981; 141:184-6.

116. Hastings MJG, Easmon CSF, Neill J, et al. Group B streptococcal colonization and the outcome of pregnancy. J Infect 1986;12:23-39.

117. Bobbitt JR, Damato JD, Sakakini J. Perinatal complications in group B streptococcal carriers: a longitudinal study of prenatal patients. Am J Obstet Gynecol 1985; 151:711-7.

118. Lamont RF, Taylor-Robinson D, Newman M, et al. Spontaneous early preterm labour associated with abnormal genital bacterial colonization. Br J Obstet Gynaecol 1986;93:804-10.

119. Martin DH, Koutsky L, Eschenbach DA, et al. Prematurity and perinatal mortality in pregnancies complicated by maternal *Chlamydia trachomatis* infections. JAMA 1982;247:1585-8.

120. Harrison HR, Alexander ER, Weinstein L, et al. Cervical *Chlamydia trachomatis* and mycoplasmal infections in pregnancy: epidemiology and outcomes. JAMA 1983;250:1721-7.

121. Ross SM, Windsor IM, Robins-Browne RM, et al. Microbiological studies during the perinatal period: an attempt to correlate selected bacterial and viral infections with intrauterine deaths and preterm labour. S Afr Med J 1984;86:598-603.

122. Sweet RL, Landers DV, Walker C, et al. *Chlamydia trachomatis* infection and pregnancy outcome. Am J Obstet Gynecol 1987;156:824-33.

123. Klein JO, Buckland D, Finland M. Colonization of newborn infants by mycoplasmas. N Engl J Med 1969;280:1025-30.

124. Foy H, Kenny GE, Wentworth BB, et al. Isolation of *Mycoplasma hominis*, T-strains, and cytomegalovirus from the cervix of pregnant women. Am J Obstet Gynecol 1970;106:635-43.

125. Braun P, Yhu-Hsiung L, Klein JO, et al. Birth weight and genital mycoplasmas in pregnancy. N Engl J Med 1971;284:167-71.

126. Harrison RF, Hurley R, DeLouvois J. Genital mycoplasmas and birth weight in offspring of primigravida women. Am J Obstet Gynecol 1979;133:201-3.

127. Ross JM, Furr PM, Taylor-Robinson D, et al. The effect of genital mycoplasmas on human fetal growth. Br J Obstet Gynaecol 1981;88:749-55.

128. Kass EH, McCormack WM, Lin JS, et al. Genital mycoplasmas as a cause of excess premature delivery. Trans Assoc Am Physicians 1981;94:261-6.

129. Upadhyaya M, Hibbard BM, Walker SM. The role of mycoplasmas in reproduction.

Fertil Steril 1983;39:814-8.

130. McCormack WM, Rosner B, Yhu-Hsiung L, et al. Effect on birth weight of erythromycin treatment of pregnant women. Obstet Gynecol 1987;69:202-7.

131. Shurin PA, Alpert S, Rosner B, et al. Chorioamnionitis and colonization of the newborn infant with genital mycoplasmas. N Engl J Med 1975;293:5-8.

132. Dische MR, Quinn PA, Czegledy-Nagy E, et al. Genital mycoplasma infection: intrauterine infection, pathologic study of the fetus and placenta. Am Soc Clin Pathol 1979;72:167-73.

133. Embree JE, Krause VW, Embil JA, et al. Placental infection with *Mycoplasma hominis* and *Ureaplasma urealyticum:* clinical correlation. Obstet Gynecol 1980;56:475-81.

134. Kundsin RB, Driscoll SG, Pelletier PA. *Ureaplasma urealyticum* incriminated in periantal morbidity and mortality. Science 1981;213:474-6.

135. Kundsin RB, Driscoll SG, Monson RR, et al. Association of *Ureaplasma urealyticum* in the placenta with perinatal morbidity and mortality. N Engl J Med 1984;310:941-5.

136. Zlatnik FJ, Burmeister LF, Swack NS. Chorionic mycoplasmas and prematurity. J Reprod Med 1986;31:1106-8.

137. Mason PR, Brown MT. Trichomonas in pregnancy. Lancet 1980;II:1025.

138. Ross SM, Middelkoop AV. Trichomonas infection in pregnancy—Does it affect perinatal outcome? S Afr Med J 1983;63:566-7.

139. Hardy PH, Hardy JB, Nell EE, et al. Prevalence of six sexually transmitted disease agents among pregnant inner-city adolescents and pregnancy outcome. Lancet 1984;II:333-7.

140. Watts DH, Eschenbach DA. Treatment of chlamydia, mycoplasma, and group B streptococcal infections. Clin Obstet Gynecol 1988;31:435-52.

141. Gravett MG, Nelson HP, DeRouen T, et al. Independent associations of bacterial vaginosis and *Chlamydia trachomatis* infection with adverse pregnancy outcome. JAMA 1986;256:1899-1903.

142. Toth M, Witkin S, Ledger W, et al. The role of infection in the etiology of preterm birth. Obstet Gynecol 1988;71:723-6.

143. Tambyraja RL, Salmon JA, Karim SMM, et al. F prostaglandin levels in amniotic fluid in premature labor. Prostaglandins 1977;13:339-48.

144. Mitchell MD, Flint APF, Bibby JG. Plasma concentrations of prostaglandins during late human pregnancy: influence of normal and preterm labor. J Clin Endocrinol Metabol 1978;46:947-51.

145. Sellers SM, Mitchell MD, Bibby JG, et al. A comparison of plasma prostaglandin levels in term and preterm labour. Br J Obstet Gynaecol 1981;88:362-6.

146. Karim SMM, Devlin J. Prostaglandin content of human amniotic fluid. Br J Obstet Gynaecol 1966;74:230-4.

147. Romero R, Emamian M, Wan M, et al. Prostaglandin concentrations in amniotic fluid of women with intra-amniotic infection and preterm labor. Am J Obstet Gynecol 1987;157:1461-7.

148. Weitz CM, Ghodgaonkar RB, Dubin NH, et al. Prostaglandin F metabolite concentration as a prognostic factor in preterm labor. Obstet Gynecol 1986;67:496-9.

149. Nieder J, Augustin W. Concentrations of prostaglandins in amniotic fluid in premature labor. Z Geburtshilfe Perinatol 1984;188:7-11.

150. Romero R, Wu YK, Mazor M, Hobbins JC, Mitchell MD. Amniotic fluid prostaglan-

din E_2 in preterm labor. Prostaglandins, Leukotrienes, and Essential Fatty Acids 1988;34:141-5.

151. Romero R, Wu YK, Sirtori M, Oyarzun E, Mazor M, Hobbins JC, Mitchell MD. Amniotic fluid concentrations of prostaglandin $F_{2\alpha}$,13,14-dihydro-15-keto-11,16-cyclo prostaglandin E_2 (PGEM-II) in preterm labor. Prostaglandins 37;1989:149-61.

152. Romero R, Emamian M, Wan M, et al. Increased concentrations of arachidonic acid lipoxygenase metabolites in amniotic fluid during parturition. Obstet Gynecol 1987;70:849-51.

153. Romero R, Wu YK, Mazor M, et al. Increased amniotic fluid leukotriene C_4 concentration in term human parturition. Am J Obstet Gynecol 1988;159:655-7.

154. Ritchie DM, Hahn DW, McGuire JL. Smooth muscle contraction as a model to study the mediator role of endogenous lipoxygenase products of arachidonic acid. Life Sci 1984;34:509-13.

155. Bennett PR, Elder MG, Myatt L. The effects of lipoxygenase metabolites of arachidonic acid on human myometrial contractility. Prostaglandins 1987;33:837-44.

156. Carraher R, Hahn DW, Ritchie DM, et al. Involvement of lipoxygenase products in myometrial contractions. Prostaglandins 1983;26:23-32.

157. Romero R, Wu YK, Mazor M, Hobbins JC, Mitchell. Amniotic fluid 5-hydroxyeicosatetraenoic acid in preterm labor. Prostaglandins 1988;36:179-87.

158. Romero R, Wu YK, Mazor M, et al. Amniotic fluid arachidonate lipoxygenase metabolites in women with preterm labor. Prostaglandins, Leukotrienes, and Essential Fatty Acids 1989;36:69-75.

159. Bejar R, Curbelo V, Davis C, et al. Premature labor: bacterial sources of phospholipase. Obstet Gynecol 1981;57:479-82.

160. McGregor JA, Lawellin D, Franco-Buff A. Phospholipase A_2 activity of genital tract flora detected with two substrates. Presented at the 32nd Annual Meeting of the Society for Gynecologic Investigation. Phoenix, AZ, 1985.

161. Lamont RF, Rose M, Elder MG. Effects of bacterial production prostaglandin E production by amnion cells. Lancet 1985;II:1131-3.

162. Bennett PR, Rose MP, Myatt L. Preterm labor: stimulation of arachidonic acid metabolism in human amnion by bacterial products. Am J Obstet Gynecol 1987; 156:649-55.

163. Romero R, Kadar N, Hobbins JC, et al. Infection and labor: the detection of endotoxin in amniotic fluid. Am J Obstet Gynecol 1987;157:815-9.

164. Romero R, Hobbins JC, Mitchell MD. Endotoxin stimulates prostaglandin E_2 production by human amnion. Obstet Gynecol 1988;71:227-8.

165. Romero R, Roslansky P, Oyarzun E, et al. Labor and infection, II. Bacterial endotoxin in amniotic fluid and its relationship to the onset of preterm labor. Am J Obstet Gynecol 1988;158:1044-9.

166. Lamont RF, Anthony F, Myatt L, et al. Production of PGE_2 by human amnion in vitro in response to addition of media conditioned by micro-organisms associated with chorioamnionitis and preterm labor (submitted).

167. Romero R, Edwin S, Avila C, Foster J, Wu YK, Mitchell MD. Prostaglandin production by amnion and decidual cells in response to bacterial products. Presented at the 36th Annual Meeting of the Society for Gynecologic Investigation. San Diego, CA, 1989.

168. Dinarello CA. Interleukin-1. Rev Infect Dis 1984;6:51-95.

169. Romero R, Wu YK, Brody DT, Oyarzun E, Duff GW, Durum SK. Human decidua: a

source of interleukin-1. Am J Obstet Gynecol 1989;73:31-4.

170. Romero R, Durum S, Dinarello C, et al. Interleukin-1: a signal for the initiation of labor in chorioamnionitis. Presented at 33rd Annual Meeting of the Society for Gynecologic Investigation. Toronto, March 19–22, 1986.

171. Romero R, Wu YK, Brody DT, Oyarzun E, Duff GW, Durum SK. Human decidua: a source of interleukin-1. Obstet Gynecol 1989;73:31-4.

172. Romero R, Brody DT, Oyarzun E, et al. Infection and labor, III. Interleukin-1: a signal for the onset of parturition. Am J Obstet Gynecol 1989;160:1117-23.

173. Ito A, Hiro D, Ojima Y, et al. Spontaneous production of interleukin-1-like factors from pregnant rabbit uterine cervix. Am J Obstet Gynecol 1988;159:261.

174. Romero R, Manogue KR, Murray MD, et al. Infection and labor, IV. Cachectin-tumor necrosis factor in the amniotic fluid of women with intraamniotic infection and preterm labor. Am J Obstet Gynecol 1989;161:336-41.

175. Casey ML, Cox SM, Beutler B, Milewich L, MacDonald PC. Cachectin/tumor necrosis factor-α formation in human decidua. J Clin Invest 1989;83:430-6.

176. Romero R, Manogue K, Oyarzun E, Wu YK, Cerami A. Human decidua: a source of tumor necrosis factor. Eur J Obstet Gynecol Reprod Biol 1989;33:55-60.

177. Gauldie J, Richards C, Harnish D, Lansdcorp P, Baumann H. Interferon β₂/B-cell hepatocyte-stimulatory factor type 2 shares identity with monocyte-derived hepatocyte stimulating factor and regulates the major acute phase protein response in liver cells. Proc Natl Acad Sci USA 1987;84:7251-5.

178. May LT, Ghrayeb J, Santhanam U, et al. Synthesis and secretion of multiple forms of β₂-interferon/B cell differentiation factor-2-hepatocyte stimulating factor by human fibroblasts and monocytes. J Biol Chem 1988;263:7760-6.

179. May LT, Torcia G, Cozzolino F, et al. Interleukin-6 gene expression in human endothelial cells: RNA start sites, multiple IL-6 proteins and inhibition of proliferation. Biochem Biophys Res Commun 1989;159:991-8.

180. Zhang Y, Lin Y, Vilcek J. Synthesis of interleukin-6 (interferon-β₂/B cell stimulatory factor 2) in human fibroblasts is triggered by an increase in intracellular cyclic AMP. J Biol Chem 1988;263:6177-82.

181. Kupper T, Min K, Sehgal PB, et al. Production of IL-6 by keratinocytes: implications for epidermal inflammation and immunity. Ann NY Acad Sci 1989;557:454-65.

182. Tabibzadeh SS, Santhanam U, Sehgal PB, May LT. Cytokine-induced production of interferon-β₂/interleukin-6 by freshly-explanted human endometrial stromal cells: modulation by estradiol-17β. J Immunol 1989;142:3134-9.

183. Evans MI, Hajj SN, Devoe LD, Angerman NS, Moawad AH. C-reactive protein as a predictor of infectious morbidity with premature rupture of membranes. Am J Obstet Gynecol 1980;138:628-52.

184. Romero R, Avila C, Santhanam U, Sehgal PB. Amniotic fluid interleukin-6 in preterm labor: association with infection. J Clin Invest (in press).

185. Hoffman DR, Romero R, Johnston JM. Detection of platelet-activating factor in amniotic fluid of complicated pregnancies. Am J Obstet Gynecol 1990;162:525-8.

186. Romero R, Oyarzun E, Nores J, et al. The prevalence, microbiology and clinical significance of intraamniotic infection in spontaneous parturition at term. Presented at the 37th annual meeting of the Society for Gynecologic Investigation. St. Louis, MO, 1990.

187. Romero R, Avila C, Callahan R, Mazor M, Hobbins JC, Dinarello C. Interleukin-1α and interleukin-1β in preterm labor and preterm premature rupture of membranes.

Presented at the 10th annual meeting of the Society of Perinatal Obstetricians. Houston, TX, 1990.

188. King JF, Grant A, Keirse MJNC, Chalmars I. β-mimetics in preterm labour: an overview of the randomized controlled trials. Br J Obstet Gynaecol 1988;95:211.

189. Romero R, Salafia C. Unpublished observations.

190. Arias F. Placental insufficiency: an important cause of preterm labor and preterm premature ruptured membranes. Presented at the 10th annual meeting of the Society of Perinatal Obstetricians. Houston, TX, 1990.

191. Garfield RE. Uterine mast cells: immunogenic control of myometrial contractility. Presented at the 36th annual meeting of the Society of Gynecologic Investigation. San Diego, CA, 1989.

25

Uterine Stimulation with Oxytocin

M. Yusoff Dawood

Department of Obstetrics, Gynecology and Reproductive Sciences,
University of Texas Medical School, Houston

F ollowing the demonstration by William Blair Bell in 1909 (1) that human uterine contractions were induced by posterior pituitary extracts given at cesarean section, Hofbauer used posterior pituitary extract for *therapy of delayed labor* in 1911 (2). Subsequently, in 1927 Hofbauer (3) introduced the use of posterior pituitary extract for *induction of labor*. After du Vigneaud et al. (4) identified the structure of oxytocin and subsequently synthesized it in 1953 (5), oxytocin as opposed to posterior pituitary extract became commonly used by obstetricians for induction or augmentation of labor. Buccal pitocin was first reported for induction of labor by Dillon et al. in 1960 (6).

This chapter considers the use of oxytocin to stimulate the pregnant uterus. The indication, route of administration, dose, and regimen of oxytocin employed for stimulating the pregnant uterus will be discussed.

INDICATIONS

Oxytocin is employed to stimulate the pregnant uterus for augmentation of inadequate uterine contractions or treatment of dysfunctional labor, induction of labor, or abortion, and promotion of strong uterine contractions in the immediate postpartum period to prevent or treat excessive hemorrhage. Induction of labor, which is the initiation of labor by artificial means, should no longer be carried out for elective or convenience purposes other than because of medical reason requiring termination of the pregnancy. Thus, induction of labor using oxytocin may be indicated in pregnancies complicated by pre-eclampsia, hypertension, renal disease, diabetes mellitus, intrauterine growth retardation, postdatism, and postmaturity. Intravenous oxytocin, either as a slow bolus dose or as an intravenous infusion drip, is commonly given during the third stage of labor with, or immediately after, delivery of the placenta, both at vaginal and cesarean deliveries. This application of oxytocin promotes increase in uterine tone and thereby reduces blood loss during the third stage of labor and the immediate postpartum period. While labor can be effectively induced either surgically or with an oxytocin, often combined amniotomy and administration of oxytocin are frequently used.

TIMING OF OXYTOCIN ADMINISTRATION

For active management of labor, oxytocin is commonly started as soon as it is deemed that the completion of labor and delivery must be rapidly coaxed along. Under such circumstances, oxytocin is administered, with or without amniotomy, as soon as this decision is reached. The aim of active management of labor is to shorten the duration of labor, and often the latent phase of labor may be compressed, thus contributing to the shortening of the time of labor. Based on percentages of successful amniotomy alone in bringing about labor, oxytocin may be started 6 to 12 h after and should be started by 12 h following rupture of membranes if uterine contractions are not established yet. About 60% will have successfully gone into labor 6 h after amniotomy, and about 80% will have done so 12 h after amniotomy. For augmenting inadequate uterine contractions, oxytocin should be administered as soon as there is evidence of inadequate uterine activity as reflected by reliable tocographic monitoring and abnormal deviation of the labor curve. If used for active management of the third stage of labor or to reduce postpartum hemorrhage during the third stage of labor and thereafter, oxytocin is given immediately after delivery of the infant or after delivery of the placenta.

ROUTE OF ADMINISTRATION

Oxytocin has been administered through four different routes: intranasally as a snuff, transbuccally with buccal pitocin, intramuscularly, and intravenously. Although all these routes have been employed in the past to stimulate uterine contractions in women, at present only the intravenous route of administration should be considered when stimulating the pregnant uterus and for induction of labor in women. However, in veterinary practice, intramuscular injection of oxytocin (40–60 U) at 340 days' gestation or 1 month before term in the mare will induce delivery of a normal foal. A rapid bolus dose of oxytocin should never be given intravenously because of the risk of severe hypotension, reduced coronary perfusion, and cardiac arrest especially if the patient is under anesthesia.

DOSE OF OXYTOCIN

Currently there are two schools of thought regarding the dose of oxytocin to be employed for stimulating uterine contractions in late pregnancy. On the one hand, *physiological doses* of oxytocin (2–4 mU/min) as originally suggested by Theobald et al. (7) are consistent with normal physiology, while *pharmacological doses* of oxytocin for induction of labor have been advocated by those who believe in being guided by the clinical and tocographic end points of strong uterine activity (8, 9). Logical conclusion as to which is the more preferred dose range to be employed when giving oxytocin to stimulate the gravid uterus requires a critical exploration and understanding of both the normal endogenous maternal and fetal circulating levels of oxytocin as well as the factors regulating uterine sensitivity to oxytocin and cervical ripening.

Endogenous Levels of Oxytocin

Although maternal circulating levels of oxytocin increase during pregnancy from its prepregnant levels, there is no further increase in such levels between late pregnancy and the first stage of labor (10–12). The circulating levels of oxytocin in the mother during the first stage of labor are consistent with the levels produced by an oxytocin infusion rate of 2–4 mU/min (13, 14). However, with spontaneous labor, fetal secretion of oxytocin is increased during the first stage of labor (15, 16). We have calculated that the transfer of oxytocin from the fetal compartment toward the maternal side (placenta and uterus) is approximately 2–3 mU/min. These endogenous levels are consistent with, and support the use of physiological doses of oxytocin (2–6 mU/min).

Uterine Sensitivity to Oxytocin

Relatively insensitive to oxytocin in early pregnancy, the human uterus becomes increasingly more responsive to this neuropeptide as pregnancy progresses toward term. Caldeyro-Barcia and Sereno (17) found that uterine sensitivity to oxytocin reaches a maximum at 32 to 36 weeks' gestation in women with no further change in oxytocin sensitivity thereafter. However, Theobald et al. (18) reported that during the last days of pregnancy and before labor, the uterine sensitivity to oxytocin increased by as much as 200- to 1000-fold. In spite of these seemingly different observations just before labor, clinical experience indicates that the uterus becomes highly sensitive to oxytocin as term is approached. This increase in uterine sensitivity to oxytocin is mediated by, and consistent with, the rise in oxytocin receptor concentration in the pregnant human uterus as pregnancy progresses toward term (19). Data obtained both by Caldeyro-Barcia and Theobald indicate that the human uterus at term is very sensitive to physiological doses of oxytocin (2–6 mU/min) and adequate contractions will occur.

Cervical Ripeness

For successful induction of labor, the balance between uterine quiescence and cervical resistance must be shifted toward a balance favoring strong myometrial contractions and reduced cervical resistance or increased cervical ripeness. Thus, while physiological doses of oxytocin may be able to establish good, strong contractions, failure on the part of the cervix to ripen (soften and efface) and thereby decrease its resistance will either prevent or slow the progress of labor. Because traditionally clinical endpoints of uterine stimulation with oxytocin during pregnancy are judged by not only the frequency and strength of uterine contractions, but also the progress of labor as reflected by cervical dilatation and descent of the fetal presenting part, pharmacological doses may be unwittingly resorted to by those who advocate the use of pharmacologic doses of oxytocin. That cervical preparedness as clinically assessed is an important determinant is reflected by the direct correlation between the outcome of induction of labor and Bishop's score of the cervix; induction failure increases from none with a Bishop's score of 9, to 5% with a score of 5 to 8, and to 22% with a score of 4 or less (20).

Evidence from Oxytocin Infusion

Measurements of circulating maternal plasma levels of oxytocin indicate that mean plasma levels of about 50 pg/ml were obtained with 4–6 mU/min of oxytocin infusion during oxytocin-induced labor in women, as well as in pregnant baboons at term (13, 14). These maternal plasma levels are consistent with, and similar to, the levels found in women during the first stage of spontaneous labor.

Based on the dose of oxytocin required for augmentation of labor, Theobald et al. (7) found that 94% of multiparous and 93% of nulliparous women required only up to 5 mU/min of oxytocin for establishment of labor. More recently Seitchik and Castillo (21), using more sophisticated computer-defined uterine contractile activity to assist with titration of the dose of oxytocin given to establish labor, found that 91% of nulliparous and 92% of multiparous women required ≤5 mU/min of oxytocin, a strikingly similar finding to the clinical observations of Theobald et al. (7). Similarly using the automated loop feedback infusion system, which calibrates the dose of oxytocin infused based on active contraction area or uterine activity integral (UAI) over the previous 15 min, Steere et al. (22) also found that labor and delivery were achieved in most women with ≤6 mU/min of oxytocin. From all these various lines of evidence, there is much persuasive data to support the use of physiological doses of oxytocin when given to stimulate uterine contractions in the pregnant uterus during late pregnancy.

REGIMENS FOR ADMINISTRATION OF OXYTOCIN

When given to stimulate the uterus, oxytocin is administered continuously as an intravenous infusion. A variety of regimens exists for the rate and frequency at which the dose is increased, as well as the methods employed for determining effective uterine contractions as an index of response to uterine stimulation. Until recently, the rate of increment of the dose infused was usually every 20 min. Recents pharmacokinetic studies in both pregnant and nonpregnant women and men using constant infusion of oxytocin and reaching steady-state plasma levels indicate that the metabolic clearance rate of oxytocin is unchanged during pregnancy and is about 20–25 ml/kg body weight (23, 24). The half-life of oxytocin is about 10–12 min, which is much longer than the half-life previously estimated based on indirect assessment rather than direct pharmacokinetic determinations. Measurements of plasma oxytocin during constant infusion with incremental doses of oxytocin at intervals of 20–40 min indicate that a minimum duration of 20 min and more, usually 30 min, is necessary to reach a steady-state plasma oxytocin concentration. Using uterine contractions as the index, Caldeyro-Barcia and Heller (25) estimate that it takes about 14 to 60 min to achieve a steady state of uterine response while Seitchik and Castillo (21) suggest 30 min or more. Thus, when giving oxytocin it is probably more valid to increase the dose at a rate not faster

Table 1. Physiological dose of oxytocin required for augmentation of labor.

Investigator	Parity	Number of Patients	Oxytocin (mU/min)		
			<3 (%)	3–5 (%)	>5 (%)
Theobald et al., 1948 (7)	0	61	30 (49)	27 (44)	4 (7)
Seitchik and Castillo, 1983 (21)*	0	45	15 (33)	26 (58)	4 (9)
Theobald et al., 1948 (7)	≥1	49	23 (47)	23 (47)	3 (6)
Seitchik and Castillo, 1983 (21)	≥1	34	20 (59)	12 (35)	2 (6)
Theobald et al., 1948 (7)	All	110	53 (48)	50 (46)	7 (6)
Seitchik and Castillo, 1983 (21)	All	79	35 (44)	38 (48)	6 (8)

*Used computer-defined uterine contractile activity.

than every 30 min. The balance of evidence (see above) currently favors using a physiological dose of oxytocin when stimulating the pregnant uterus. The studies of Theobald et al. (7), Seitchik and Castillo (21), and Steere et al. (22) have clearly established that more than 90% of women at term can have their uteri successfully stimulated with ≤6 mU/min of oxytocin to achieve delivery. Nevertheless, the advocates of pharmacologic doses of oxytocin (8) and active management of labor (26) recommend increasing the dose of oxytocin to significantly higher levels that are unquestionably pharmacologic. Pharmacological doses of oxytocin are probably appropriate for those gravid women whose uteri will not respond to physiological doses of oxytocin, but are not necessary in all term pregnant women. To be able to reliably separate those women who require pharmacological doses of oxytocin from those who require physiological doses, it is necessary to employ well-defined, sensitive indices of uterine contractility, as well as other clinical parameters of uterine sensitivity to oxytocin. While the Bishop's score of the cervix is often employed to show correlation with successful outcome of induction of labor, there is insufficient or no published data to show a correlation between the amount of oxytocin required to stimulate the term uterus and cervical ripeness.

Of equal importance is the starting dose of oxytocin employed to initiate uterine contractions at term. Clearly, a higher starting dose is more likely to end up with a much larger peak or maintenance dose given a regime with similar rates of dose increments. Wein (27) found that if the starting dose is high (3.3 mU/min), the maintenance dose increased to higher levels than when the initial dose is low (0.7 mU/min). Likewise, if the dose is doubled with every increment, as opposed to a fixed number of milliunits, the peak or maintenance dose of oxytocin reached will also be higher and more likely to be in the pharmacological dose range. The studies that have shown that the physiological doses of oxytocin are adequate indicate that the rate of oxytocin to be increased with each increment should not exceed 1.0 mU/min. The starting dose currently employed in many protocols is either 0.5 mU/min, or 1.0 mU/min. Data available from oxytocin challenge tests suggests that 0.5 mU/min may be able to produce tocographically detectable uterine contractions, but these contractions are likely to be effective to bring about labor unless the patient was already in labor on her own initiative. Furthermore, very few patients will successfully go into labor when induced with 0.5 mU/min of oxytocin (21). Thus, an initial dose of 1.0 mU/min is preferable, but it is difficult to justify recommending initial doses of 6 mU/min or more (26, 28).

In the computer-defined uterine contractility studies of Seitchik and his colleagues (21) and in the closed-loop automatic uterine activity defined feedback loop system employed by Steere (22), the dose of oxytocin necessary to bring about uterine contractions is 6 mU or less. Much higher doses were given in the group monitored with internal tocography, but without a computer-defined, or integrated uterine-response feedback protocol system. Therefore, in spite of uterine contractility monitoring with open-ended intrauterine pressure catheters, there is a tendency to increase the dose of oxytocin when the uterine contraction information is processed only clinically, as opposed to being constantly and mathematically defined. Furthermore, the initial uterine response to oxytocin stimulation is an incremental phase during which uterine contractions progressively increase in frequency and strength, followed by a stable phase during which time any further increase in oxytocin dose will not lead to further normal changes in the contraction (29). The clinical assessment or interpretation of nonmathematically defined uterine contractions accounts for the higher doses of oxytocin being given by overshooting the stable phase of the uterine response to oxytocin. This curvilinear response of the uterus to oxytocin stimulation allows for the forgiving nature of oxytocin and the side effects being less frequently observed than expected.

Table 2 summarizes the intravenous oxytocin dose regimen to be used for induction of labor as suggested by the American College of Obstetricians and Gynecologists Technical Bulletin (30). Based on many of the above considerations, we suggest the regimen outlined in Table 3. An initial starting dose of 1.0 mU/min rather than 0.5 mU/min is preferred, while the dose increment should be 1.0 mU/min until 8 mU/min, followed by 2–4 mU/min until 24 mU/min. The greater increments after 8 mU/min take into consideration the fact that most women will

Table 2.   Intravenous oxytocin regimen for induction of labor.

Initial dose:	0.5 mU/min
Increments:	To 1 mU/min; then 1–2 mU/min
Rate of increment:	Every 30–60 min
Objective:	Uterine contractions
	Lasting 40–90 sec
	Every 2–3 min
	Intensity 40–90 mmHg
Resting tone:	≤15–20 mmHg
Endpoint:	Adequate progress of labor

Source: Derived from American College of Obstetrics and Gynecologists, Induction and augmentation, Technical Bulletin No 110, Am Coll Obstet Gynecol, Washington, DC, 1987.

Table 3. Suggested regimen for continuous intravenous infusion of oxytocin for induction of labor.

Initial dose:	1 mU/min
Increments:	1 mU/min until 8 mU/min
	Then 2–4 mU/min until 20 mU/min
Rate of increment:	Every 30 min
Objective:	Uterine contractions
	Lasting 40–90 sec
	Every 2–3 min
	Intensity 40–90 mmHg
	150–250 Montevideo units
Resting tone:	≤15–20 mmHg
Endpoint:	Adequate progress of labor

have responded to doses of oxytocin within the physiological range, and the few who will not have established adequate uterine contractions probably may have uterine sensitivity or cervical ripeness significantly different from normal. The rate of increment is 30 min rather than up to 60 min because a steady state is readily achieved during this interval. It might be preferable to add a better defined mathematical endpoint than the Montevideo units as suggested in Table 2, but the computer formulation employed by Seitchik and his colleagues (21) is not readily available for clinical use and the active contraction area of uterine activity integral (UAI) as employed by other investigators (31) has widely differing normal values that have to be established for each population or center.

A noteworthy clinical observation is the continuing maintenance of sustained good uterine contractions once labor is established even when the maintenance dose of oxytocin is reduced. The mechanisms responsible for such a maintenance in the face of a reduced dose of exogenous oxytocin could be due to (*a*) increased enodgeonous oxytocin release, be it from the mother or fetus, (*b*) increased uterine sensitivity to oxytocin by changes in either uterine oxytocin receptors or the receptor binding kinetics, and (*c*) oxytocin-induced release of prostaglandins that further maintains the uterine contractions. Oxytocin can induce release of prostaglandins (32–34), but whether this is the mechanism accounting for the above observation remains to be proven. Nevertheless, the ability to reduce the oxytocin maintenance dose once labor is established without significantly altering uterine contractions is worthy of consideration when stimulating the uterus with oxytocin.

Pulsatile Administration of Oxytocin

Many neuropeptides are secreted in pulses or episodically. Consequently, some neurohormones are administered in a pulsatile fashion. Whereas endogenous oxytocin is secreted in pulses or spurts during human labor (11, 35, 36), exogenous oxytocin is given as a continuous intravenous infusion to stimulate uterine contractions. Continuous administration of oxytocin intravenously appears to be inconsistent with our understanding of the physiology and metabolism of oxytocin. Oxytocin exerts its uterotonic effect through a receptor-mediated mechanism, specific receptors for which have been shown to be present in the smooth-muscle cells of the uterus and mammary gland. When oxytocin binds to its myometrial receptors, the duration of its inavailability, replenishment, or recycling is not known. Therefore, when oxytocin is given as a continuous intravenous infusion and especially in supraphysiologic doses, the myometrial oxytocin receptors are bound, become temporarily not available to more oxytocin, which is being continuously infused, or the receptors may progressively become saturated and unable to bind more oxytocin temporarily. With these considerations, it appears that pulsed administration, similar to pulsatile endogenous oxytocin release, may be a more physiologic regimen, provide a more rational and safer way of administering oxytocin, and reduce the total dose of oxytocin given. In a preliminary study on women undergoing amniotomy followed by pulsed administration of oxytocin given 1 min of every 10 min, Pavlou et al. (37) found that it lowered the total dose of oxytocin given and was just as effective as the continuous intravenous infusion method. In the last 4 years, we have conducted three separate randomized studies (38–40) to compare the efficacy and safety of pulsatile administration of oxytocin with a standard continuous intravenous administration.

Regimen for Pulsatile Administration of Oxytocin. In our regimen, oxytocin was delivered in pulsatile boluses every 8 min by an intermittent infusion pump (Model AS-2C, Autosyringe, Hooksett, NH) with each bolus given over a 10-sec period. The starting dose was 1.0 mU/pulse, and the pulse dose was doubled every 24 min (after every 3 pulses) as needed to obtain adequate uterine activity, which was defined as at least 3 uterine contractions of 160 or more Montevideo units in a 10-min period.

Continuous intravenous infusion of oxytocin was administered via an IMED 927 pump (IMED Corporation, San Diego, CA) starting with a dose of 1.0 mU/min and increased by 1.0 mU/min every 30 min for the induction group (38, 40), but 1.0 mU/min every 20 min for the uterine augmentation group (39). The dose was increased as needed to attain adequate uterine activity. All patients in all the three studies had an intrauterine pressure catheter placed upon starting oxytocin for the study on augmentation of labor (39), and as soon as membranes could be ruptured for the induction of labor studies (38, 40). For each of the three studies, the clinical characteristics of patients receiving either pulsed or continuous oxytocin infusion within each study were not significantly different.

Augmentation of Labor with Pulsed Administration of Oxytocin

In a recently reported study (39), we examined 94 patients with term pregnancies who underwent augmentation of labor with either continuous (n = 48) or pulsed (n = 46) intravenous oxytocin infusion (see Fig. 1). To compare the mean dose of oxytocin required, the pulsed doses were converted to milliunits per minute. With

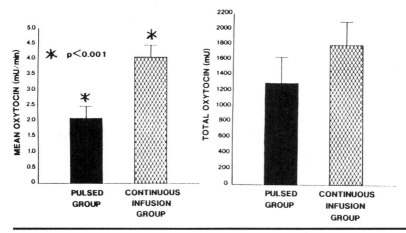

Fig. 1. Mean or average dose of oxytocin (left panel) and total dose of oxytocin (right panel) used for pulsed administration (46 patients) versus continuous intravenous infusion of oxytocin (48 patients). The bar graphs show the mean ± SEM.

pulsed administration, a significantly lower mean dose of oxytocin (2.1 ± 0.4 mU/ min) was required than with the continuous administration (4.1 ± 0.4 mU/min; P = < 0.001). The total dose of oxytocin required was also lower with pulsed administration (1300 ± 332 mU) than with continuous administration (1803 ± 302 mU). Even when controlled for gravidity, the mean dose of oxytocin was significantly lower with pulsed administration than with continuous administration. However, the mean rate of increase in uterine contractions in Montevideo units (calculated by subtracting the baseline uterine activity from the adequate uterine activity reached, divided by the number of hours between these two activities for each subject) receiving pulsed oxytocin was higher than in patients receiving continuous oxytocin regardless of the route of fetal delivery.

Hyperstimulation—defined as 5 or more uterine contractions in succession without return to baseline tonus, or prolonged uterine contraction that caused fetal bradycardia—did not occur with either method of oxytocin administration. There were no significant differences with respect to the labor characteristics of patients who received either pulse or continuous oxytocin infusion for augmentation of their labor (Table 4). The incidence of cesarean section was not significantly different between the two methods of oxytocin administration. The mean birth weight of the infants delivered in the pulsed oxytocin group (3327 ± 68 g) was not significantly different from that in the continuous oxytocin group (3288 ± 74 g). Although 43 of 46 infants in the pulsed oxytocin group had Apgar scores of 7 or more at 1 min, while only 41 of 48 in the continuous oxytocin group had similar Apgar scores, the difference was not significant.

Pulsatile Oxytocin for Induction of Labor

In a prospective, pilot, randomized study, we compared the efficacy and safety of pulsed administration of oxytocin with continuous intravenous oxytocin infusion in

Table 4. Labor characteristics of patients who had augmentation of labor with either pulsed or continuous oxytocin infusion.

Augmentation of Labor	Pulsed-Oxytocin Group (n = 46)	Continuous Oxytocin Group (n = 48)	Differences Between Treatment Groups
Onset of oxytocin to delivery	401.8 ± 43.9 min[a]	386.0 ± 36.6 min	NS
Onset of oxytocin to adequate labor[b]	198.2 ± 27.4 min[c]	157.3 ± 12.1 min[d]	NS
Pain medication during labor	34.8%	35.4%	NS
Epidural anesthesia during labor	23.9%	22.9%	NS
Contraction pattern			
Normal	78.3%	79.2%	NS
Dysfunctional[e]	21.7%	20.8%	NS

Source: From Cummiskey KC, Gall SA, Dawood MY, Pulsatile administration of oxytocin for augmentation of labor, Obstet Gynecol 1989;74:869-72.

NS = Not significant.

[a]Mean ± SEM.   [b]Regular uterine contractions ≥160 Montevideo units.

[c]n = 40.   [d]n = 45.

[e]Defined as coupling or tripling of uterine contractions for 1 h or more during labor.

20 term pregnant women who had medical indication for induction of labor (38). We found no significant difference between the two methods of giving oxytocin with respect to the time interval until adequate labor, the induction-delivery interval, the vaginal delivery rate, the change in hemoglobin, the pain medications needed, and the Apgar scores at 1 min and 5 min. Significant, however, was the finding that pulsed administration of oxytocin halved both the total dose and highest dose of oxytocin infused per minute (Fig. 2). The peak, or highest, dose of oxytocin, was only 5.2 ± 0.8 mU/min with pulsed administration, but 9.2 ± 1.8 mU/min with continuous intravenous infusion (P = <0.05).

Because the number of subjects in this pilot study was small, we conducted another labor induction study with a new set of patients: 106 women who needed induction of labor for medical indications and who received either pulsed administration (n = 50) or continuous intravenous infusion of oxytocin (n = 56) in a randomized prospective study (40). The maternal characteristics (gestational ages, age at induction), induction-delivery interval analgesia for labor, cesarean section rates, and most of the newborn characteristics were similar with both methods of giving oxytocin. However, several differences emerged with respect to the dose of oxytocin used, the relationship between Bishop's score, and the amount of oxytocin for each method of oxytocin administration and jaundice in the newborn. We found that the total dose of oxytocin given (3564 ± 487 mU for pulsed oxytocin vs. 7684 ± 844 mU for continuous oxytocin), the average dose per minute (3.9 ± 0.3 mU/min for pulsed oxytocin vs. 7.8 ± 0.4 mU/min for continuous oxytocin) and the peak dose administered (9.6 ± 0.8 mU/min for pulsed oxytocin vs. 14.1 ± 0.7 mU/min for continuous oxytocin) were significantly lower in all instances with pulsed oxytocin.

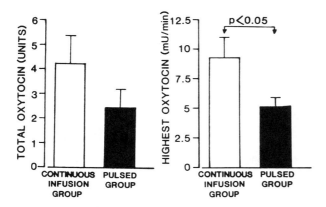

Fig. 2. Doses (mean ± SEM) required for induction of labor using pulsed or continuous intravenous infusion of oxytocin. (From Odem RR, Work BA, Dawood MY, Pulsatile oxytocin for induction of labor: a randomized prospective controlled study, J Perinat Med 1988;16:31-7.)

The differences persisted even when controlled for parity so that in primagravida as well as multigravida, pulsed administration of oxytocin resulted in a much lower dose than with continuous infusion. Similarly, the difference persisted even when controlled for the number of days induction was carried out (1, 2, or 3 days) and for Bishop's score of the cervix. It is noteworthy that we found with both continuous infusion and pulsed administration of oxytocin, the dose of oxytocin required was directly related to the Bishop's score, but was always significantly lower with pulsed administration than with continuous administration. The incidence of uterine hyperstimulation was infrequent and was similar with both methods of giving oxytocin infusion. Noteworthy is the finding that pulsed administration required a significantly smaller infusion fluid volume than the continuous group. This is an advantage in high-risk conditions requiring close monitoring or restriction of fluids, as in patients with pre-eclampsia, pulmonary edema, cardiac, and renal diseases. Cesarean section rate was 6% in the pulsed group and 12.5% in the continuous oxytocin group. Even when the patients who required cesarean section were excluded, the pulsed group continued, receiving significantly less total mean and peak doses of oxytocin than the continuous infusion group.

ADVERSE EFFECTS OF OXYTOCIN

When given to stimulate the pregnant uterus, oxytocin can potentially produce adverse effects on the mother, including uterine hypertonus, tetany, uterine rupture, water intoxication, and on the fetus, including fetal distress, fetal hypoxia, and an increased incidence of neonatal hyperbilirubinemia.

Fetal Effects

The risk of developing neonatal hyperbilirubinemia is dependent on both the total dose of oxytocin given to the mother and the maturity of the fetus (38–40). Thus, giving a lower total dose of oxytocin using physiological doses and administering it in a pulsatile fashion should widen the margin of safety for, and reduce the risk of, developing neonatal hyperbilirubinemia. Although the number of patients recently studies by us (40) may be considered to be still small, we found three infants in the pulsed oxytocin group and five infants in the continuous oxytocin group developed clinically recognizable and biochemically confirmed neonatal hyperbilirubinemia. It is particularly noteworthy that the three infants in the pulsed oxytocin group were preterm with lower birth weights and lower maximum levels of pretreatment serum bilirubin than the five infants in the continuous-oxytocin group, who were larger and had higher bilirubin levels.

Buchan (43) found an increased incidence of neonatal hyperbilirubinemia when more than 4500 mU of oxytocin was given to the mother. Because pulsed administration of oxytocin for induction of labor delivers only 3200–3600 mU, the incidence of hyperbilirubinemia should not increase with such a regimen. Oxytocin increases osmotic swelling and deformability of erythrocytes in a time- and dose-dependent manner to induce hemolysis, an effect similar to that of vasopressin (44), as well as increased osmotic fragility of erythrocytes due to transplacental hyponatremia and hyposmolality to bring about neonatal hyperbilirubinemia (43, 45, 46).

Although some still believe that oxytocin increases the incidence of fetal distress (47), a recent randomized study of oxytocin for correction of active-phase abnormalities of labor did not find any increase in the need for cesarean delivery for fetal distress (48). In a long-term follow-up study of children delivered after oxytocin-induced or spontaneous labors, no significant differences could be uncovered in either the neurologic or developmental indices between the two groups (49).

Maternal Effects

Because of the potential risk of uterine rupture, there has been much reticence in using oxytocin to stimulate uterine contractions in patients with previous cesarean sections and twins. There is no clear data to support this contention. On the contrary, careful studies have concluded that there is no contraindication to the use of oxytocin to stimulate the multigravid uterus, or the uterus with twin pregnancy, or a previous cesarean section scar as long as there is no insuperable fetopelvic disproportion, and there is adequate monitoring of uterine contractions and fetal heart (50–54).

To avoid or detect oxytocin-associated uterine hyperstimulation, electronic monitoring of the uterine response is essential. While the latent phase of labor can be effectively shortened by as much as 50% with oxytocin (55), the characteristics of the uterine contraction are not uniformly agreed upon. There is an incremental phase of 1.5–2.0 h in uterine activity in oxytocin induced labor, after which there is no further increase in uterine activity in the subsequent stable phase of 3.5–4.0 h (29). Thus, once the stable phase is reached, further augmentation in uterine activity cannot be produced with oxytocin, but there is an increased risk of hypretonus. In one study, the frequency, intensity, and amplitude of oxytocin-induced contractions as well as the variability between contractions were found to be similar to those in spontaneous labor (55). With computer analysis, oxytocin-induced uterine contractions had higher rates of increase in uterine pressure and shorter duration of contraction, but the analysis also included dysfunctional labor treated with oxytocin (56, 57).

Most of the maternal adverse effects of oxytocin can be avoided by appropriate administration of oxytocin, ensuring no overdosing and starting with low doses of oxytocin (1 mU/min), adequate supervision, sensitive monitoring of uterine pressure, and increasing the dose at sufficient intervals. Water intoxication can be avoided by use of physiological saline rather than sodium-free infusion fluids, and also with pulsed administration of oxytocin requiring significantly less infusion fluid volume.

REFERENCES

1. Blair-Bell W. The pituitary body and the therapeutic value of the infundibular extract in shock, uterine atony and intestinal paresis. Br Med J 1909;2:1609-10.
2. Hofbauer J. Hypophysenextrakt als Wehenmittel. Zentralbl Gynaekol 1911;35:137-8.
3. Hofbauer J, Hoerner JK. The nasal application of pituitary extract for the induction of labor. Am J Obstet Gynecol 1927;14:137-48.
4. du Vigneaud V, Ressler C, Trippett S. The sequence of amino acids in oxytocin, with a proposal for the structure of oxytocin. J Biol Chem 1953;205:949-57.
5. du Vigneaud V, Ressler C, Swan JM, et al. The synthesis of an octapeptide amide with the hormonal activity of oxytocin. J Am Chem Soc 1953;75:4879-80.
6. Dillon TF, Douglas RG, du Vigneaud V, et al. Transbuccal administration of oxytocin for induction and stimulation of labor. Obstet Gynecol 1960;15:587-92.
7. Theobald GW, Graham A, Campbell J, et al. The use of posterior pituitary extracts in physiological amounts in obstetrics: a preliminary report. Br Med J 1948;2:123-7.
8. Turnbull AC, Anderson ABM. Induction of labor: results with amniotomy and oxytocin titration. J Obstet Gynaecol Br Commonw 1968;75:32-41.
9. Toaff ME, Hexroni J, Toaff R. Induction of labor by pharmacological and physiological doses of intravenous oxytocin. Br J Obstet Gynaecol 1978;85:101-8.
10. Dawood MY, Raghavan K, Pociask C. Radioimmunoassay of oxytocin. J Endocrinol 1978;76:261-70.
11. Dawood MY, Ylikorkala O, Trivedi D, et al. Oxytocin in maternal circulation and amniotic fluid during pregnancy. J Clin Endocrinol Metab 1979;49:429-34.
12. Dawood MY, Raghavan K, Pociask C, et al. Oxytocin in human pregnancy and parturition. Obstet Gynecol 1978;51:138-43.
13. Dawood MY, Lauersen NH, Trivedi D, et al. Studies on oxytocin in the baboon during pregnancy and delivery. Acta Endocrinol 1979;91:704-18.
14. Fuchs A-R, Fuchs F, Husslein P, et al. Oxytocin receptors in the human uterus during pregnancy and parturition. Am J Obstet Gynecol 1984;150:734-41.
15. Dawood MY, Wang CF, Gupta R, et al. Fetal contribution to oxytocin in human labor. Obstet Gynecol 1978;52:205-9.
16. Chard T, Hudson CIV, Edwards CRW, et al. Release of oxytocin and vasopressin by the human fetus during labor. Nature 1971;234:352-4.
17. Caldeyro-Barcia R, Sereno JA. The response of the human uterus to oxytocin

throughout pregnancy. In: Caldeyro-Barcia R, Heller H, eds. Oxytocin. New York: Pergamon Press, 1961:177.

18. Theobald GW, Robards MF, Suter PEN. Changes in myometrial sensitivity to oxytocin in man during the last six weeks of pregnancy. Br J Obstet Gynaecol 1969; 76:385-93.

19. Fuchs A-R, Goeschen K, Husslein P, et al. Oxytocin and initiation of human parturition, III. Plasma concentrations of oxytocin and 13, 14-dihydro, 15-keto-prostaglandin $F_{2\alpha}$ in spontaneous and oxytocin-induced labor at term. Am J Obstet Gynecol 1983;147:497-502.

20. Bishop EH. Pelvic scoring for elective induction. Obstet Gynecol 1964;24:266-8.

21. Seitchik J, Castillo M. Oxytocin augmentation of dysfunctional labor, II. Uterine activity data. Am J Obstet Gynecol 1983;145:526-9.

22. Steere PJ, Carter MC, Choong K, et al. A multicenter prospective randomized controlled trial for induction of labor with an automatic closed-loop feedback controlled oxytocin infusion system. Br J Obstet Gynaecol 1985;92:1127-33.

23. Dawood MY, Ylikorkala O, Trivedi D, Fuchs F. Oxytocin levels and disappearance rate and plasma follicle-stimulating hormone and luteinizing after oxytocin infusion in man. J Clin Endocrinol Metab 1980;50:397-400.

24. Leake RD, Weitzman RE, Fisher DA. Pharmacokinetics of oxytocin in the human subject. Obstet Gynecol 1980;56:701-4.

25. Caldeyro-Barcia R, Heller H. Oxytocin. New York: Pergamon Press, 1961:129-30.

26. O'Driscoll K, Jackson RJA, Gallagher JT. Prevention of prolonged labor. Br Med J 1969;2:447-80.

27. Wein P. Efficacy of different starting doses of oxytocin for induction of labor. Obstet Gynecol 1989;74:863-8.

28. Barber HRK, Graber EA, Orlando A. Augmented labor. Obstet Gynecol 1972;39:933-41.

29. Woolfson J, Steere PJ, Bashford CC, et al. The management of uterine activity in induced labour. Br J Obstet Gynaecol 1976;83:934-7.

30. American College of Obstetricians and Gynecologists. Induction and augmentation. Technical Bulletin No 110. Washington, DC: Am Coll Obstet Gynecol, 1987.

31. Steere PJ, Carter MC, Beard RW. normal levels of active contraction area in spontaneous labour. Br J Obstet Gynaecol 1984;91:211-9.

32. Roberts JS, McCracken JA, Gavagan JE, et al. Oxytocin stimulated release of prostaglandin $F_{2\alpha}$ in vitro: correlation with estrus cycle and oxytocin binding. Endocrinology 1976;99:1107-14.

33. Chan WY. Relationship between the uterotonic action of oxytocin and prostaglandins: oxytocin action and release of PG activity in isolated nonpregnant and pregnant rat uteri. Biol Reprod 1977;17:541-8.

34. Fuchs A-R, Fuchs F, Husslein P, et al. Oxytocin receptors and human parturition: a dual role for oxytocin in the initiation of labor. Science 1982;215:1396-8.

35. Chard T. Boyd NRH, Forsling ML, McNeilly AS, Landon J. The development of a radioimmunoassay for oxytocin: the extraction of oxytocin from plasma and its measurement during parturition in human and goat blood. J Endocrinol 1970;48: 223-34.

36. Chard T, Gibbens GL. Spurt release of oxytocin during surgical induction of labor in women. Am J Obstet Gynecol 1983;147:678-80.

37. Pavlou C, Barker GH, Roberts A, et al. Pulsed oxytocin infusion in the induction of

labour. Br J Obstet Gynaecol 1978;85:96-100.

38. Odem RR, Work BA, Dawood MY. Pulsatile oxytocin for induction of labor: a randomized prospective controlled study. J Perinat Med 1988;16:31-7.

39. Cummiskey KC, Gall SA, Dawood MY. Pulsatile administration of oxytocin for augmentation of labor. Obstet Gynecol 1989;74:869-72.

40. Cummiskey KC, Dawood MY. Induction of labor with pulsatile oxytocin. Am J Obstet Gynecol (submitted).

41. Beazley JM, Alderman B. Neonatal hyperbilirubinemia following use of oxytocin in labour. Br J Obstet Gynaecol 1975;82:265-71.

42. D'Souza SW, Black P, MacFarlane T, Richards B. The effect of oxytocin in induced labour on neonatal jaundice. Br J Obstet Gynaecol 1979;86:133-8.

43. Buchan PC. Pathogenesis of neonatal hyperbilirubinemia after induction of labour with oxytocin. Br Med J 1979;1:1255-57.

44. Singhi S, Singh M. Pathogenesis of oxytocin-induced neonatal hyperbilirubinemia. Arch Dis Child 1979;15:399-402.

45. Singhi S, Singh M. Transplacental asymptomatic hyponatremia following oxytocin infusion during labour. Indian J Med Res 1979;70:55-7.

46. D'Souza SW, Lieberman B, Cadman J, Richards B. Oxytocin induction of labour: hyponatraemia and neonatal jaundice. Eur J Obstet Gynecol Reprod Biol 1976;22:309-17.

47. Friedman EA, Sachtleben, MR. High risk labor. J Reprod Med 1971;7:28-32.

48. Cardozo L, Pearce JM. Oxytocin in active-phase abnormalities of labor: a randomized study. Obstet Gynecol 1990;75:152-7.

49. Friedman EA, Sachtleben, MR, Wallare AK. Infant outcome following labor induction. Am J Obstet Gynecol 1979;133:718-22.

50. Horenstein JM, Phelan JP. Previous cesarean section: the risks and benefits of oxytocin usage in a trial of labor. Am J Obst Gynecol 1985;151:564-9.

51. Flamm BL, Dunnett C, Fischerman E, Quilligan EJ. Vaginal delivery following cesarean section: use of oxytocin augmentation and epidural anesthesia with internal tocodynamic and internal fetal monitoring. Am J Obstet Gynecol 1984;148:759-63.

52. Silver RK, Gibb RS. Predictors of vaginal delivery in patients with a previous cesarean section who require cesarean section. Am J Obstet Gynecol 1987;156:57-60.

53. Dawood MY, Lim YL, Ratnam SS. Twin pregnancy in Singapore. Aust NZ J Obstet Gynecol 1975;15:93-8.

54. Dawood MY, Ratnam SS, Ng R. Oxytocin stimulation and uterine rupture in the grandmultipara. Singapore Med J 1974;15:40-4.

55. Lindmark G, Nilsson BA. A comparative study of uterine activity in labor induced with prostaglandin $F_{2\alpha}$ or oxytocin and in spontaneous labor. Acta Obstet Gynecol Scand 1977;56:87-94.

56. Seitchick J, Chakoff ML. Oxytocin-induced uterine hypercontractility pressure wave forms. Obstet Gynecol 1976;48:436-41.

57. Seitchik J, Chatkoff ML, Hayashi RH. Intrauterine pressure waveform characteristics of spontaneous and oxytocin- or prostaglandin $F_{2\alpha}$-induced active labor. Am J Obstet Gynecol 1977;127:223-7.

26

Preterm Inhibition of Myometrial Contractility: Clinical Considerations

Robert K. Creasy

Department of Obstetrics, Gynecology and Reproductive Sciences, University of Texas Medical School, Houston

T here appears to be little question that preterm labor and delivery is the most serious reproductive problem, in terms of perinatal mortality and morbidity, and adverse economic and social impact, facing obstetricians in the 1990s. Our understanding of parturition, as outlined elsewhere in this book has seen progress in recent years but is still not complete. Until we fathom the age-old question of what initiates parturition, we must try to use effectively all of the clinical modalities we have in the most prudent manner to decrease the size of the problem of preterm delivery.

PREVENTION OF PRETERM LABOR

There are obviously two main ways to prevent spontaneous preterm delivery. First is the prevention of the initiation of labor, and the second is the successful inhibition of spontaneous preterm labor. To clinically attack the first issue (i.e., the prevention of the initiation of preterm labor), we must be able to predict that spontaneous preterm labor will subsequently occur in a given patient with a degree of discrimination that warrants some sort of preventive intervention, such as behavioral modification or drug therapy. Most of the current modalities have at best a positive predictive value of only 20%–35% and a sensitivity of 40%–70% (1-3). A sensitive and inexpensive method of predicting preterm labor, such as a colorimetric dipstick to check morning saliva or urine, with a positive predictive value of over 75%, is needed, but awaits further scientific knowledge. For the present, any prevention trial needs to suffer a high possibility of a patient not having the problem the trial is designed to prevent, and makes proper analysis difficult.

INHIBITION OF PRETERM LABOR

A series of difficulties confronts our attempts at inhibiting preterm labor. These include the method to diagnosis preterm labor, the early detection of the process in order to be able to use tocolysis, and the agent or agents by which to achieve satisfactory inhibition.

Diagnosis of Preterm Labor

It is axiomatic when considering tocolytic agents that one must be able to make a correct diagnosis of preterm labor. Unfortunately, the accurate diagnosis of preterm labor continues to be an enigma for the clinical obstetrician. The first component that creates difficulty is that the duration of a gestation is frequently unknown, although the widespread application of ultrasound mensuration has decreased this part of the problem. The issue of whether or not true preterm labor is present is not easy unless the process is far advanced, a time when tocolytic therapy is less efficacious. In preterm patients with regular contractions every 2–5 min, there is a 35%–60% chance that placebo therapy alone can achieve a term birth if this is the only criteria used (4, 5). The incorporation of cervical change into the criteria lowers the possibility of a false diagnosis to 10%–20% (6). Difficulties in making an accurate diagnosis obviously compound the problem of analyzing results of tocolytic trials. It is important that appropriate power calculations, with this error in mind, be done before such trials are undertaken. Once again, further basic and clinical research is needed to provide a method by which a rapid and accurate diagnosis can be made. In the meantime, the criteria for a diagnosis of preterm labor should include regular uterine contractions and ruptured membranes. If the membranes are intact, cervical change should also be documented, or the cervix should be well-effaced or more than 2 cm dilated.

Early Detection of Preterm Labor

Most reports of a decade or more showed that approximately only 10% of patients with spontaneous preterm birth were actually candidates for the use of labor-inhibiting drugs (7, 8). Various programs that have given some hope of decreasing the incidence of preterm birth have focused upon improving the early diagnosis of preterm labor and increasing the number of patients who are candidates for a trial of tocolysis (9–11). Results of these early diagnosis programs have been mixed, with poorer results noted in particular in patients of lower socioeconomic status. In general, the various components of these programs consist of risk evaluation of patients and then weekly or biweekly visits stressing education of warning signs, possible cervical evaluation, and daily sampling of uterine activity by palpation or instrumental monitoring in the home setting.

Controversy has existed over whether the home programs for daily monitoring of uterine activity, which in essence consist of instrumental monitoring of uterine activity and daily contact by a trained nurse, are associated with a decrease in preterm births. Both the Diagnostic and Therapeutic Technology Assessment panel of the Journal of the American Medical Associates (12) and a recent National Institute of Health workshop on the subject have concluded that this approach is associated with a decreased incidence of preterm birth in high-risk patients, but that the relative contributions of the daily nursing contact and the instrumental monitoring remain to be determined.

Interestingly, approximately 30%–45% of the control patients in these recent trials, patients who had only special education and more frequent visits, and perhaps phone contact 2 times per week, were candidates for tocolysis (11, 13, 14). This is a marked improvement over the 10% candidacy rate previously reported, indicating that improvement in early diagnosis can be made with somewhat simple approaches. The tocolytic agents used in these randomized controlled trials demonstrating decreased preterm births were generally β-adrenergic compounds or magnesium sulfate for initial tocolysis and oral β-adrenergics for long-term maintenance therapy.

β-ADRENERGIC TOCOLYSIS

The β-adrenergic compounds and magnesium sulfate are currently the most widely utilized agents for tocolytic therapy in the United States. Considerable controversy continues concerning the efficacy of these agents in regard to decreasing preterm birth and the sequelae of preterm delivery. Beneficial results obtained in association with some early preterm labor detection programs, both historically based and in prospective randomized trials, and in placebo controlled trials have not been reproduced in other centers with similar studies (9–11, 14). Potential explanations for these disparate findings include the following: a high potential for a false diagnosis of preterm labor, rigid rather than malleable treatment protocols resulting in a lack of treating an individual patient's need, a lack of knowledge of pharmacokinetics of agents used, risk and benefit considerations, variable definition of side effects that can lead to treatment cessation, potential of preselection bias, difficulty in recruitment of patients leading to protracted studies inviting entry of confounding variables over time, etc. There appears to be little controversy over their ability to initially inhibit myometrial activity, but the duration of effect is widely questioned (15).

Although these compounds have been in extensive use for over two decades, uniformity of opinion remains minimal as to appropriate dosage and optimal route and method of delivery. Indeed, it has only been in the past few years, that good pharmacokinetic data has become available concerning the use of β-adrenergic compounds in pregnant patients (16, 17). It has been shown that there is wide variability in plasma concentrations of ritodrine in pregnant women who receive similar infusion rates, even with correction for body weight or surface area. This variability is mainly due to major differences in clearness. Although plasma ritodrine is cleared rapidly, over 2 h is required for the concentration in plasma to be reduced by half, indicating extreme binding in extravascular spaces (16). The basis of these differences in clearances of ritodrine is poorly understood, but they can lead either to failure to achieve therapeutic concentrations or to potential toxicity. Moreover, because the half-life of ritodrine is more than 2 h, and plasma concentrations of most drugs continue to rise at constant infusion rates for at least four half-lives, a steady state is not reached for at least 8–10 h, and the end result may well be a plasma concentration significantly above the target.

Because of the reported myometrial tachyphylaxis that can occur with β-adrenergic tocolysis, there has been an intensified investigation of β-adrenergic receptor function in both animals and humans. Continued β-adrenergic exposure reduces both myometrial receptor number or density in human myometrial strips as well intracellular cylic adenosine monophosphate (cAMP) (18, 19), and this is associated with decreased tocolytic efficacy (20). At the same time, it has been reported that phosphodiesterase activity is increased with continued β-adrenergic exposure, which can lead to inactivation of cAMP (19). The concomitant use of dexamethasone and ritodrine, to reverse the receptor effects, seen with continued exposure of the agonist (21), has prevented a significant loss in receptor density and maintained adenylate cylase activity, but not the decreased tocolytic efficacy supporting the concept of increased cAMP degradation by phosphodiesterases. This has raised the suggestion that phosphodiesterase drugs such as papaverine or theophylline may have a role alone or in combination with β-adrenergics (22).

The above concepts of downregulation and densitization of β-adrenergic receptor function have led to newer approaches in the clinical setting. Caritas et al. have suggested, based upon their pharmacokinetic data, that lower infusion rates, increased over longer periods of time and then decreased after tocolysis is achieved, be used (20). Spatling and colleagues have reported that intermittent intravenous pulses of the β-agonist fenoterol, as compared to continuous infusions leads to one-fifth of the drug being used, and this is associated with decreased length of intravenous treatment, increased birth weights, and greater prolongation of pregnancy (23). In similar fashion, intermittent intramuscular injections of ritodrine as compared to continuous intravenous infusions result in similar effective short-term prophylaxis using one-third of the medication and at lower serum concentrations (24). Studies in sheep, which demonstrated myometrial desensitization to continuous but not to intermittent β-adrenergic infusions, have been supported by studies in the human (25–27). Lam has suggested the intermittent use of subcutaneous terbutaline administered by pump. A low basal rate providing low serum concentrations of terbutaline is maintained, and boluses are programmed to be administered during peak periods of uterine activity (27). The preliminary reports indicate that lower doses of medication can be associated with significant improvement in prolongation of pregnancy. Serum concentrations again show some significant variability following a bolus injection (28).

MAGNESIUM SULFATE

Although magnesium sulfate has been used extensively for years for the treatment of pre-eclampsia, the dosages needed for the treatment of preterm labor have not been clearly identified. The therapeutic range is reportedly 5–8 mg/100 ml (22). Rigid protocols to stay within this broad range do not permit individualization of treatment. We have seen a number of patients who fail to achieve tocolysis at 6.5

mg/100 ml and who cease contracting when 7.0 mg/100 ml is reached, and restart contracting when serum levels are permitted to fall again to the previous range. There is little question that significant clinical effort, close observation, and individualization of patient treatment is needed to optimize results.

Side Effects

Maternal side effects, some of which are potentially life-threatening, such as pulmonary edema or myocardial ischemia, can be associated with the β-adrenergic compounds. An improved understanding of fluid dynamics and close attention to fluid management have decreased the incidence of pulmonary edema, a problem reported with both β-adrenergic drugs and magnesium sulfate. Patients' acceptance of prolonged high serum concentrations of magnesium has also been poor in our experience. Less worrisome side effects such as nausea and palpitations seen with β-adrenergic can also introduce poor patient acceptance.

EMERGENT TOCOLYTICS

Because of the continuing controversy over efficacy, the need for significant clinical effort, and the presence of potentially serious side effects and patient acceptance problems, there continues to be a search for alternative approaches to clinical tocolysis. Emergent candidates as tocolytic agents include the following: a re-examination of the prostaglandin synthesis inhibitors (PGSIs); the calcium-channel antagonists; the antihypertensive agent diazoxide, which is believed to activate adenyl cyclate; phosphodiesterase inhibitors such as aminophylline and theophylline; and the oxytocin analogs that are thought to provide competitive inhibition of oxytocin.

Prostaglandin Synethesis Inhibition

Various nonsteroidal anti-inflammatory agents such as indomethacin can inhibit the cyclo-oxygenase enzyme leading to a decreased synthesis of prostaglandins $F_{2\alpha}$ and E_2. Since prostaglandins can have a stimulatory action during parturition, there has been interest in the use of PGSIs as tocolytic agents. A small placebo-controlled trial and larger observational reports have reported that indomethacin is as efficacious as the β-adrenergic agents and magnesium sulfate, with prevention of preterm delivery in 80% of patients with intact membranes and preterm labor (30, 31).

Various maternal diseases, such as coagulation disorders, drug-induced asthma, and peptic ulcers, contraindicate the use of PGSIs, but the major clinical concern has been the potential serious adverse effect upon the fetal ductus, namely, its constriction. Constriction of the human fetal ductus arteriosus has been clearly detected in at least 50% of fetuses, at 26–31 weeks, whose mothers were receiving indomethacin (32). Resolution of the constriction resolves within 24 h of discontinuing drug treatment of the mother. Others have proposed that at this gestational age the ductus arteriosus of the fetus might not respond so readily to the

PGSIs (33). The interesting feature is that in two large observational trials, there were only 3 perinatal deaths in 367 patients, 2 of which were not related to treatment (31, 34). It may well be that partial ductal constriction of a normal fetus is well tolerated. However, theoretically, if ductal constriction occurred in a growth-retarded fetus whose umbilical blood flow is already compromised, that ductal constriction would be more problematic. Also worrisome are inconsistent reports of severe oligohydramnios, thought to be secondary to decreased fetal glomerular filtration. Thus, the use of these agents currently indicate a need for close and repetitive fetal observation.

Calcium Channel Antagonists

Because of the known role of free intracellular calcium in promoting smooth-muscle contractility, there is interest that one of the calcium channel antagonists may be a useful tocolytic drug, as well as therapeutic for angina, etc. In animals and the human, there can be a tocolytic effect. Little information has been published to date on their use in clinical trials of patients with preterm labor. In general, these reports suggest efficacy at least equal to β-adrenergics (35). Maternal side effects seen in these few patients studied have been mild flushing, etc. Although no adverse fetal effects have been reported clinically, fetal hypercapnea, acidosis, hypoxia, and demise have been reported in studies in the monkey and sheep. These animal experiments have led to appropriate caution in their use clinically.

Other Agents.   Aminophylline and theophylline have been suggested as tocolytic agents due to their phosphodiesterose-inhibiting effects, the resultant increase in cAMP leading to smooth-muscle relaxation (36, 37). The latter report indicated that unacceptable maternal side effects may be achieved before effective tocolysis. Adverse maternal effects have also been a concern with the use of the potent antihypertensive drug diazoxide as a tocolytic agent. One observational report used pretreatment volume expansion to prevent serious maternal hypotension before administering the drug for tocolysis (38). The tocolytic effect was rapid in onset. It would seem that although the drug may be a potent tocolytic agent, the potential for serious maternal hypotension will hinder widespread clinical usage.

Alkylated analogs of oxytocin and vasopressin were shown to have myometrial inhibitory effects a decade ago. The possibility that oxytocin analogs might act as a competitive inhibitor of oxytocin is based on the concept that there are increased numbers of oxytocin receptors in the uterus of some women who enter spontaneous preterm labor. One appealing aspect of the use of oxytocin analogs is that theoretically they should affect only target sites having oxytocin receptors, namely, the uterus and the breast; however, there has been no close examination of other tissues for these receptors, and such analogs could affect vasopressin sites of action. In two preliminary studies, involving patients between 27 and 36 weeks with short-term infusions, there was a significant tocolytic effect in 19 of 22 patients (39, 40). There were no observable maternal or fetal effects in these short-duration studies.

SUMMARY

In summary, although prevention of preterm labor is preferable to attempts at inhibition of preterm labor, in order to decrease preterm delivery at its morbid sequelae, prediction of preterm labor is still in its infancy, and we must therefore maximize our clinical efforts at the inhibition site. Prevention of preterm labor must await further scientific advances so that prediction can be enhanced.

Inhibition of preterm labor has been hampered by a lack of early detection of preterm labor, a lack of pharmacologic information, and concerns over adverse side effects of treatment on both mother and fetus. Early detection programs have increased the number of patients in whom tocolysis can be tried, but they are not widespread. Improvements in basic knowledge should enhance the use of current tocolytics, while new agents with the same or different mechanisms of action can be developed and assessed.

REFERENCES

1. Creasy RK, Gummer BA, Liggins GC. A system for predicting spontaneous preterm birth. Obstet Gynecol 1980;55:692-5.
2. Holbrook RH Jr, Laros RK Jr, Creasy RK. Evaluation of a risk-scoring system for prediction of preterm labor. Am J Perinatol 1989;6:62-8.
3. Main DM, Gabbe SG. Risk scoring for preterm labor: Where do we go from here? Am J Obstet Gynecol 1987, 157:789-93.
4. Wesselius-deCasparis A, Thiery M, Yole S, et al. Results of a double-blind multicentre study with ritodrine in premature labour. Br Med J 1971;3:144-7.
5. Steer CM, Petrie RH. A comparison of magnesium sulfate and alcohol for the prevention of premature labor. Am J Obstet Gynecol 1977;129:1-4.
6. Ingemarsson I. Effect of terbutaline on premature labor. A double-blind placebo-controlled study. Am J Obstet Gynecol 1976, 125:520-4.
7. Zlatnik FJ. The applicability of labor inhibition to the problem of prematurity. Am J Obstet Gynecol 1972;113:704-6.
8. Stubblefield PG. Causes and prevention of preterm birth: an overview. In: Fuchs F, Stubblefield PG, eds. Preterm birth: causes, prevention and management. New York: Macmillan, 1984:3-20.
9. Herron M, Katz M, Creasy RK. Evaluation of a preterm birth prevention program: preliminary report. Obstet Gynecol 1982:59:452-6.
10. Main DM, Gabbe SG, Richardson D, et al. Can preterm deliveries be prevented? Am J Obstet Gynecol 1985;151:892-8.
11. Morrison JC, Martin JN, Martin RW, et al. Prevention of preterm birth by ambulatory assessment of uterine activity: a randomized study. Am J Obstet Gynecol 1987;156:536-43.
12. Diagnostic and therapeutic technology assessment, home monitoring of uterine activity. J Am Med Assoc 1989;261:3027-9.
13. Katz M, Gill PJ, Newman RB. Detection of preterm labor by ambulatory monitoring of uterine activity: a preliminary report. Obstet Gynecol 1986;68:773-8.
14. Iams JD, Johnson FF, O'Shaughnessy RW. A prospective random trial of home uterine activity monitoring in pregnancies of increased risk of preterm labor, II. Am J Obstet Gynecol 1988;159:595-603.

15. King JF, Grant A, Keirse MJNC, et al. Beta-mimetics in preterm labour: an overview of the randomized controlled trials. Br J Obstet Gynaecol 1988;95:211-22.

16. Caritas SN, Venkataramanan R, Darby MJ, et al. Pharmacokinetics of ritodrine administered intravenously: recommendations for changes in the current regimen. Am J Obstet Gynecol 1990;162:429-37.

17. Lyrenas S, Grahnen A, Lindberg B, et al. Pharmacokinetics of terbutaline during pregnancy. Eur J Clin Pharmacol 1986;29:619-23.

18. Berg G, Andersson RGG, Ryden G. β-adrenergic receptors in human myometrium during pregnancy: changes in the number of receptors after β-mimetic treatment. Am J Obstet Gynecol 1985;151:392-6.

19. Berg G, Andersson RGG, Ryden G. Effects of selective beta-adrenergic agonists in spontaneous contractions, cAMP levels and phosphodiesterase activity in myometrial strips from pregnant women treated with terbutaline. Gynecol Obstet Invest 1982;14:56-64.

20. Caritas SN, Chiao JP, Moore JJ, et al. Myometrial desensitization after ritodrine infusion. Am J Physiol 1987;253:E410-7.

21. Ward SM, Caritas SN, Chiao JP, et al. Dexamethasone effects on ritodrine induced changes in myometrial contracility and β-adrenergic receptor function. Am J Obstet Gynecol 1988;159:1461-6.

22. Berg G, Andersson RGG, Ryden G. In vitro study of phosphodiesterase-inhibiting drugs: a compliment to β-sympathomimetic drug therapy in premature labor. Am J Obstet Gynecol 1983;145:802-6.

23. Spatling L, Fallenstein F, Schneider H, et al. Bolus tocolysis: treatment of preterm labor with pulsatile administration of a β-adrenergic agonist. Am J Obstet Gynecol 1989;160:713-7.

24. Gonik B, Benedetti T, Creasy RK, et al. Intramuscular versus intravenous ritodrine hydrochloride for preterm labor management. Am J Obstet Gynecol 1988;159:323-8.

25. Casper RF, Lye SJ. Myometrial desensitization to continuous but not to intermittent β-adrenergic agonist infusion in the sheep. Am J Obstet Gynecol 1986;154:301-5.

26. Ke R, Vohra M, Casper RF. Prolonged inhibition of human myometrial contractility by intermittent isoproterenol. Am J Obstet Gynecol 1984;149:841-4.

27. Lam F, Gill P, Smith M, et al. Use of the subcutaneous terbutaline pump for long-term tocolysis. Obstet Gynecol 1988;72:810-3.

28. Lam F. Personal communication 1990.

29. Petrie RH. Tocolysis using magnesium sulfate. Semin Perinatol 1981;5:266-73.

30. Niebyl J, Blake DA, White RD, et al. The inhibition of premature labor with indomethacin. Am J Obstet Gynecol 1980;136:1014-9.

31. Dudley DKL, Hardie MJ. Fetal and neonatal effects of indomethacin used as a tocolytic agent. Am J Obstet Gynecol 1985;151:181-4.

32. Moise KJ, Huhta JC, Sharif DS, et al. Indomethacin in the treatment of premature labor: effects on the fetal ductus arteriosus. N Engl J Med 1988;319:327-31.

33. Niebyl J. Prostaglandin synthetase inhibitors. Semin Perinatol 1981;5:274-87.

34. Amy JJ, Theiry M. The prevention of preterm labour. Prostaglandin Perspectives 1985;1:9-11.

35. Read MD, Wellby DE. The use of calcium antagonist (nifedipine) to suppress preterm labour. Br J Obstet Gynaecol 1986;93:933-7.

36. Liu DTY, Blackwell RJ. The value of a scoring system in predicting outcome of

preterm labour and comparing efficacy of treatment with aminophylline and salbutamol. Br J Obstet Gynaecol 1978;85:418-22.

37. Lipshitz J. Uterine and cardiovascular effects of aminophylline. Am J Obstet Gynecol 1978;131:716-8.

38. Adamsons K, Wallach RC. Treating preterm labor with diazoxide. Contemp Ob/Gyn 1988;131:161-77.

39. Akerlund M, Stromberg P, Hauksson A, et al. Inhibition of uterine contractions of premature labour with an oxytocin analogue. Results from a pilot study. Br J Obstet Gynaecol 1987;94:1040-4.

40. Andersen LF, Lyndrup J, Akerlund M, et al. Oxytocin receptor blockade: a new principle in the treatment of preterm labor? Am J Perinatol 1989;6:196-9.

Author Index

A
Anwer, K., 69
Avila, C., 319

B
Beier, S., 153
Boshier, D. P., 143
Brekus, C. A., 319

C
Calder, A. A., 283
Casey, M. L., 43
Challis, J. R. G., 143
Chaouat, G., 267
Cheung, P. Y. C., 143
Chwalisz, K., 153
Crankshaw, D. J., 85
Creasy, R. K., 371

D
Dawood, M. Y., 355
Do Khac, L., 123
Downing, S. J., 237

E
Elger, W., 153

F
Fähnrich, M., 153
Fraher, L. J., 143
Fuchs, A.-R., 177

G
Garfield, R. E., 21, 153
Goureau, O., 123
Grover, A. K., 53
Guilbert, L., 267

H
Han, V. K., 143
Harbon, S., 123
Hasan, S. H., 153

Hayashi, R. H., 309
Hertelendy, F., 221
Hwang, J.-J., 237

J
Jacobs, R. A., 143

K
Kamm, K. E., 43
Khan, I., 53
Kinsky, R., 267

L
Langlois, D., 143
Lao Guico-Lamm, M., 237
Laurent, D., 153
Leiber, D., 123
Lundin-Schiller, S., 205

M
Marc, S., 123
Marshall, J. M., 3
Mazor, M., 319
Mironneau, J., 9
Mitchell, M. D., 205
Mokhtari, A., 123
Molnár, M., 221

N
Neef, G., 153

O
Ottow, E., 153

P
Papka, R. E., 253
Pulkkinen, M., 295

R
Riemer, R. K., 103, 113
Riley, S. C., 143
Roberts, J. M., 113

Subject Index

A23187 (ionophore), 34, 56, 228
Abortion, 158-173, 267-271, 277, 296, 307, 319, 320, 355
Acetylcholine, 9, 16, 17, 46, 71, 76, 107, 108, 110, 196
ACTH, 149, 177
Actin, 43-45, 47
Action potential, 3-7, 9, 10, 22-24, 26, 33, 35-37, 43, 44, 296; *see also* Membrane potential
Adenosine diphosphate, 17, 60, 118-120, 134
Adenosine monophosphate, cyclic (cAMP), 17, 27, 34, 37, 73, 75-78, 113-121, 123-138, 205, 206, 374, 376; *see also* cAMP-dependent protein kinase
Adenosine triphosphate, 9, 15-17, 27, 44, 55-60, 70, 76, 118, 196, 228; *see also* ATPase
Adenylate cyclase/adenylyl cyclase, 34, 113-121, 124, 126, 130-138, 198, 206, 374, 375; *see also* Adenosine monophosphate, cyclic
Adrenergic agonist/receptor, 34, 37, 54, 62, 76, 87, 110, 113-121, 133, 134, 177, 206, 259, 373-375
Adrenocorticotropic hormone, 149, 177
AF-DX116 (and subtypes of muscarinic receptor), 130-132
Amniotic fluid, 207-212, 223, 278, 287, 319-343
Amniotomy, 277, 278, 288-292, 298, 356
Angiotensin, 49, 54, 107, 108, 213
Antiestrogen, 33, 170
Antiprogesterone, 29, 31, 153-173
Arachidonic acid, 33, 103, 106, 129, 146, 147, 149, 186, 188, 205-215, 221, 233-235, 331-333
ATPase, 36, 44, 57-61, 70, 74, 76, 77, 96, 106 192, 196, 197; *see also* Myosin phosphorylation
Atropine, 16, 124, 132, 257, 258

Baboon, 358
Bacteria in amniotic cavity, 319-343
Benzyl ester, 34
Beta adrenergic agonist/receptor, 34, 37, 62, 76, 87, 113-121, 133, 134, 206, 373-375
Bird, 221
Birth control, 311, 312
Bishop score, 290, 358, 359, 365
Bradykinin, 54
Brain, 55, 59, 61, 62, 134
Braxton Hicks contraction, 284, 298
Buccal pitocin, 355, 356

Ca++
  -dependent protein kinase, 58
  and myosin phosphorylation, 43-51
  -pump, 55-63, 70, 76, 77, 106, 107, 196
  and smooth-muscle contraction, 43-51, 53-63
  see also Calcium/calcium ion and Calcium channel
Cachectin, 209, 328, 335-340, 342
Caffeine, 17, 55
Calciosome, 55
Calcium/calcium ion, 3-7, 9, 11-17, 22-24, 27, 34-37, 43-51, 53-63, 69-78, 92, 93, 96, 103-114, 123, 127-130, 136-138, 192, 195-198, 205, 207, 221, 228-235, 376; *see also* Ca++ and Calcium channel
Calcium channel
  blockers, 5, 7, 11, 12, 48, 71, 196, 311, 312, 375, 376; *see also* particular calcium blockers
  types, 9, 12, 54
  see also Ca++ and Calcium/calcium ion
Calmodulin, 43-45, 48, 59, 60, 62, 63, 69, 70, 76, 107, 114, 197
Calsequestrin, 55
cAMP, 17, 27, 34, 37, 73, 75-78, 113-121, 123-138, 205, 206, 374, 376; *see also* cAMP-dependent protein kinase